A U.S. Army
Medical Base in
World War I France

A U.S. Army Medical Base in World War I France

Life and Care at Bazoilles Hospital Center, 1918–1919

Peter Wever

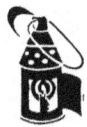

McFarland & Company, Inc., Publishers
Jefferson, North Carolina

ISBN (print) 978-1-4766-7618-0
ISBN (ebook) 978-1-4766-3562-0

LIBRARY OF CONGRESS and BRITISH LIBRARY
CATALOGUING DATA ARE AVAILABLE

Library of Congress Control Number 2019943097

© 2019 Peter Wever. All rights reserved

No part of this book may be reproduced or transmitted in any form or by any means, electronic or mechanical, including photocopying or recording, or by any information storage and retrieval system, without permission in writing from the publisher.

Front cover images: Installation of a Carrel-Dakin apparatus for irrigation of a wound above the right knee of a soldier admitted to Base Hospital No. 18 (National Archives). Personal items recovered at the former site of Bazoilles Hospital Center, *left to right* a U.S. Army Medical Corps collar disk, an Army Nurse Corps pin and an identification tag of patient Frederick Loeffel (author collection).

Printed in the United States of America

McFarland & Company, Inc., Publishers
Box 611, Jefferson, North Carolina 28640
www.mcfarlandpub.com

In honor of those who needed care
and the ones who cared for them
at Bazoilles Hospital Center

Table of Contents

Preface   1

Introduction   3

ONE. The Evacuation Chain of the American Expeditionary Forces: From Frontline to Bazoilles Hospital Center   7

TWO. Bazoilles Hospital Center in Operation: 63,769 Treated in Ten Months   18
   The Sound of the Siren   35

THREE. "With the Wounded": Wound Care at Bazoilles Hospital Center   38
   Gas! Gas! Treatment of Gas Cases   54

FOUR. Patients of Bazoilles Hospital Center: Three Soldiers Admitted Because of Battle Injuries   57
   Treatment of Wounded German Prisoners of War   65

FIVE. Spanish Flu: The Toll of Influenza and Secondary Pneumonia   68
   Convalescent Camp No. 2   76

SIX. "Dear Mother": Letters from Bazoilles Hospital Center   79

SEVEN. The Ministering Angels of Base Hospital No. 60: The Spanish Flu Outbreak on Board the USS *Leviathan*   86
   War Is Over   94

EIGHT. A Medical Officer's Photo Album: Pictures of Daily Life   96
   Christmas Overseas   104

NINE. Patients of Bazoilles Hospital Center: Three Soldiers Admitted Because of Physical and Mental Disease   108
   Review of the Personnel by General Pershing   118

TEN. Capital Punishment at Bazoilles-sur-Meuse: The Execution
of Two American Soldiers 122

ELEVEN. Traces of Medical Care at Bazoilles Hospital Center: Items
from Institutional and Personal Collections 132

Appendix 155

Chapter Notes 161

Bibliography 169

Index 175

Preface

In 1999, my parents-in-law moved from the Netherlands to Bazincourt-sur-Saulx in the *département* Meuse in Northern France. Their new home was some 50 miles south of the much fought-over village of Montfaucon-d'Argonne which was among the first-day objectives of the U.S. Army in the 1918 Meuse-Argonne Offensive at the end of World War I. Having repeatedly read the Illustrated Classics cartoon *The First World War* as a child, I had remained somewhat fascinated by the Great War. Still, it was not until 2010 that I made my first battlefield trip to the Meuse-Argonne region among a group of four friends. Returning to our roadside parked car from a forest near Cunel, we, almost literally, stumbled upon several U.S. Army objects from World War I, uncovered by recent road work. Among the recovered items were a capped glass vial for anti-tetanus serum, a glass tube filled with iodine and a roll of wire gauze for splints, presumably all remnants of an American field hospital. In the years after, I regularly returned to the Meuse-Argonne region for battlefield trips. On the side, as a result of my initial finds, I developed an interest in medical aspects of World War I focusing on the U.S. Army Medical Department and its overseas hospitals. This resulted in medical-historical publications in the *British Medical Journal, Military Medicine, Medical Humanities, Influenza and Other Respiratory Viruses* and the *Journal of the Royal Army Medical Corps*.

In the spring of 2015, I downloaded an image from online auction site eBay showing an aerial view of Base Hospital No. 18. Looking for the location of this hospital, I found it had been situated at Bazoilles-sur-Meuse in the *département* Vosges, some 45 miles south-east of my parents-in law's place. Base Hospital No. 18 had been part of a large U.S. Army hospital center consisting at the height of its operation of eight base hospitals (Nos. 18, 42, 46, 60, 66, 79, 81 and 116), a convalescent camp and a military cemetery, collectively known as Bazoilles Hospital Center. On May 16, 2015, I made my first trip to Bazoilles-sur-Meuse to discover that, at first glance, nothing in the small village bears witness to the presence of Bazoilles Hospital Center. But in subsequent trips, I was able to recover numerous items illustrative of daily life at the center. In addition, I searched the internet for information on Bazoilles Hospital Center and found that there is as much to discover online as there is on site.

In the spring of 2016, I purchased the World War I photo album of Major Theodore J. Abbott, Chief of Medical Service at Base Hospital No. 116. The album contains over 200 pictures illustrating daily life and medical care at Bazoilles Hospital Center. The antiquarian bookseller brought me in contact with Lawrence Osgood, the son of First Lieutenant Howard Osgood, who had been in charge of the wound bacteriology division at the center laboratory of Bazoilles Hospital Center. Lawrence Osgood generously allowed me to quote from the unpublished transcript of World War I letters and diary entries from his father written in part at Bazoilles Hospital Center. Likewise, Sanders Marble (Senior Historian, Army Medical Department Center of History and Heritage, San Antonio, Texas) provided a transcript of the unpublished war memoirs of Louise Kalkman, nurse at Base Hospitals Nos. 60 and 81. Greg Donaldson generously donated items from the estate of his great aunt Eleanor Donaldson, Chief Nurse of Base Hospital No. 46, and provided details about her army service.

Gradually, the idea emerged to write a book about Bazoilles Hospital Center. A book that intends to illustrate daily life and medical care at one of the largest U.S. Army hospital centers during World War I providing the reader with a vivid picture of what conditions were like for both patients and medical personnel. In November 2016, I took a two-week research leave and visited the Historical Collections & Archives of the Oregon Health & Science University in Portland, Oregon, which keeps archival records of Base Hospital No. 46. Subsequently, I visited the Edward Jones Research Center at the National World War I Museum and Memorial in Kansas City, Missouri, and the National Archives at Kansas City. I want to thank Meg Langford (Public Services Coordinator, Historical Collections & Archives, Oregon Health & Science University) and Jonathan Casey (Archivist and Edward Jones Research Center Manager) for their warm reception.

While writing the book, I received transatlantic help on many occasions. Foremost, I want to thank Bernadine Lennon (Veterans History Project Coordinator, Greene-Dreher Historical Society, Greentown, Pennsylvania; like a dog with a bone) and Jim Shetler (no mission beyond reach) for their dedication and support in too many ways to mention. Likewise, I owe thanks to Dustin Farris, Susi Adler and Nancy Schaff (President 314th Infantry Descendants & Friends, Commissioner Maryland World War I Centennial Commission). Dave McQuigg provided details about the life of his grandfather Private Harry H. McQuigg. I am proud that his identification tag was returned to the McQuigg family some hundred years after he lost it at Bazoilles Hospital Center. Michele McCarthy (St. John's Cemetery, Worcester, Massachusetts) supported me in my research into Private Michael J. O'Connor. Le Anne Loesel (Gilmanton American Legion Auxiliary, Gilmanton, Wisconsin) and Diane Lisowski (Administrative Assistant, Gilmanton School District) provided details about Nurse Eileen L. Forrest from Base Hospital No. 60. Karen Seeman aided with information on her great-great-uncle Private Delbert D. Graves.

On this side of the Atlantic, I received help from Wim "Mudra" Degrande, Rogier van de Hoef and Emma Wever. Support with photos and illustrations was provided by Arno Vingerhoets, Ronald Flisijn and Anneliek Holland. I especially want to thank Maarten and Didi Otte (B&B 14–18 Nantillois, Meuse-Argonne 1918 Museum, Nantillois, France) for lasting friendship, support and shelter while finishing this book.

In my search for a publisher, I was assisted by Sanders Marble, Maarten Otte and Christina Holstein. I want to express my gratitude to Natalie Foreman and her colleagues at McFarland for confidence in a book about World War I written by a non-native English speaker from an at-the-time neutral country.

I owe the most thanks to Chaja, Lisa and Haye for their continuing love regardless of the fact I was writing a book I promised not to write. I will not say never again.

Introduction

Although World War I might be considered the neglected world war, much has been written about the advances in medicine made possible by the slaughter of 1914–1918. Facial surgery, prosthetic limb technology, blood transfusion, mobile radiology, evacuation of casualties, wound disinfection and anesthesia have all benefited from the injuries brought about by new heavy artillery and machine guns. Yet, hardly any contemporary books have been published about daily life and routine medical care at field, evacuation and base hospitals of the U.S. Army in France where these advances were put into practice. Recommended among the few published war memoirs are *Lamp for a Soldier: The Caring Story of a Nurse in World War I* by Nurse Sarah Sand of Base Hospital No. 60 (published 1976), *Dear Ginny: Letters to my Wife* by Captain Verne R. Mason of Base Hospital No. 18 (published 2005) and, in particular, *Finding Helen: The Letters, Photographs and Diary of a World War I Battlefield Nurse* about Nurse Helen Bulovsky's service at Base Hospital No. 22 and Evacuation Hospital No. 5 (published 2014). Recently published descriptions of U.S. Army medical units include *A Grateful Heart: The History of a World War I Field Hospital* about the 103rd Field Hospital, 26th Sanitary Train, 26th Division (published 2002), *Skilled and Resolute: A History of the 12th Evacuation Hospital and the 212th MASH, 1917–2006* (published 2013) and *History of 318 Field Hospital* in recognition of the men of the 318th Field Hospital, 305th Sanitary Train, 80th Division (published 2017). However, there seem to be no contemporary publications on U.S. Army hospital centers, although, in retrospect, the U.S. Army Medical Department recognized the formation of such centers among the most important of its enterprises in World War I.

The United States entered World War I on April 6, 1917, when President Woodrow Wilson signed the declaration of war on Germany. Within a year, America assembled an army of nearly four million men and women. With the arrival in June 1917 of the first American troops in France emerged the need to provide adequate hospital facilities. Therefore, the American Red Cross raised and equipped base hospitals, which became part of the U.S. Army when called into active duty. To reduce staff and overhead demands, it was planned as early as September 1917 to group from 2 to 20 base hospitals in hospital centers. On November 11, 1918, Armistice Day, around 20 hospital centers were in operation with a total bed capacity of over 180,000. Other hospital centers were being constructed and additional ones projected adding towards a planned total bed capacity in hospital centers of 500,000 should the war continue until April 1919.

The first U.S. Army hospital center in operation was located at Bazoilles-sur-Meuse in the *département* Vosges. It was simply referred to as Bazoilles Hospital Center. The 412 inhabitants of the small village would be outnumbered by 63,769 patients treated at

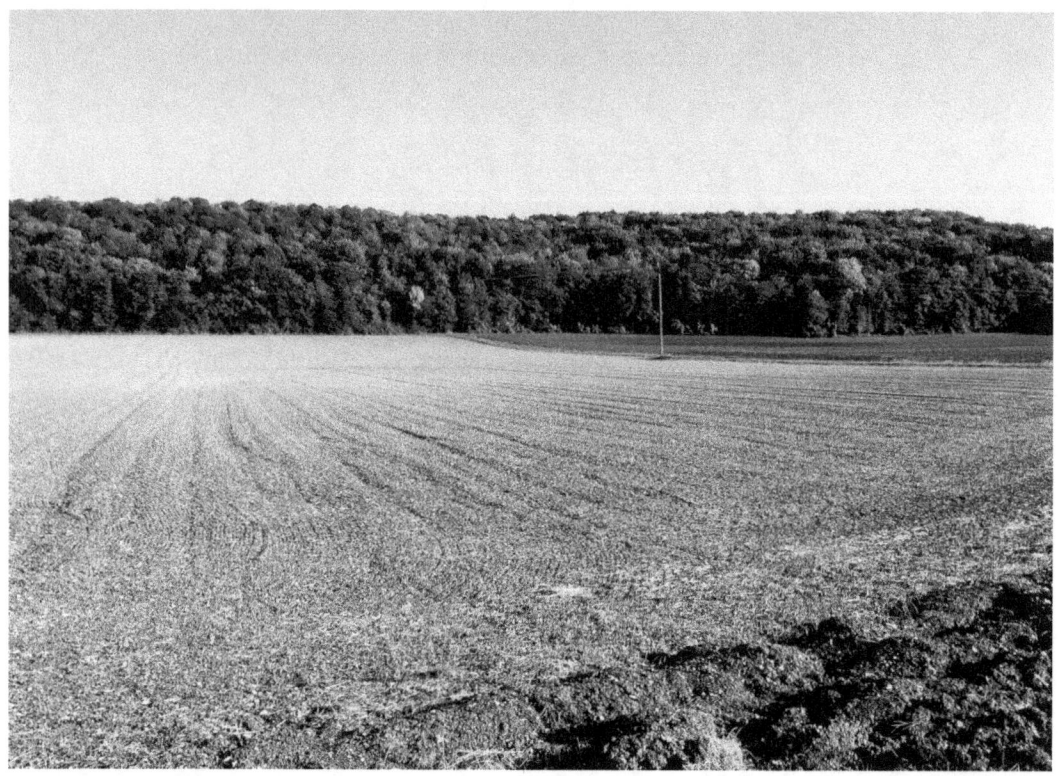

Present-day view of the fields at Bazoilles-sur-Meuse where Base Hospitals Nos. 81 and 116 were in operation in 1918–1919 as part of Bazoilles Hospital Center. More than 18,000 American soldiers received treatment in these two base hospitals (photograph by author).

the center in its ten months of operation. Because of its location in the so-called Advance Section, Bazoilles Hospital Center received far more casualties directly from the frontline than hospital centers located further from the front. This book sets out to describe daily life and medical care at Bazoilles Hospital Center providing the reader with a vivid picture of what conditions were like for both patients and medical personnel. Emphasis will be on aspects of wound care, wound infection and the Spanish flu, which raged on the Western Front during the large U.S. Army offensives of September–November 1918. Bazoilles Hospital Center was also the site where two American soldiers (out of a total of eleven in France) were executed by hanging after court martial conviction for rape. One chapter of this book deals with rumors that surfaced in 1921 of illegal hangings of American soldiers during and after the First World War at, among other places, Bazoilles-sur-Meuse. These chapters alternate with sections in which medical care for specific patient groups (prisoners of war, gas patients, convalescent patients) as well as certain key events (air raid alarms, Armistice Day, Christmas 1918, inspection by Commander-in-Chief Pershing) are highlighted using transcriptions of hospital histories and letters and diary entries of personnel of the center.

One hundred years after World War I, crops grow on the fields where the base hospitals of Bazoilles Hospital Center were located in 1918–1919. It is nowadays difficult to imagine that over 63,000 injured or ill American soldiers suffered, healed or died in wooden barracks and canvas tents hastily erected alongside the still existent rail track.

Objects recovered from the fields and the edge of the forest are silent witnesses of their one-time presence. As names—and faces—can be more confronting than admission numbers and casualty figures, personal stories of medical personnel and individual soldiers who worked, were treated—or died—at Bazoilles Hospital Center are provided throughout the book. Such stories include the histories of six patients treated at the center who were identified after the author recovered their identification tags in 2016 at the former site of the center. Herewith, the book provides recognition to the men and women who served at Bazoilles Hospital Center and the soldiers treated there. This book tries to tell—if at all possible—their story and sacrifice.

One

The Evacuation Chain of the American Expeditionary Forces
From Frontline to Bazoilles Hospital Center

Even before the American declaration of war on Germany, the United States had acknowledged the need for medical preparedness. In fact, the first unit of the American Expeditionary Forces to arrive in France was Base Hospital No. 4 which was organized at the Lakeside Hospital in Cleveland, Ohio. The U.S. Army Medical Department established an evacuation chain for the hospitalization and evacuation of the wounded and sick from the front line. To reduce staff and overhead demands, base hospitals and a convalescent camp were grouped in large hospital centers. In retrospect, the U.S. Army Medical Department recognized the formation of these hospital centers among the most important of its enterprises in World War I.

Early American Hospital Initiatives in World War I

On April 6, 1917, President Woodrow Wilson signed the American declaration of war on Germany. The Great War had been raging in a large part of the world following Austria-Hungary's declaration of war on Serbia on July 28, 1914, in response to the assassination of Archduke Franz Ferdinand, heir to the throne of Austria-Hungary, and his wife Sophie in the streets of Sarajevo on June 28, 1914.[1] In September 1914, as part of its charter to provide war relief, the American National Red Cross had sent eleven hospital units to Europe, followed by two more in November 1914. These hospitals provided medical care on both sides of the conflict for approximately one year, employing 75 surgeons and 255 nurses and treating approximately 30,000 patients. The hospital units were withdrawn when donations to the Red Cross declined and it was decided to use the money that was saved to purchase medical supplies for the combatants.[2]

At the very start of the war, the 1906-founded American Hospital of Paris was offered use of the nearby *Lycée Pasteur* (Pasteur Lyceum) to organize a fully outfitted military hospital. This hospital became known as the American Ambulance Hospital, but was officially named the *Ambulance de l'Hôpital Américain de Paris, section des blessés* (the Ambulance of the American Hospital of Paris, Wounded Section; *ambulance* designates a military hospital). It was entirely financed by the generosity of American donors. In

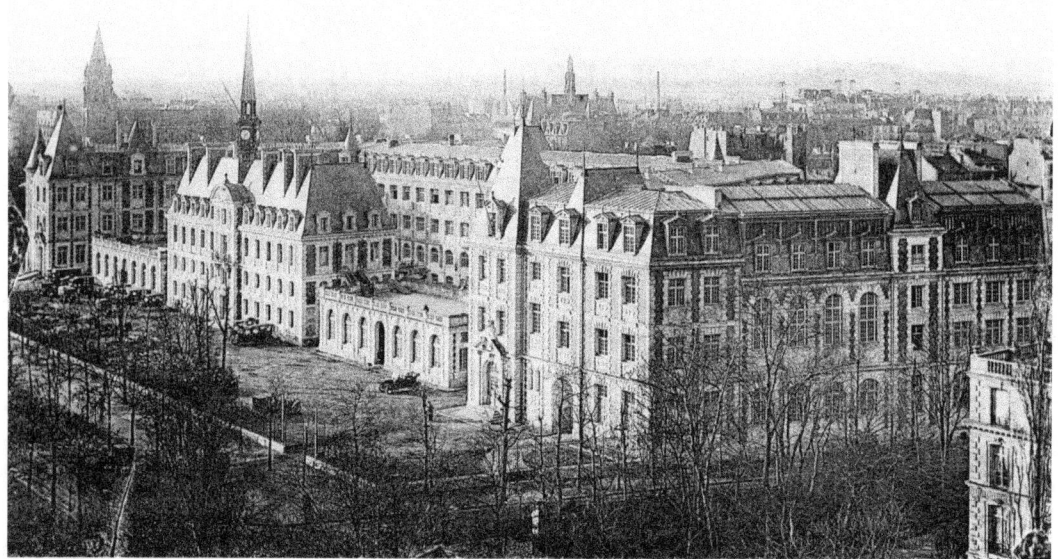

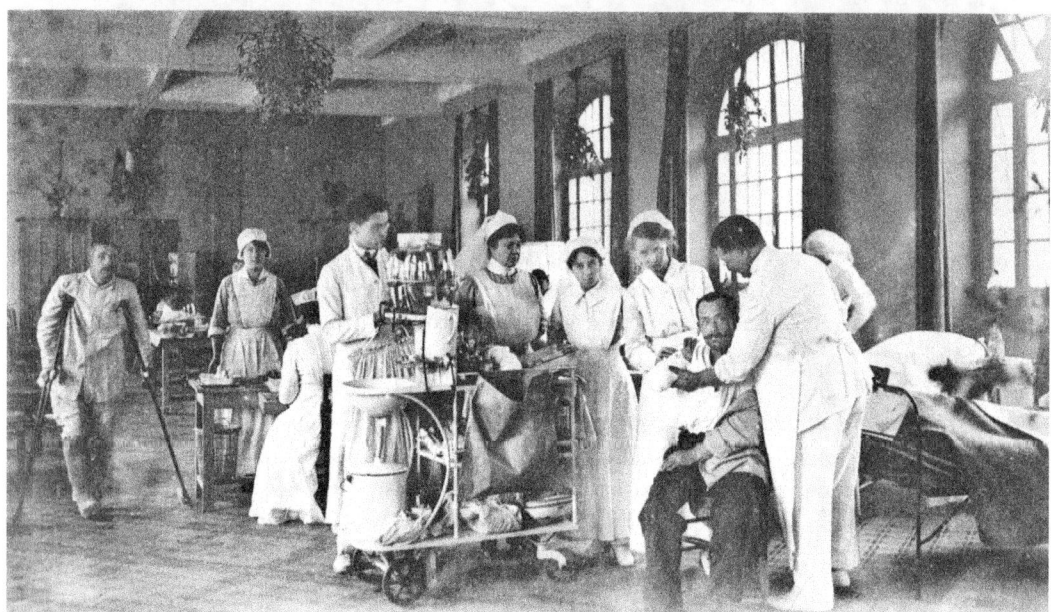

Top: This postcard depicts the *Ambulance de l'Hôpital Américain de Paris, section des blessés* which became known as the American Ambulance Hospital in Paris (author's collection). *Bottom*: A postcard showing the morning rounds at the American Ambulance Hospital in Paris. The soldier receiving medical attention has an amputated right forearm (U.S. National Library of Medicine. Digital Collections. http://resource.nlm.nih.gov/101669232; accessed January 13, 2018).

January 1915, a number of American medical schools began a series of rotations of medical teams at the American Ambulance Hospital: the Lakeside Hospital Unit from the Western Reserve University in Cleveland, Ohio, from January to March 1915, the Harvard University Medical Center from Boston, Massachusetts, from April to June 1915 and the University of Pennsylvania Medical Center from Philadelphia, Pennsylvania, from July 1915 to June 1917. By December 1916, the American Ambulance Hospital was treating 1,600 wounded men daily. Under the auspices of the American Hospital of Paris, several "auxiliary" hospitals were established closer to the front, the first of which at Juilly. The American Ambulance Hospital was served by fully equipped Ford Model T ambulances of the American Ambulance Field Service, which later also offered help to other military hospitals. Several other American initiatives also organized volunteer units of motorized ambulances in France.[3]

Raising Base Hospitals

One of the doctors involved in the organization of the American Ambulance Hospital was the surgeon George W. Crile from Cleveland, Ohio. It was Crile who brought forward the idea of raising the American Ambulance Hospital's personnel from universities for which he made a deal with the trustees of the Lakeside Hospital. After their return from France, both Crile and neurosurgeon Harvey Cushing from the Harvard University Medical Center gave speeches about their experiences and their views on the necessity for medical preparedness. The Surgeon General of the U.S. Army, William C. Corgas, heard Crile's address at the American First Aid Conference, where he "advocated well-organized hospital units of men who have trained together." Impressed by Crile's remarks, Corgas asked him in a letter dated August 25, 1915, how the U.S. Army Medical Department should establish a base hospital if war was declared. Crile answered that "the heads of surgery in the American medical colleges in good standing would form an excellent nucleus from which such reserve organizations may be built." This set the stage for the raising of the Red Cross base hospitals two years later.[4]

The leadership of the American Medical Association, American Surgical Association, the Congress of American Physicians and Surgeons, the American College of Surgeons and the Clinical Congress of Surgeons in North America met in Chicago in April 1916 to form a Committee on Medical Preparedness. This committee petitioned President Wilson to increase medical readiness in the army. The committee proved instrumental in integrating the medical community with the armed services. It adopted Crile's base hospital plan and recommended it to Surgeon General Corgas. The correspondence with Crile convinced the Surgeon General and he asked Crile, Cushing and internist J. M. Swan to proceed with organizing base hospitals. It was agreed upon that the Red Cross would raise and equip the base hospital units along military lines. However, when the hospitals were called into active duty, they would become part of the army. It was initially planned by the army and Red Cross to raise 38 base hospitals of 500 beds each. Shortly after the declaration of war, the Medical Department expanded this to 50 units. The Red Cross visited medical schools throughout the country to encourage the organization of base hospitals.[5]

In March 1916, the Red Cross and the Lakeside Hospital agreed that Crile would form a base hospital unit, which came to be known as Base Hospital No. 4. It was to remain ready for service as required by the Red Cross or the Surgeon General. Planning

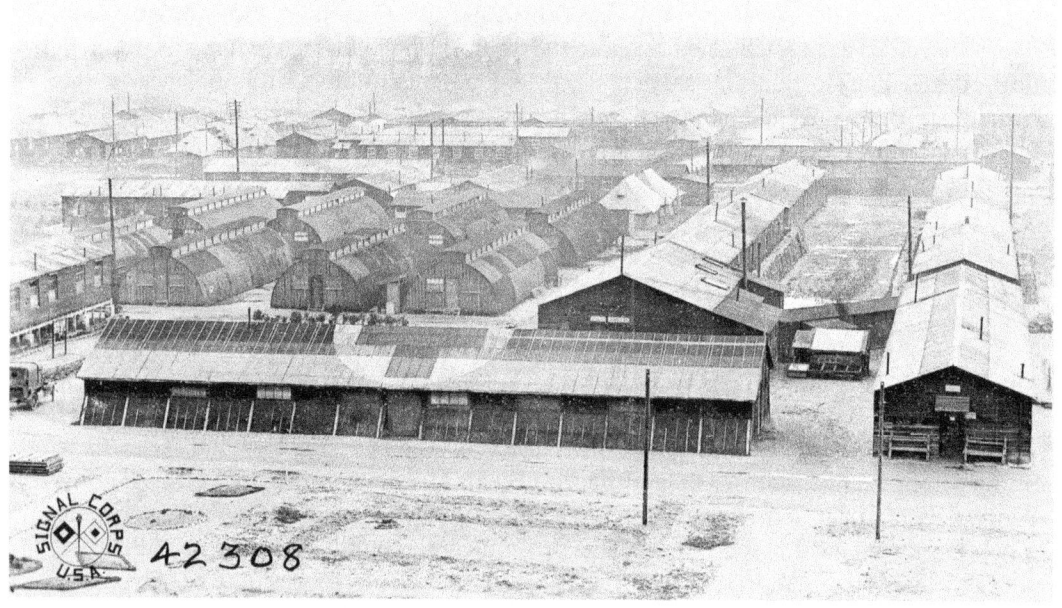

Base Hospital No. 4 in Rouen, France. This hospital was the first unit of the American Expeditionary Forces to arrive in France (National Archives at College Park, Maryland [Record Group 111: Records of the Office of the Chief Signal Officer, 1860–1985, Photographs of American Military Activities, ca. 1918–ca. 1981, National Archives Identifier 530707: photograph no. 111-SC-42308]).

for their upcoming Passchendaele Offensive,[6] a British medical liaison officer to the United States requested six base hospitals from the new ally on April 27, 1917. The following day, only 22 days after President Wilson signed the declaration of war, Crile received orders to mobilize Base Hospital No. 4. Ten days later, on May 8, it sailed from New York and arrived in England on May 17. King George welcomed the American nurses and doctors on the steps of Buckingham Palace on May 23.[7] After a week in England, the unit embarked for France arriving in Rouen on May 25. There, it took over operation of British General Hospital No. 9 and received its first patients on May 28. It was the first unit of the American Expeditionary Forces to arrive in France and it was already treating casualties on the day that its Commander-in-Chief, General John J. Pershing, embarked for Europe in New York. In the two-and-a-halve weeks after Base Hospital No. 4 sailed, it was followed by Base Hospital No. 5, organized at Harvard University, Base Hospital No. 2, organized at the Presbyterian Hospital, New York, New York, Base Hospital No. 10, organized at the Pennsylvania Hospital, Philadelphia, Pennsylvania, Base Hospital No. 21, organized at the Washington University, St. Louis, Missouri, and Base Hospital No. 12, organized at the Northwestern University, Chicago, Illinois. All these units took over operation of British General Hospitals.[8] Eventually, on November 12, 1918, the day after the Armistice was signed, there were 153 overseas base hospitals in operation.[9] Bed

One. The Evacuation Chain of the American Expeditionary Forces 11

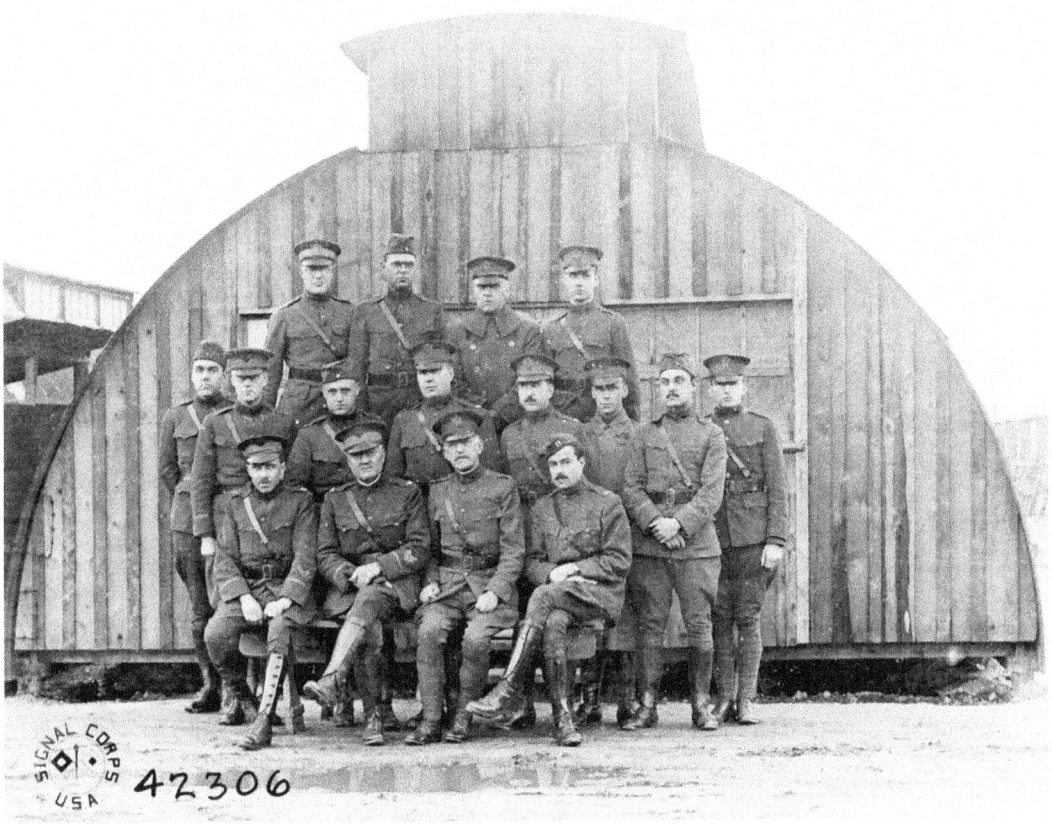

Officers of Base Hospital No. 4, with Colonel George W. Crile seated second from the left in the front row (National Archives at College Park, Maryland [Record Group 111: Records of the Office of the Chief Signal Officer, 1860–1985, Photographs of American Military Activities, ca. 1918–ca. 1981, National Archives Identifier 530707: photograph no. 111-SC-42306]).

capacity of base hospitals, which originally had been 500 beds, had been expanded to 1,000 and hospital staff consisted of 35 medical officers, 100 nurses and 200 enlisted men.[10] In general, the two most important departments in a base hospital were the surgical department which took care of the wounded and the medical department which handled cases of gas poisoning and cases with disease.[11]

The Base, Intermediate and Advance Sections

Transport and evacuation of the wounded and sick presented the U.S. Army with difficulties in many ways different from the problems which had confronted the French and British Armies. For the French and British, there was no need for long lines of evacuation to home ports. The short route to England made it possible for British wounded to rapidly reach military home hospitals. For the U.S. Army, it was impracticable to send home its wounded and sick, except for a relatively small number, who were permanently disabled. The American Expeditionary Forces was compelled to hospitalize almost all its sick and wounded in France, and to some extent in England. Therefore, large hospitals

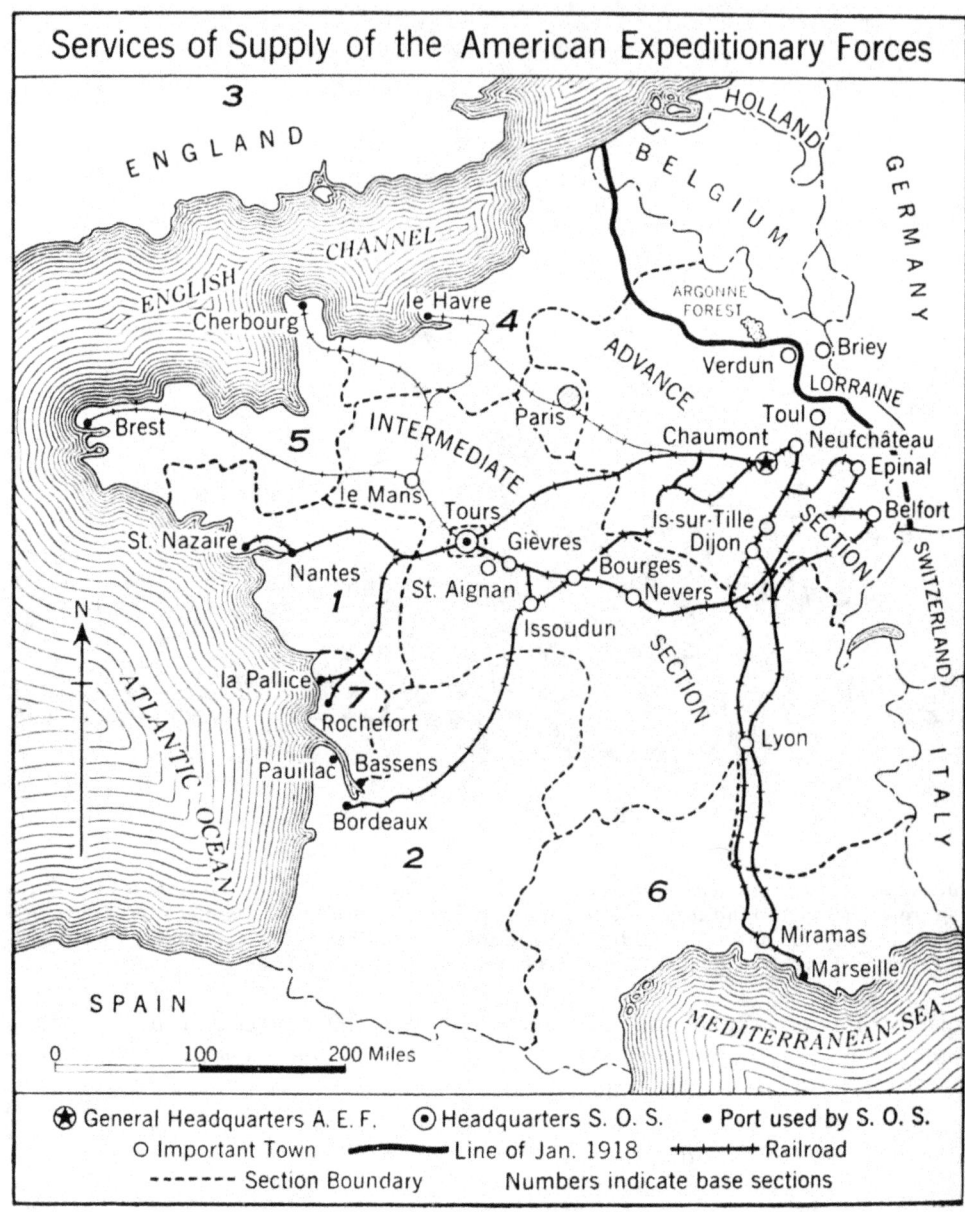

Map of the Services of Supply of the American Expeditionary Forces showing its Base Sections, Intermediate Section, Advance Section, headquarters at Tours and ports and railroads used (American Battle Monuments Commission. *American Armies and Battlefields in Europe: A History, Guide and Reference Book*. Washington, D.C.: Government Printing Office, 1938: 438).

and hospital groups were situated on its supply lines. Patients were moved there by train which made ample hospital train service one of the prime elements of a successful evacuation service.[12]

The evacuation of wounded to the rear as well as the handling of enormous volumes of supplies and the moving of units from one point to another were performed by an organization known as the Services of Supply or more generally the S.O.S. In essence, the Services of Supply began in the United States and extended across the Atlantic Ocean to Europe. It entered France mainly at ports along its western coast from Brest southward, as ports farther north were already heavily used by the French and British Armies. The railway lines which ran northeastward from these ports bypassed the congested region near Paris where the greater part of the French war factories and large supply depots were located. For purposes of administration, the Services of Supply was divided into several Base Sections, located around the ports of debarkation, one Intermediate Section and one Advance Section located progressively nearer the front line. Eventually, there were nine Base Sections, including six in France, one in England, one in Italy and one comprising Antwerp, Belgium, and Rotterdam, the Netherlands.[13]

The Evacuation Chain

To transport the wounded and sick from the front line to the rear ("down the line"), an evacuation chain was established. Medical Department men accompanying the fighting troops dressed the wounded, applied splints and placed them at any sheltered point accessible.[14] Stretcher bearers (litter bearers) carried the wounded from the front line to a battalion aid station.[15] Each battalion normally had one battalion aid station, which was situated as near to the front as possible. In the trenches, battalion aid stations consisted in general of a series of adjoining rooms. In open warfare, battalion aid stations were much simpler, occupying any spot affording some protection from hostile fire, such as a shell hole, cellar, culvert, quarry, dugout, or behind a ruined wall.[16] Medical services at a battalion aid station included first aid, application or readjustment of dressings and splints, hemorrhage control, administration of anti-tetanus serum and morphine, emergency treatment of gassed cases, administration of warmth to prevent shock and preparation of a diagnosis tag.[17]

From a battalion aid station, stretcher bearers carried the wounded further back to a dressing station, which was usually made of tents affording limited shelter. As a rule, two or three dressing stations were established for one division depending on the width of its sector, availability of roads and military activity. Dressing station equipment was often limited in variety, consisting of dressings, splints, litters, blankets, anti-tetanus serum, a few drugs including morphine, instruments and anti-gas supplies. A kitchen unit was part of a dressing station making it possible to supply hot food. At the dressing station, cases were selected for transportation by ambulance to field hospitals.[18] Each division in the U.S. Army was composed of several units including a so-called Sanitary Train. This medical unit comprised a field hospital section with three motorized and one animal-drawn field hospitals, an ambulance section with three motorized and one animal-drawn ambulance companies, eight camp infirmaries, one medical supply unit and one mobile laboratory. Normal capacity of a field hospital was 216 patients. Usually, one of the field hospitals of a division cared for wounded soldiers (surgical cases), one for sick soldiers (medical cases) and one for gassed soldiers, while the fourth was held in reserve. Field hospitals used tents, but upon opportunity occupied buildings in suitable locations.[19] In open warfare, field hospitals were located three to six miles behind the front and in trench warfare even further to the rear, six to eight miles.[20] Still, field hospitals had limited equipment and could treat only the lightly wounded.[21]

From field hospitals, wounded men were taken by ambulance to evacuation hospitals

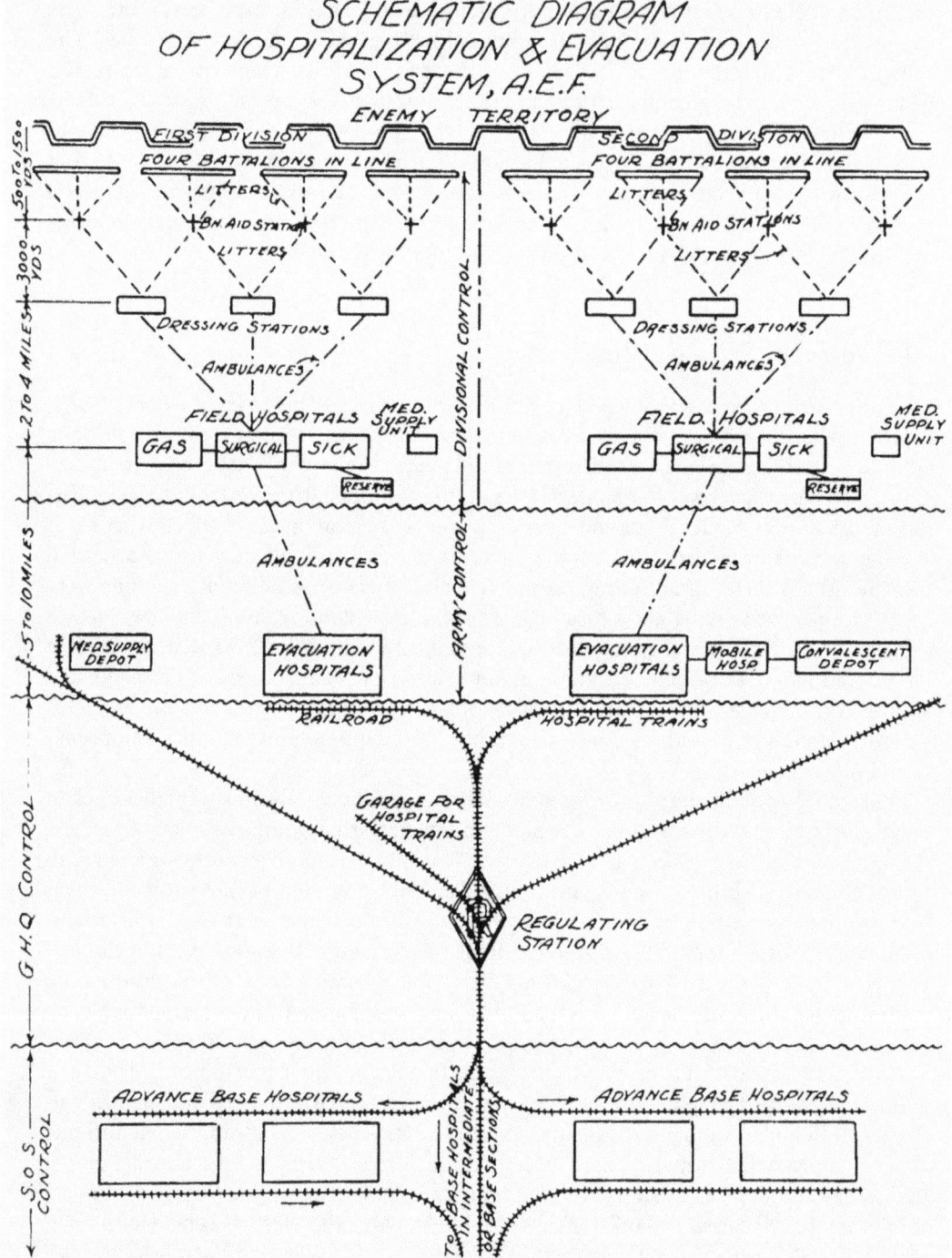

Schematic diagram of the hospitalization and evacuation system of the American Expeditionary Forces (Lynch C, Ford JH, Weed FW, *The Medical Department of the United States Army in the World War, Volume VIII: Field Operations*. Washington, D.C.: Government Printing Office, 1925: 262).

One. The Evacuation Chain of the American Expeditionary Forces 15

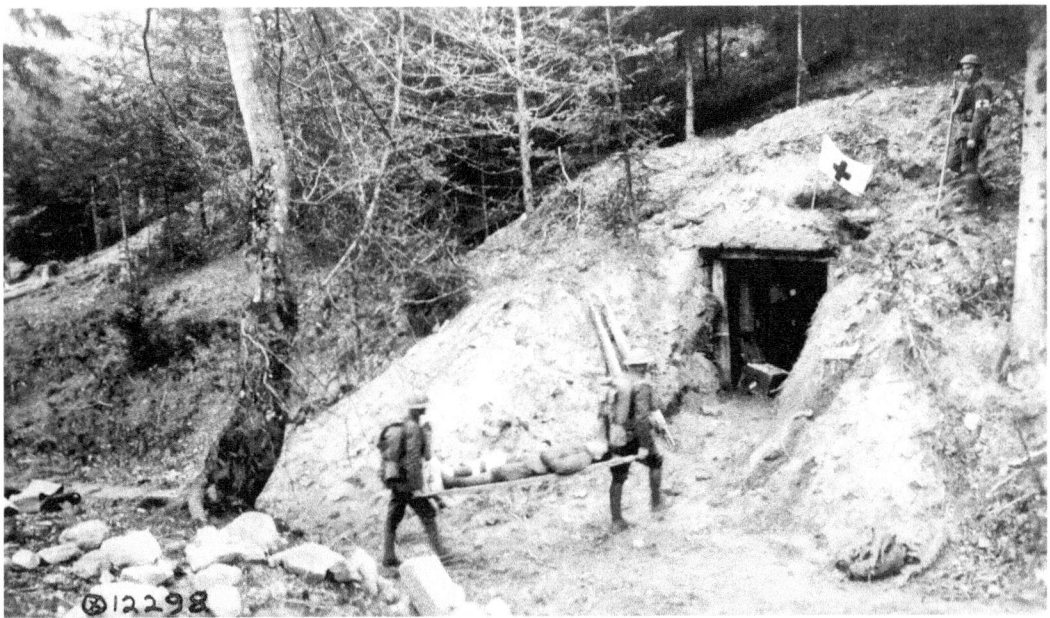

A wounded American soldier is transported by stretcher bearers to a dressing station in a dugout at Bertrichamps, France (National Archives at College Park, Maryland [Record Group 111: Records of the Office of the Chief Signal Officer, 1860–1985, Photographs of American Military Activities, ca. 1918–ca. 1981, National Archives Identifier 530707: photograph no. 111-SC-12298]).

for surgical care. They could stay there for several days to stabilize and begin recovery.[22] The preferable location of evacuation hospitals was as near to the front as possible, but safe from artillery fire, usually 9 to 15 miles from the front. They had to be accessible by good roads from the forward area and by hospital trains from the rear. Evacuation hospitals were situated in tents, barracks and existing buildings.[23] From evacuation hospitals, patients were taken by hospital trains to base hospitals, where they could receive complicated procedures and recuperate.[24]

Hospital Centers

One of the bigger problems in the U.S. Army Medical Department during World War I was a constantly increasing shortage of personnel, especially of officers and nurses.[25] As a consequence, base hospitals were stripped of officers, nurses and enlisted men to form operating and other teams for service near the front line and to staff camp hospitals serving rest and training areas.[26] To reduce staff and overhead demands, it was planned as early as September 1917 to group from 2 to 20 base hospitals and a convalescent camp in hospital centers with a capacity of up to 36,000 beds. The creation of such hospital cities required the construction of administrative and supply buildings, storehouses, garages, bakery, ice plant, post office, telegraph and telephone exchange, fire engine house, chapel, laboratory, morgue, etc., and installation of central water, sewerage and lighting systems.[27] Availability of railway facilities was an important requirement for approval of a site for construction of a hospital center. Considerations taken into account were distance from the front, proximity to main railway lines, grade and condition of trackage,

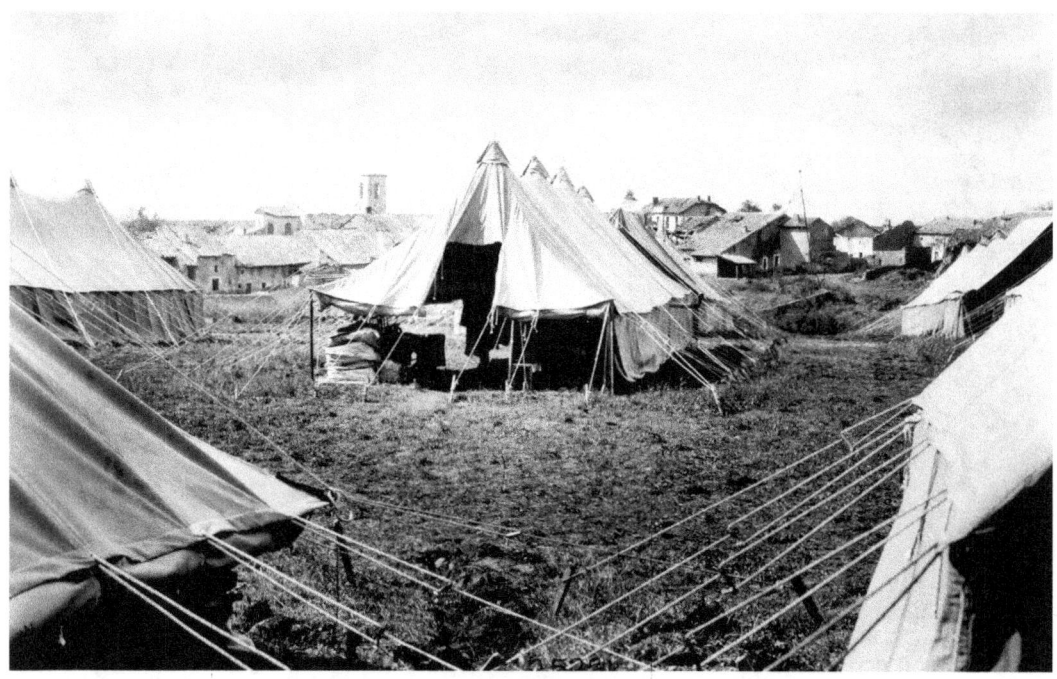

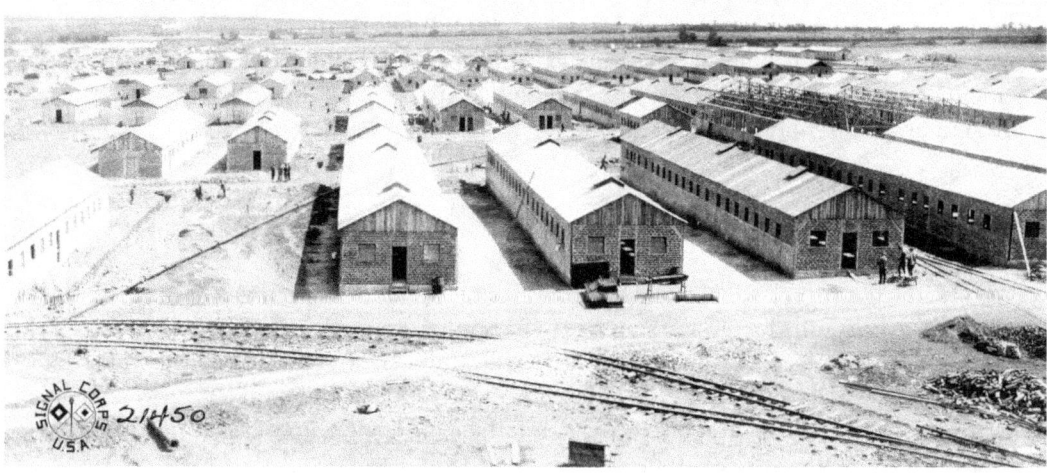

Top: Tents of Field Hospital No. 353, 314th Sanitary Train, 89th Division at Bernécourt, France (National Archives at College Park, Maryland [Record Group 111: Records of the Office of the Chief Signal Officer, 1860–1985, Photographs of American Military Activities, ca. 1918–ca. 1981, National Archives Identifier 530707: photograph no. 111-SC-25281]). *Bottom:* A view of construction work at Mars Hospital Center which was located at Mars-sur-Allier in central France (National Archives at College Park, Maryland [Record Group 111: Records of the Office of the Chief Signal Officer, 1860–1985, Photographs of American Military Activities, ca. 1918–ca. 1981, National Archives Identifier 530707: photograph no. 111-SC-21450]).

strength of bridges and existence or feasibility of railroad sidings. Buildings utilized by hospital centers were often newly constructed barracks or preexisting French buildings such as hotels or military barracks. All hospital centers had units specially equipped for treatment of surgical, orthopedic, eye, ear-nose-throat, maxillofacial (jaws and face), psychiatric, neuropsychiatric and, in some centers, contagious cases. Hospital centers were under the direct control of the commanding general of the Services of Supply. Each hospital center had a commanding officer who was given full authority in many matters.[28]

Before the Armistice commenced on November 11, 1918, around 20 hospital centers were in operation. A summary dated November 28, 1918, lists five hospital centers in the Advance Section (located at Bazoilles-sur-Meuse, Langres, Rimaucourt, Toul and Vittel-Contrexéville), eight in the Intermediate Section (located at Allerey-sur-Saône, Beaune, Clermont-Ferrand, Mars-sur-Allier, Mesves-sur-Loire, Orléans, Tours and Vichy) and seven in the Base Section (located at Angers, Beau Désert (near Bordeaux), Kerhuon (near Brest), Limoges, Nantes, Périgueux and Savenay (near St. Nazaire)). Of these, Mesves Hospital Center attained the largest size with a reported bed capacity of 25,000. Overall total bed capacity reported on November 28, 1918, was 183,483 of which 106,211 were occupied.[29] This summary excludes Riviera Hospital Center which was located at a Mediterranean coastal strip known as the *Côte d'Azur* or Riviera. This hospital center consisted of 29 convalescent hospitals, the farthest some 135 miles apart, organized in five hospital groups at and around Hyères, Saint-Raphaël, Cannes, Nice and Menton. In these places commodious hotels were leased and converted to hospitals fully equipped for the most modern work in medicine and surgery. The location of this hospital center provided stimulating atmospheric conditions like sunshine, clear skies, limited rainfall and mild climate. The first patients were received on November 7, 1918, and 13,975 cases were admitted up to April 1, 1919.[30]

At the time the Armistice was signed, a number of other hospital centers were being constructed and additional ones projected adding towards a planned total bed capacity in hospital centers of 500,000 should the war continue until April 1919.[31] In retrospect, the U.S. Army Medical Department recognized the formation of hospital centers among the most important of its enterprises in World War I.[32] The first hospital center that started as an organized center was Bazoilles Hospital Center, situated in Bazoilles-sur-Meuse.[33]

Two

Bazoilles Hospital Center in Operation
63,769 Treated in Ten Months

The first American hospital unit to arrive at Bazoilles-sur-Meuse was Base Hospital No. 18. It was functioning as an independent base hospital from July 31, 1917, onwards. Construction on Bazoilles Hospital Center began late October 1917, but progress was very slow. The center officially began operation on July 1, 1918. At the height of its operation, the center consisted of seven base hospitals located in Bazoilles-sur-Meuse, one base hospital in Neufchâteau and a convalescent camp in Liffol-le-Grand. Total hospital capacity was 7,000 beds with the possibility for crisis expansion with tents to over 13,000 beds. In the first weeks of October 1918, the number of patients treated in the center rose to over 10,000 due to admissions for Spanish flu and injuries sustained in the Meuse-Argonne Offensive. From July 1, 1918, to April 30, 1919, 63,769 patients were treated at the center indicating that 3 percent of the two million men and women that made up the American Expeditionary Forces was admitted to Bazoilles Hospital Center at some point during their overseas service.

Bazoilles-sur-Meuse

The rural village of Bazoilles-sur-Meuse is located in the *département* Vosges, named after the Vosges mountains, in the north-east of France. One U.S. Army doctor noted that Bazoilles-sur-Meuse "is a formidable name but not formidable in appearance." The town was very small, the streets were very small, there were one or two stores and people lived with cows and chickens. Yet, it was situated in a pretty little valley dotted with small forests surrounded by many hills. In all, a "picturesque" place.[1] Most houses in the village are situated on the west bank of the Meuse River, which winds its way north through the countryside towards Verdun and Belgium. The eastern railroad ran through Bazoilles-sur-Meuse and the village's train station was located on the east bank of the river. Around the time that Bazoilles Hospital Center was situated in Bazoilles-sur-Meuse, its population counted 412 people. The small city of Neufchâteau with, at that time, 4,000 inhabitants, some four miles north of Bazoilles-sur-Meuse, had a regional function. Historically, the region is of interest because of the village Domrémy-la-Pucelle, the birth place of Joan of Arc, some 11 miles to the north of Bazoilles-sur-Meuse, which proved a popular day trip for the personnel of the center.[2]

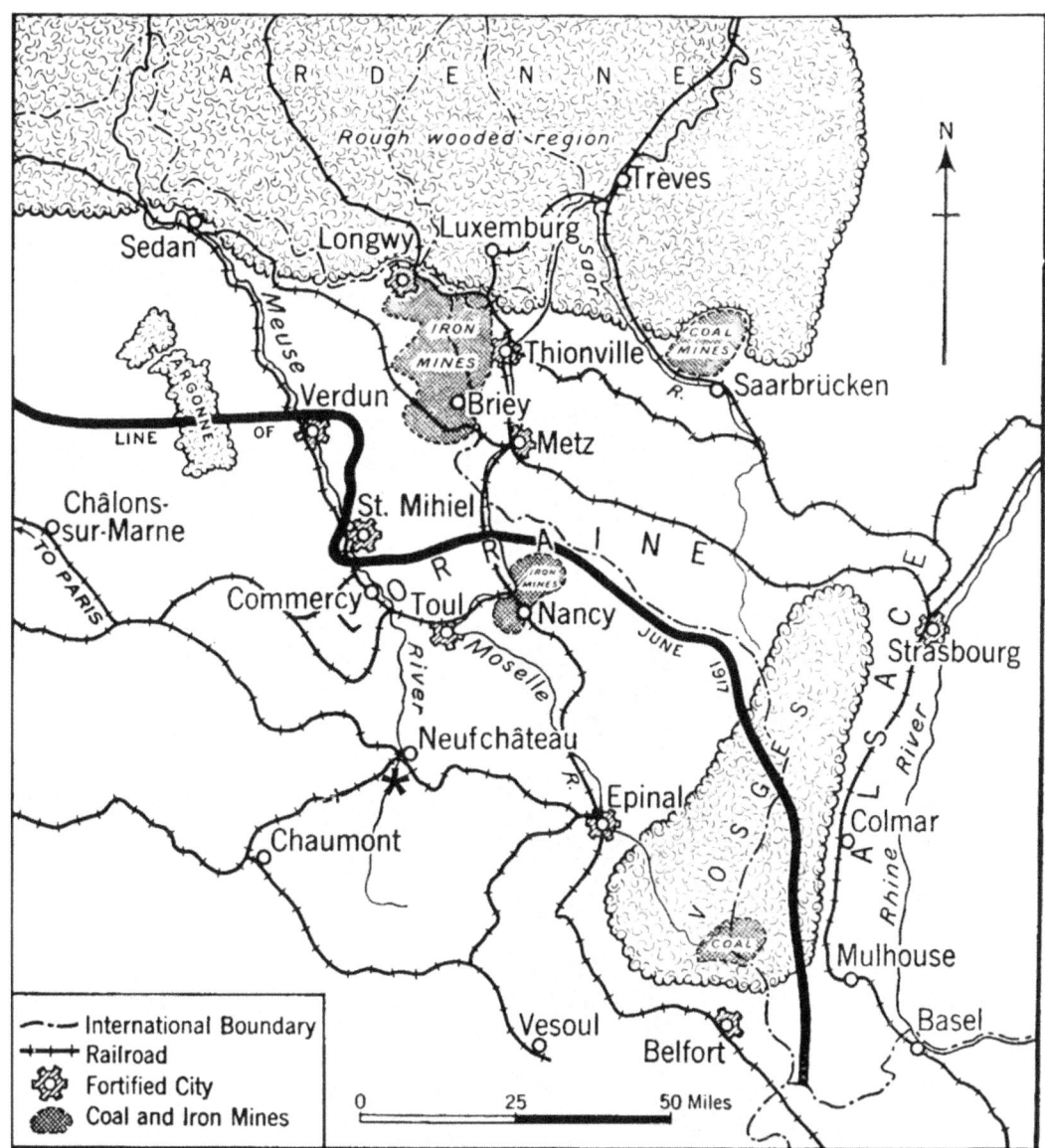

Map of the northeast of France in 1918. The location of Bazoilles-sur-Meuse, some four miles south of Neufchâteau along the Meuse River, is marked with an asterisk. The bold line designates the front line where the U.S. Army commenced large offensives in September 1918, near St. Mihiel (Battle of St. Mihiel) and the Argonne Forest (Meuse-Argonne Offensive) (American Battle Monuments Commission. *American Armies and Battlefields in Europe: A History, Guide and Reference Book*. Washington, D.C.: Government Printing Office, 1938: 16).

The name Bazoilles comes from the Latin word "basis" which stands for lowland and the old Gallic word "oye" meaning goose.[3] To the Americans, the name Bazoilles-sur-Meuse was unpronounceable, which gave way to various corrupted pronunciations and notations: Bazwillie Sure Moose, Bazwillie Submerged, Baz Eels on the Muss, Bacillus on Mush and many other variations were in vogue.[4] The local population quickly adapted to the newcomers and opened the "American Bar" which was announced by a

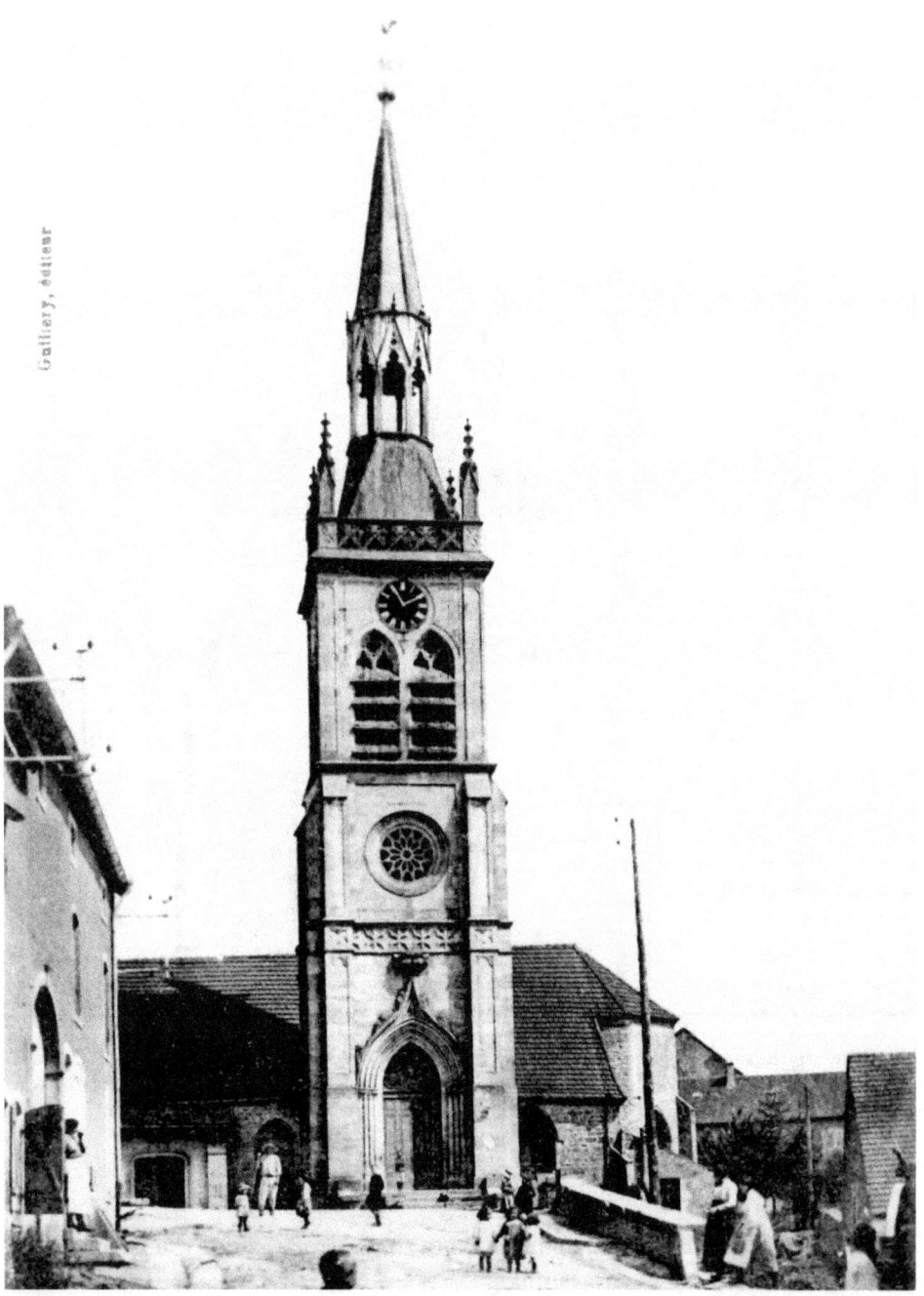

This postcard showing the church of Bazoilles-sur-Meuse was sent on February 27, 1919, by Second Lieutenant Cecil A. Carlisle from Atlanta, Georgia. He served with the Quartermaster Corps and was attached to Clothing Unit No. 310, which was presumably stationed at Bazoilles Hospital Center (author's collection).

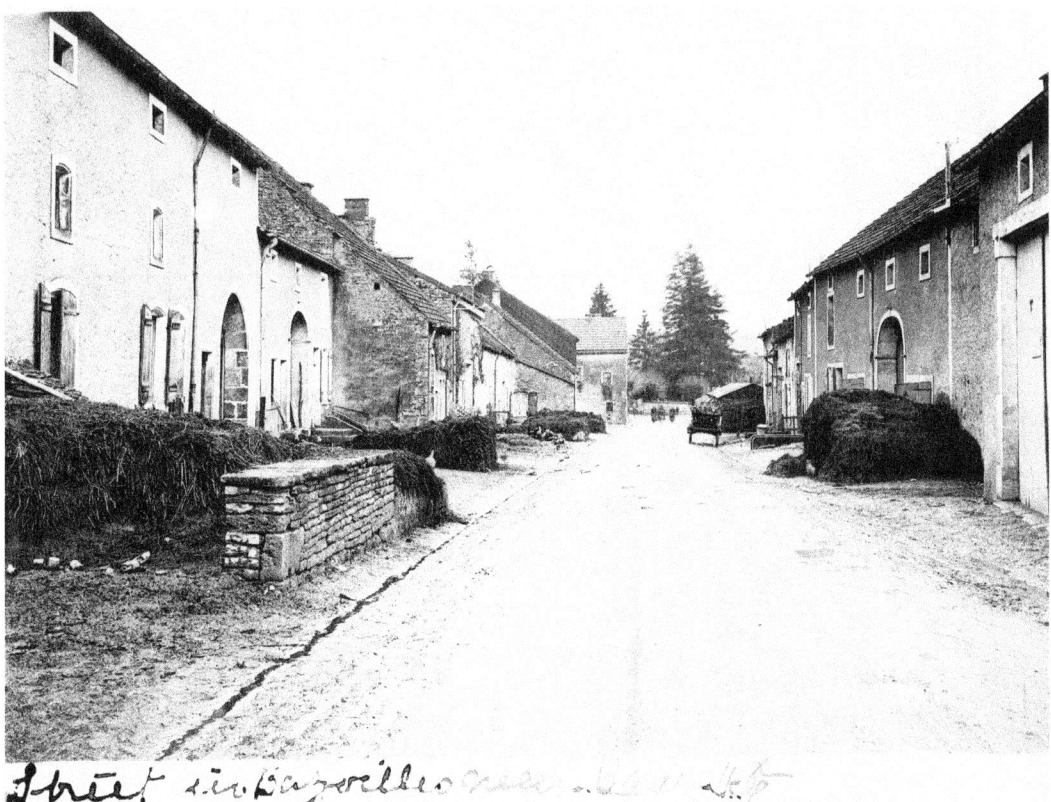

View of one of the small streets in the rural village of Bazoilles-sur-Meuse at the time of World War I. The handwritten caption reads: "Street in Bazoilles near Base [Hospital No.] 46" (courtesy Oregon Health & Science University, Portland, Oregon [Historical Collections & Archives, Eleanor Donaldson Papers, Accession No. 20080-20, box 1 folder 6 Photographic prints-Base Hospital 46]).

large road sign. As the American Bar was a cafeteria rather than a café, it never became very popular.[5]

Base Hospital No. 18

The first American hospital unit to arrive at Bazoilles-sur-Meuse, on July 26, 1917, was Base Hospital No. 18, which at that time was the farthest advanced hospital in the American Expeditionary Forces. Base Hospital No. 18 was organized in November 1916 at Johns Hopkins Hospital, Baltimore, Maryland, and, therefore, also referred to as the Johns Hopkins Unit. At Bazoilles-sur-Meuse, the unit took over the *Château de Bazoilles-sur-Meuse* (Castle of Bazoilles-sur-Meuse) from the French Medical Department. This was an estate comprising a manor, several outbuildings and a 25-acre tract of land. Additional wooden barracks were added, providing a total bed capacity of 1,000, which was later increased by tent expansion to 1,300 beds. The unit began operation on July 31, 1917, functioning independently for 11 months until July 1, 1918, when it became part of Bazoilles Hospital Center.[6]

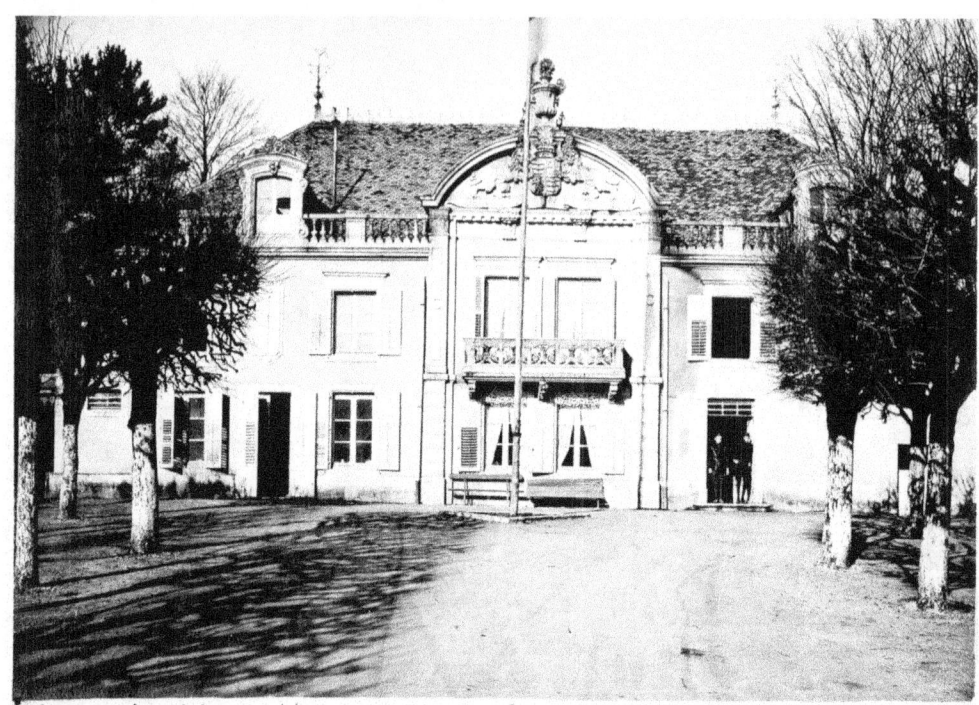

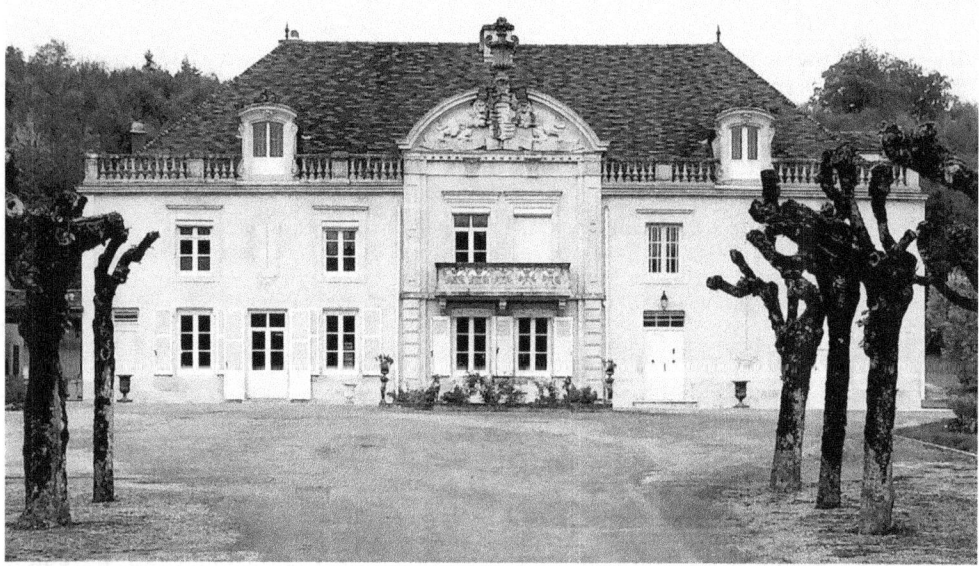

Top: View of the *Château de Bazoilles-sur-Meuse* (Castle of Bazoilles-sur-Meuse) while it was occupied by Base Hospital No. 18. The handwritten caption reads: "Johns Hopkins Hospital 1918 near Base 46" (courtesy Oregon Health & Science University, Portland, Oregon [Historical Collections & Archives, Eleanor Donaldson Papers, Accession No. 20080-20, box 1 folder 6 Photographic prints-Base Hospital 46]). *Bottom*: Present-day view of the *Château de Bazoilles-sur-Meuse* where Base Hospital No. 18 was in operation from July 31, 1917, to January 9, 1919 (photograph by author).

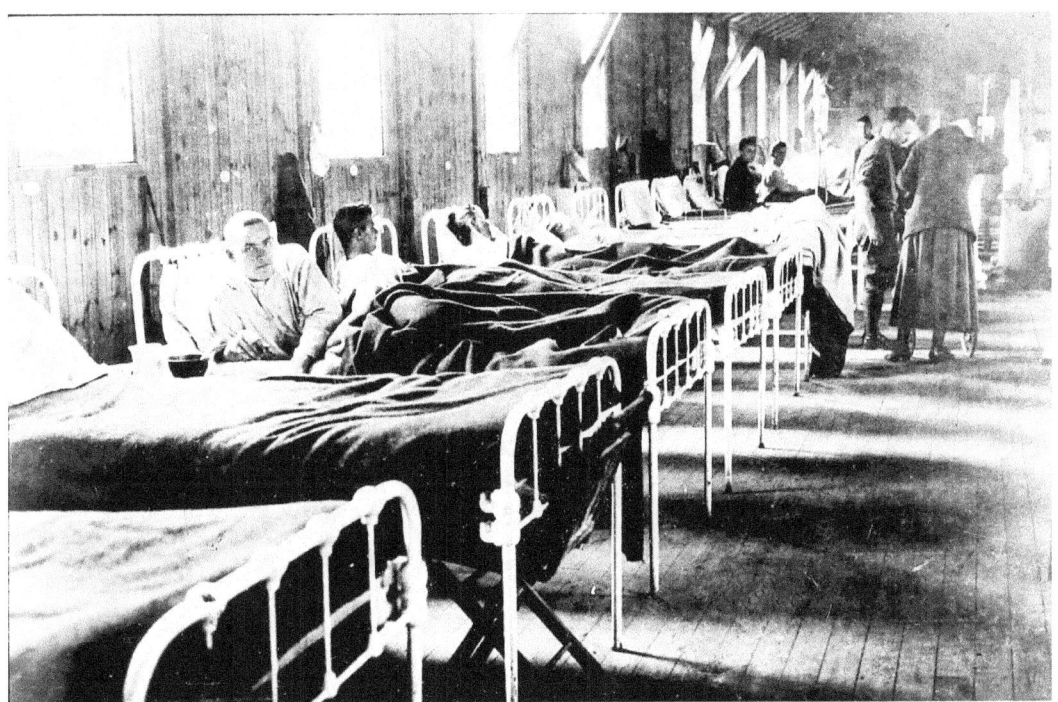

A patient ward at Base Hospital No. 18 on May 2, 1918, two months before Bazoilles Hospital Center began operation (author's collection).

In August 1917, it was ordered that Base Hospital No. 18 was to act as an evacuation hospital imposing radical changes on its system of operation. The hospital staff worked in two shifts so that the hospital could be kept running 24 hours a day. Only minimal clinical records were kept doing away with much of the clerical work, disinfestation of verminous patients was given up except in special cases and careful checking of clothes for lice was discontinued. All patients were seen by one medical officer who sent the sick directly to medical wards and the wounded to a room where their dressings were removed by orderlies and their wounds inspected by members of the surgical staff. The wounds of some patients were redressed and they were sent directly to surgical wards, while the wounds of others were merely covered and these patients were sent to the X-ray department, pre-operative room or directly to the operating room.[7]

Among the enlisted men of Base Hospital No. 18 were 32 students from the Johns Hopkins Medical School who had completed their third year in medicine. These students had been enlisted as privates in the Medical Reserve Corps with the understanding that they should be given practical training as well as organized teaching by the members of the staff. Upon completion of their course, they would be granted a degree in medicine and a commission in the U.S. Army as medical officers. The medical students' course consisted of clinical work on the patient wards and in the operating rooms as well as laboratory work. In addition, lecture courses were provided covering the practice of general medicine and surgery, the organization and administration of the U.S. Army Medical Corps and specific topics like troop sanitation, evacuation of wounded and the duties of battalion medical officers. In April 1918, degrees in medicine were granted by Johns Hopkins Medical School to 30 of the 32 students initially attached to Base Hospital No. 18.[8]

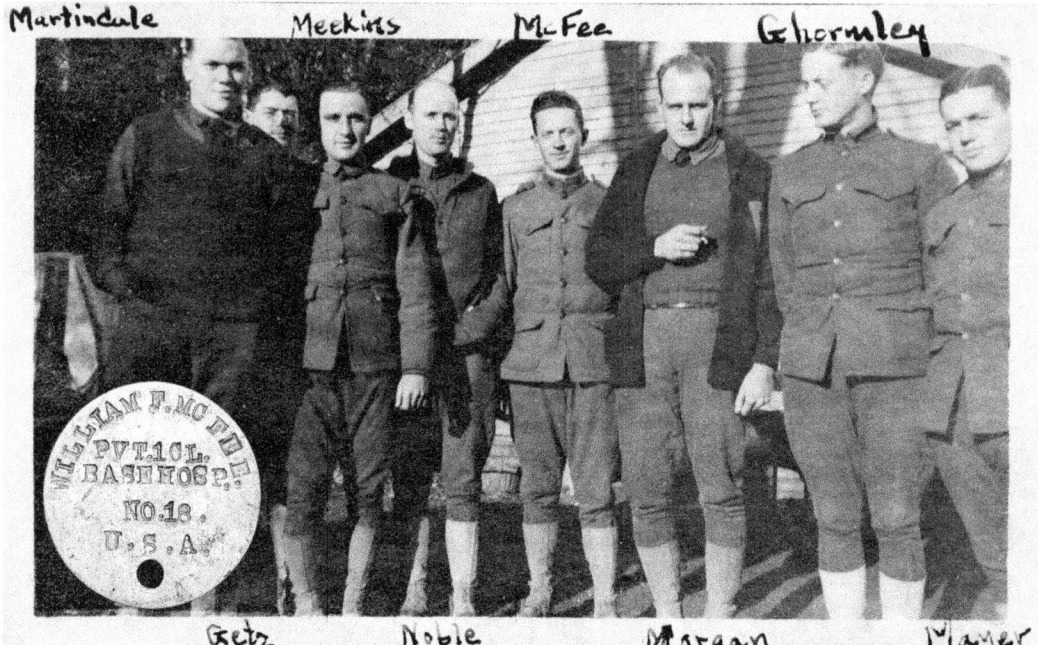

A photograph depicting eight of the 32 medical students from the Johns Hopkins Medical School who received a course of practical training and organized teaching at Base Hospital No. 18 at Bazoilles-sur-Meuse in 1917–1918. From left to right: Joseph W. Martindale, Lawrence Getz, Gilbert E. Meekins, William D. Noble, William F. McFee, Hugh J. Morgan, Ralph K. Ghormley and William F. Mayer. The inset shows the identification tag of Private First Class William F. McFee (author's collection).

A few months earlier, tragedy struck when two of the Johns Hopkins University students succumbed to an infectious disease. Private First Class Edwin Scott Linton from Washington, Pennsylvania, was attending a ward in which a case of scarlet fever developed, whereupon he contracted the disease himself. After an illness of short duration, he died, aged 24, on November 14, 1917.[9] In June 1918, Edwin Linton was posthumously awarded the medical doctor's degree from the Johns Hopkins University.[10] As a memorial to their son, the Edwin Linton Junior Fund for research in anatomy, physiology and physiological chemistry was established in 1919 by Professor and Mrs. Edwin Linton.[11] Private First Class Lyle Barnes Rich from Willow City, North Dakota, worked in the base hospital's laboratory when he contracted typhoid fever the latter part of November 1917. On December 6, his condition was complicated by a bowel perforation and he was immediately rushed to operation. Efforts were, however, unavailing and he died, aged 26, on December 8.[12] American Legion Post 112 in Willow City has been named after Lyle Rich.[13] Presumably, both students were initially interred in a small French military cemetery next to the *Château de Bazoilles-sur-Meuse*.[14] Edwin Linton and Lyle Rich were later re-buried at the Meuse-Argonne American Cemetery in Romagne-sous-Montfaucon in Plot B, Row 40, Grave 33 and Plot C, Row 39, Grave 34, respectively.[15]

The first winter in France was marked by hardship. The weather was severe, the buildings poor and fuel scarce and of inferior quality. But despite the unfavorable conditions, excellent work was accomplished. Many soldiers in the American Expeditionary Forces were certain that the Johns Hopkins Unit was the best hospital in France, in part

Washington (Pa.) Soldier With Gen. Pershing Dies

Edwin S. Linton, Son of W. & J. Professor, Succumbs to Scarlet Fever.

WASHINGTON, Nov. 16.—Private Edwin S. Linton, Medical Department, base hospital, died November 14 of scarlet fever, according to a report from Gen. Pershing today. Private Linton was a son of Prof.

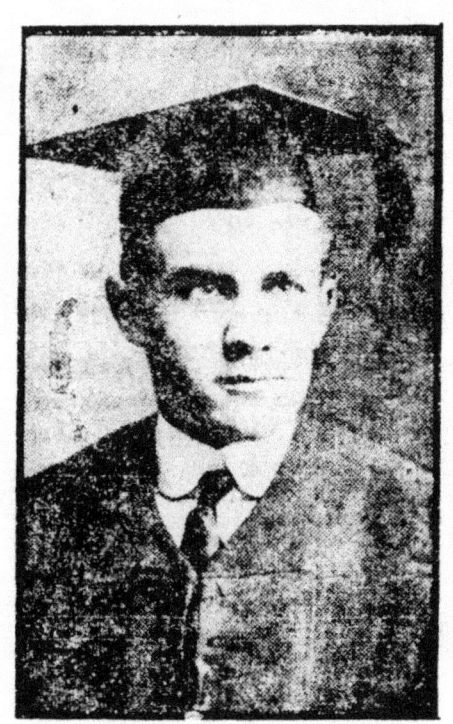

Private Edwin S. Linton.

Edward Linton of the Washington and Jefferson College (Pa.) faculty.

Newspaper item reporting the death of medical student Edwin S. Linton on November 14, 1917, at Base Hospital No 18 (Washington [Pa.] Soldier With Gen. Pershing Dies. *The Pittsburgh Gazette Times*. November 17, 1917: 5).

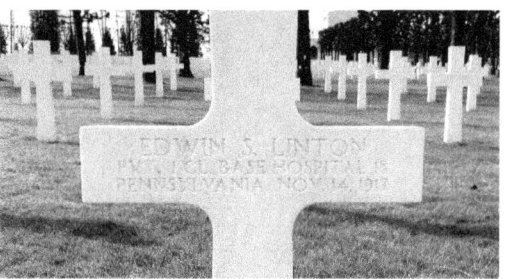

Headstone of the grave of Private First Class Edwin S. Linton at the Meuse-Argonne American Cemetery in Romagne-sous-Montfaucon (courtesy American Battle Monuments Commission [Overseas Operations Office, Paris, France; photograph by author]).

because of the reputation of its mother institution, and that one's overseas service was not complete without at least one course of treatment in Base Hospital No. 18.[16]

Construction of Bazoilles Hospital Center

In late October 1917, the Engineer Corps began construction on Bazoilles Hospital Center, but progress was very slow. The center officially began operation on July 1, 1918. At the height of its operation, Bazoilles Hospital Center consisted of eight base hospitals and a convalescent camp. Base Hospitals Nos. 18 and 116 were already in operation on July 1, followed on July 23 by Base Hospital No. 46, which was organized at the University of Oregon, Portland, Oregon, and on August 6 by Base Hospital No. 42, which was organized at the University of Maryland, Baltimore, Maryland. On October 4, Base Hospitals Nos. 60 and 81 started operation, followed on November 5 by Base Hospital No. 79. Although located at nearby Neufchâteau, Base Hospital No. 66 was also temporarily assigned to Bazoilles Hospital Center. It was first included in

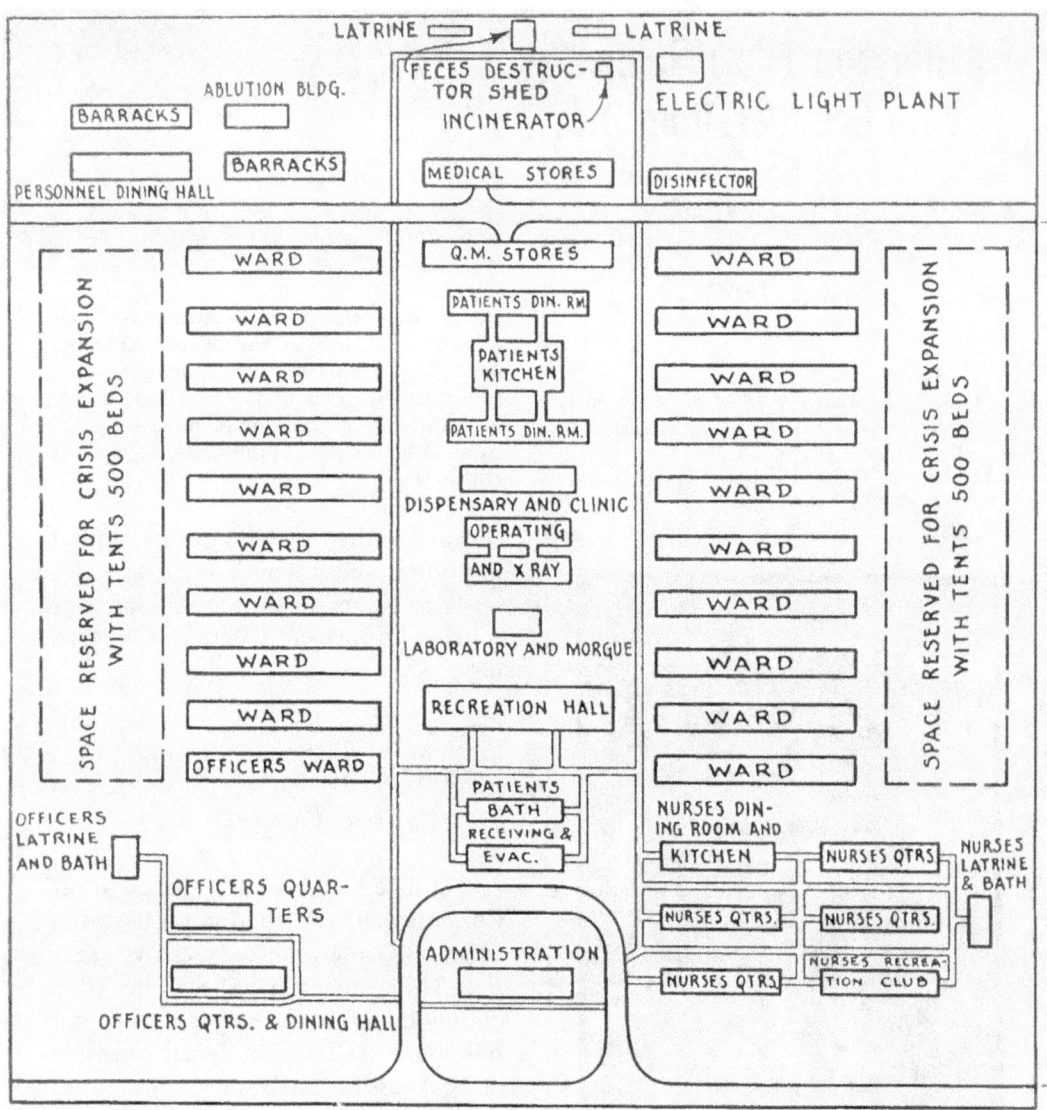

General layout of a type A hospital unit commonly used for overseas base hospitals like those at Bazoilles Hospital Center (Ford, J.H. *The Medical Department of the United States Army in the World War, Volume II: Administration American Expeditionary Forces.* **Washington, D.C.: Government Printing Office, 1927: 242).**

its bed report on August 15, but ceased to be part of the center on November 10. The convalescent camp connected to Bazoilles Hospital Center, designated Convalescent Camp No. 2, was situated in nearby Liffol-le-Grand and started operation on July 13.[17]

The work on Bazoilles Hospital Center was reported completed, with the exception of minor changes, on November 1, 1918. Its cost was approximately two million dollars. Total hospital capacity at the center was 7,000 beds with the possibility for crisis expansion with tents to over 13,000 beds. The base hospitals units at the center were so-called type A hospitals indicating that they were standard units complete in every particular and, as in most cases, built of wood. The normal layout of a type A unit comprised three

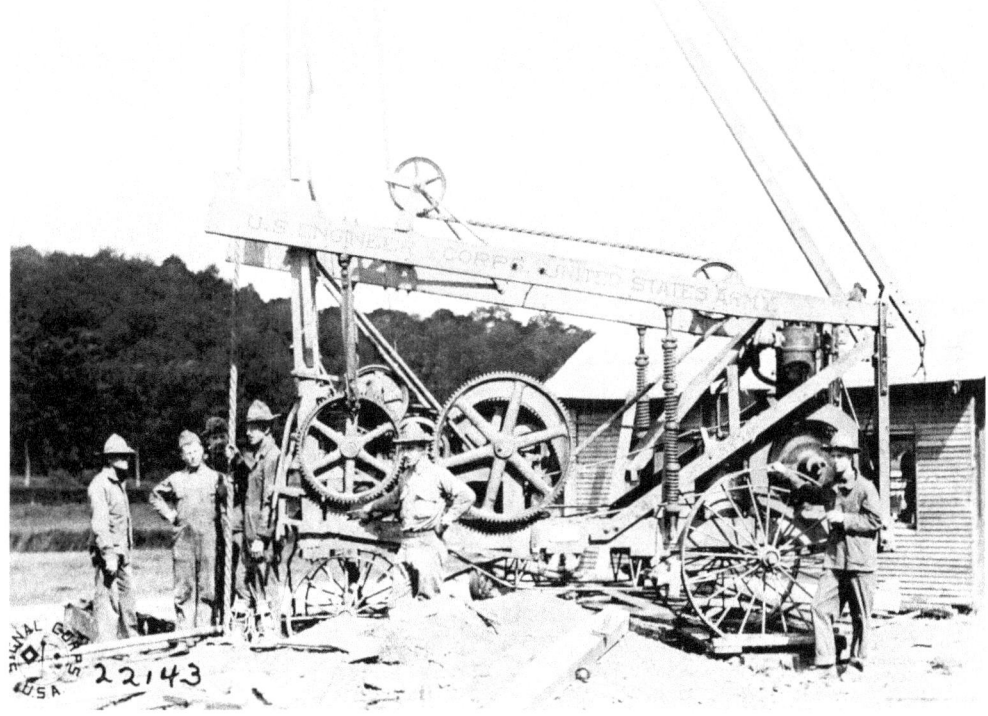

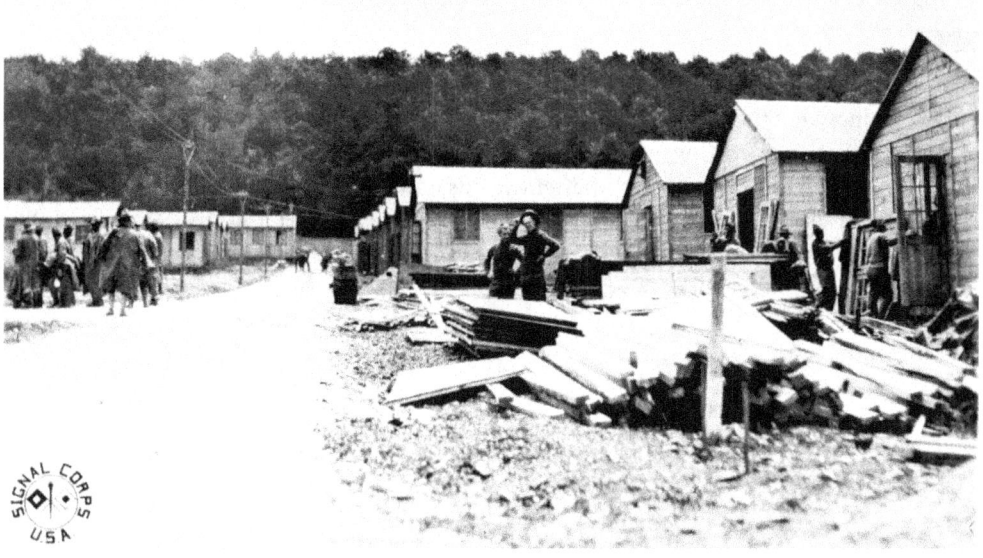

Top: A detachment of the 33rd Engineers digging wells for the water supply of Base Hospital No. 116 (National Archives at College Park, College Park, Maryland [Record Group 111: Records of the Office of the Chief Signal Officer, 1860–1985, Photographs of American Military Activities, ca. 1918c-a. 1981, National Archives Identifier 530707: photograph no. 111-SC-22143]). *Bottom:* A roadway at Base Hospital No. 116 with barracks under construction (U.S. National Library of Medicine. Digital Collections. http://resource.nlm.nih.gov/101398243; accessed December 26, 2017).

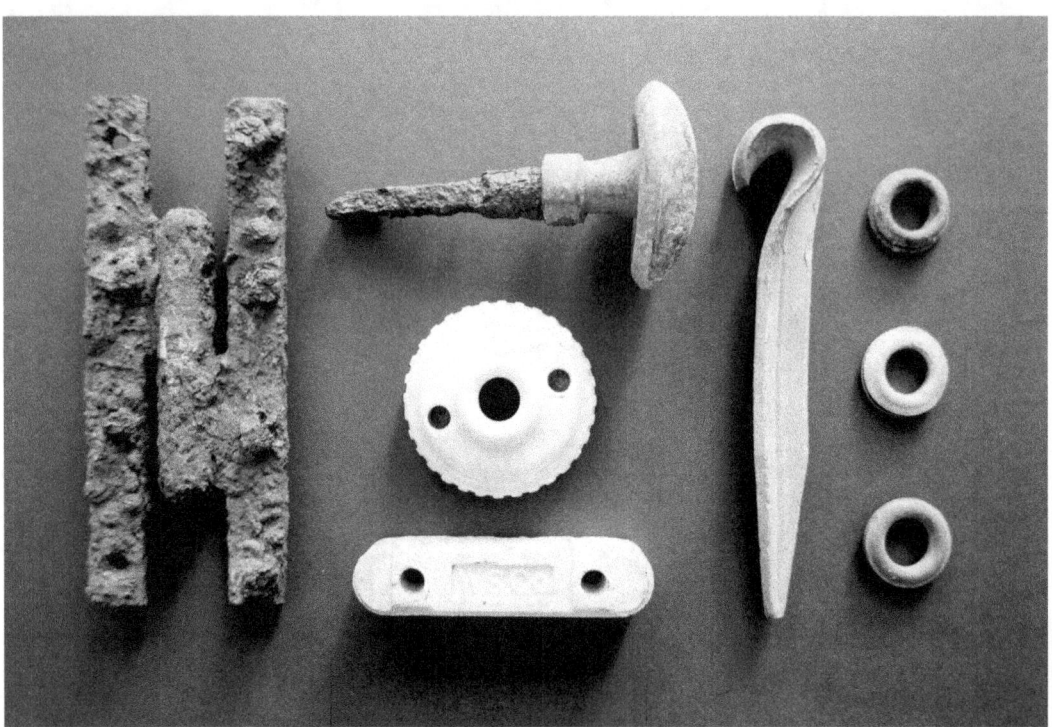

Materials recovered at the former site of Bazoilles Hospital Center illustrative of the barracks and tents erected at the site. Shown are a hinge, door knob and porcelain fixtures for electrical wiring used in barracks and a peg and eyelets from tentage (courtesy Haye Wever [private collection] and author's collection).

rows of buildings (huts or barracks) divided by roadways and walks. The central row of buildings included those pertaining to general services such as administration, reception of patients, baths, operating and X-ray sections, clinic and dining room. On each side of this central row was a block of ten patient wards and beside these sufficient space for the erection of tents as crisis expansion. The wards provided accommodation for 1,000 patients, while the crises expansion by tents doubled this capacity. In the corners of the type A hospitals, the quarters of the officers, nurses and enlisted men were located. The advantages with buildings of this type were availability, mobility, quickness of erecting and low initial cost. The first type A hospital of the American Expeditionary Forces was constructed at Bazoilles-sur-Meuse.[18]

Bazoilles Hospital Center in Operation

Bazoilles Hospital Center began operation on July 1, 1918.[19] Toward the end of July, following the Second Battle of the Marne, the number of patients rose to very near the limit of its bed capacity. Early in August, four base hospitals, with a total capacity of approximately 7,000 beds, were in operation (Base Hospitals Nos. 18, 46 and 116) or ready to operate (Base Hospital No. 42). It was feared that a large influx of casualties might entirely overflow the available capacity which was highly undesirable in a hospital center so near the front. Every opportunity was used to evacuate patients to hospitals farther

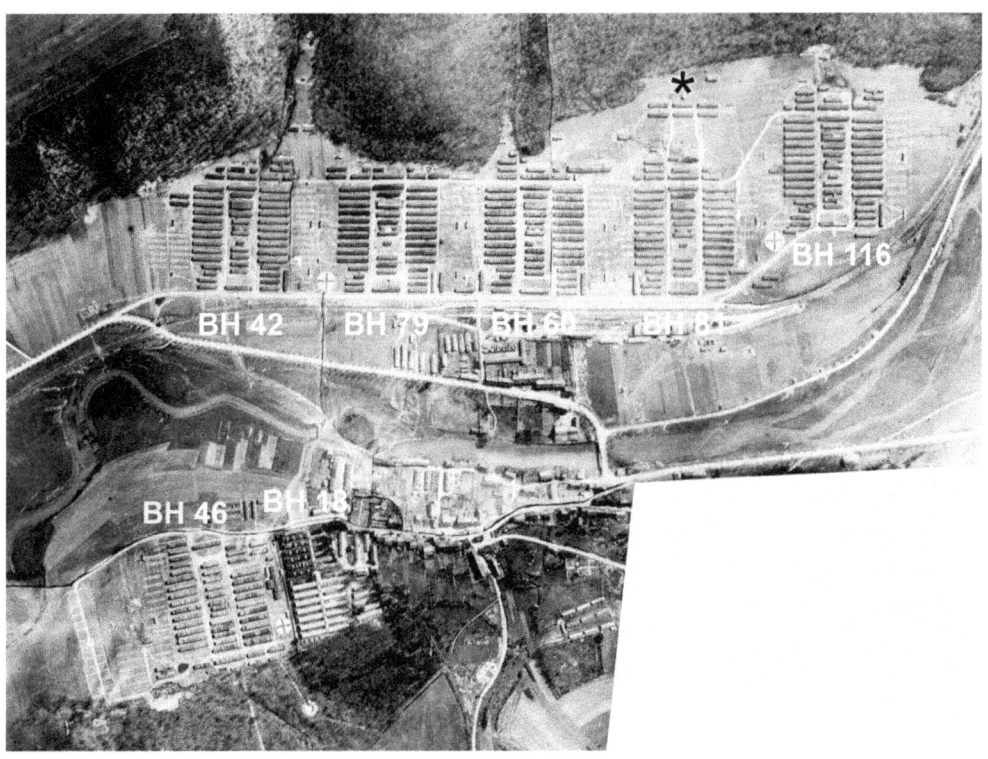

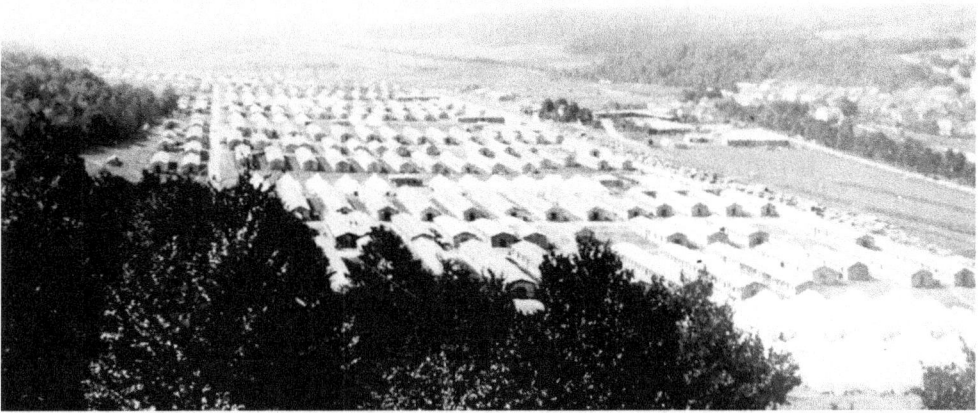

Top: Aerial view of Bazoilles-sur-Meuse showing the base hospitals of Bazoilles Hospital Center with notations of the specific location of each unit. The position of the neuropsychiatric department is marked with an asterisk. The absence of tents used for crisis expansion suggests that this photograph was taken during the later stages of operation of Bazoilles Hospital Center (author's collection). *Bottom*: Southward view on the five base hospitals of Bazoilles Hospital Center on the east bank of the Meuse River (author's collection).

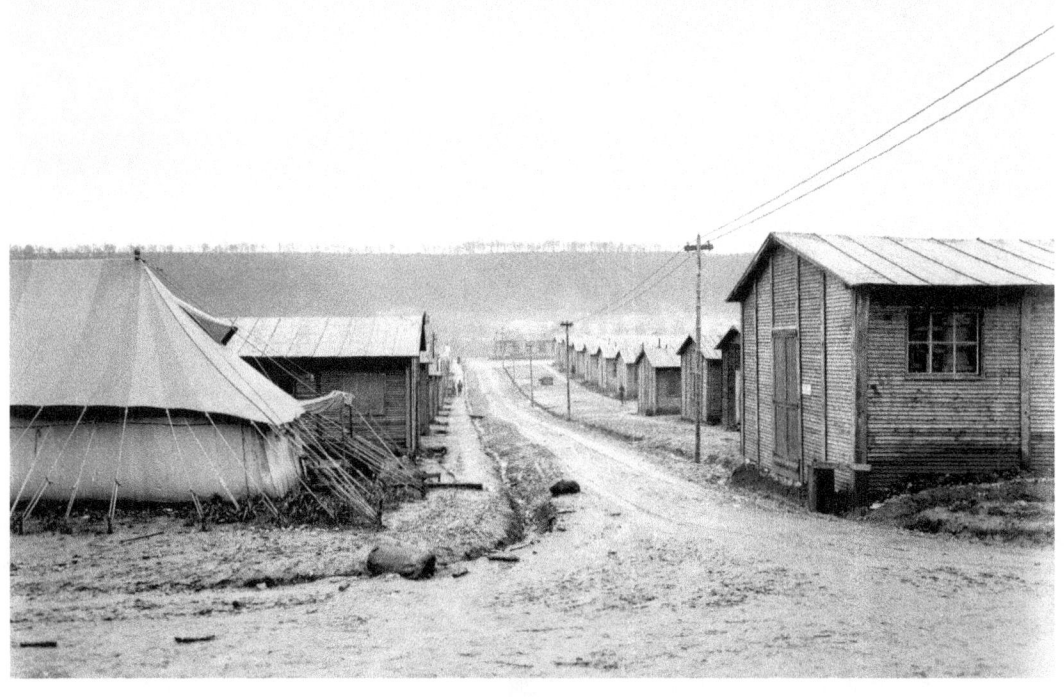

A roadway at Base Hospital No. 46 with wooden barracks and one of the tents which were used for crisis expansion (courtesy Oregon Health & Science University, Portland, Oregon [Historical Collections & Archives, Otis B. Wight–Base Hospital 46: Glass Plate Negative Collection, Accession No. 20060-12, box 1]).

to the rear. Frequently, patients were received, operated upon and evacuated within 48 hours. Thus, the base hospitals at Bazoilles Hospital Center were in reality functioning as evacuation hospitals. Consequently, despite entering into the Battle of St. Mihiel (September 12–16. 1918; 8,182 American casualties including 1,303 killed in action and 496 who died of wounds),[20] the number of patients at the center never reached 4,000 in September.[21] Captain Charles Riggs Ball from St. Paul, Minnesota, a neuropsychiatrist assigned to Base Hospital No. 60, described the operation of Bazoilles Hospital Center in the days following the start of the Battle of St. Mihiel.

> The stream of wounded at this time was so great that the Base Hospitals at Bazoilles ceased functioning as Base Hospitals and simply acted as evacuation hospitals. That is, they were unable to keep their patients and care for them over any period of time, but took them in, deloused them, changed the dressings on their wounds, allowed them a period of from 24 to 48 hours for a rest and then sent them on again to the hospitals farther back from the Front, in order to keep bed space for the steady stream of freshly wounded coming in. ... One day I selected for re-examination twenty-five patients whom I had examined within two weeks' time, in order to see what changes had occured in them since my first examination. I only found one still remaining in the hospital—all the rest had been sent on.[22]

Reconstruction aide Mia Donner Jameson from Riverside, Illinois, described Base Hospital No. 116 as an evacuation hospital "where the men came in from the field dressing stations and as soon as they were cleaned up and [their wounds] dressed, were sent to bases further removed from the front line. Only the most seriously wounded, who could

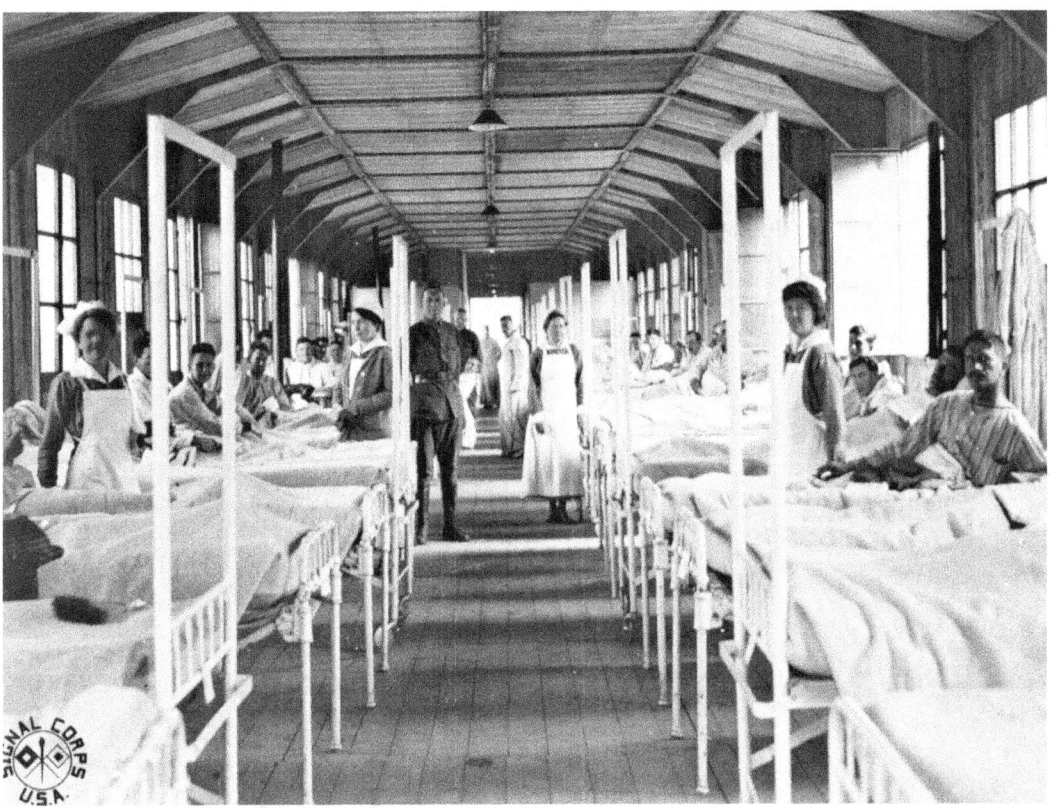

The fracture ward at Base Hospital No. 116. This unit was designated a special hospital for patients with fractures (U.S. National Library of Medicine. Digital Collections. http://resource.nlm.nih.gov/101398232; accessed February 18, 2017).

not be moved, were retained at Bazoilles."[23] At Base Hospital No. 46, roughly one-quarter of the received patients were returned to a duty status, while the remainder was evacuated to base hospitals farther in the rear.[24]

It was decided by the Commanding Officer of Bazoilles Hospital Center, Colonel Elmer Anderson Dean,[25] that the different base hospitals should assume special responsibility for specific patient groups. Base Hospital No. 18 was designated special hospital for chest and abdominal surgery. It operated an optical and ophthalmological (eye) department and received all contagious disease cases coming to the center. Base Hospital No. 42 was designated special hospital for maxillofacial (jaws and face) cases and it received all cases of mumps and measles. Base Hospital No. 46 was designated special hospital for neurosurgical cases. Base Hospital No. 116 was designated special hospital for ear, nose and throat cases and for patients with fractures and operated a neuropsychiatric department.[26]

The Meuse-Argonne Offensive (September 26–November 11, 1918; 122,063 American casualties including 26,277 deaths),[27] in combination with the Spanish flu outbreak (sickening 26 percent of the U.S. Army),[28] resulted within three weeks in admission of approximately 17,000 wounded and sick and between 11,000 and 12,000 evacuations. As a result, the number of patients in Bazoilles Hospital Center rose to over 10,000. The arrival of two additional base hospitals (Base Hospitals Nos. 60 and 81) provided the much needed property and personnel for the operation of the center. The operating staffs of the various base hospitals were pushed to the limit and in some instances worked without intermission for 24 hours or longer. Many extensive operations were made necessary by the severity of the injuries and untreated wound infections.²⁹

A marked decline in the number of admissions at Bazoilles Hospital Center occurred later in October 1918. The center was situated on the left flank of the direct line of evacuation from the Argonne region and this may have led to evacuation to large hospital

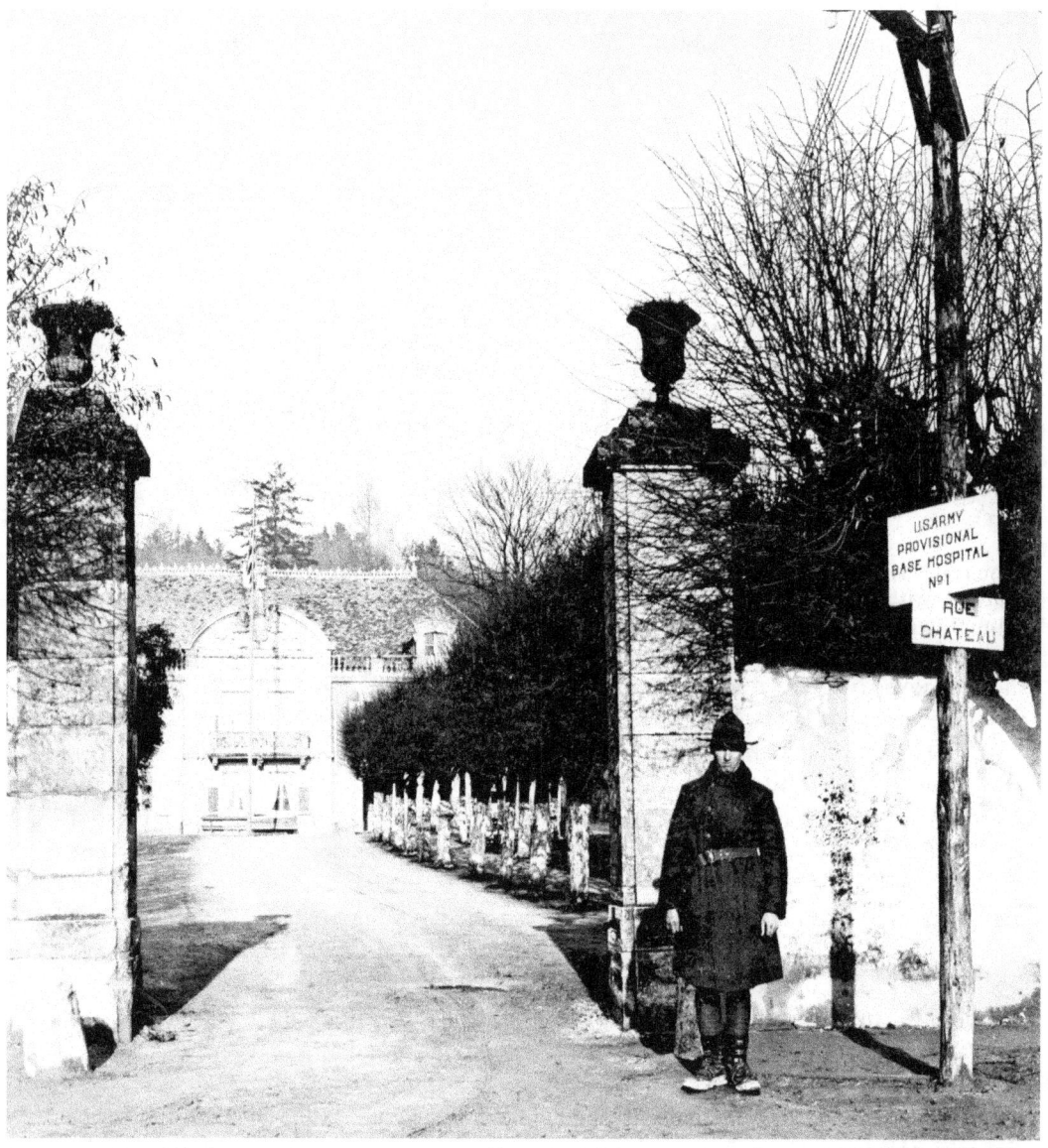

An American soldier stands guard in front of Provisional Base Hospital No. 1 which occupied the *Château de Bazoilles-sur-Meuse* after Base Hospital No. 18 had turned over its patients and property on January 9, 1919 (courtesy Oregon Health & Science University, Portland, Oregon [Historical Collections & Archives, Eleanor Donaldson Papers, Accession No. 20080-20, box 1 folder 6 Photographic prints—Base Hospital 46]).

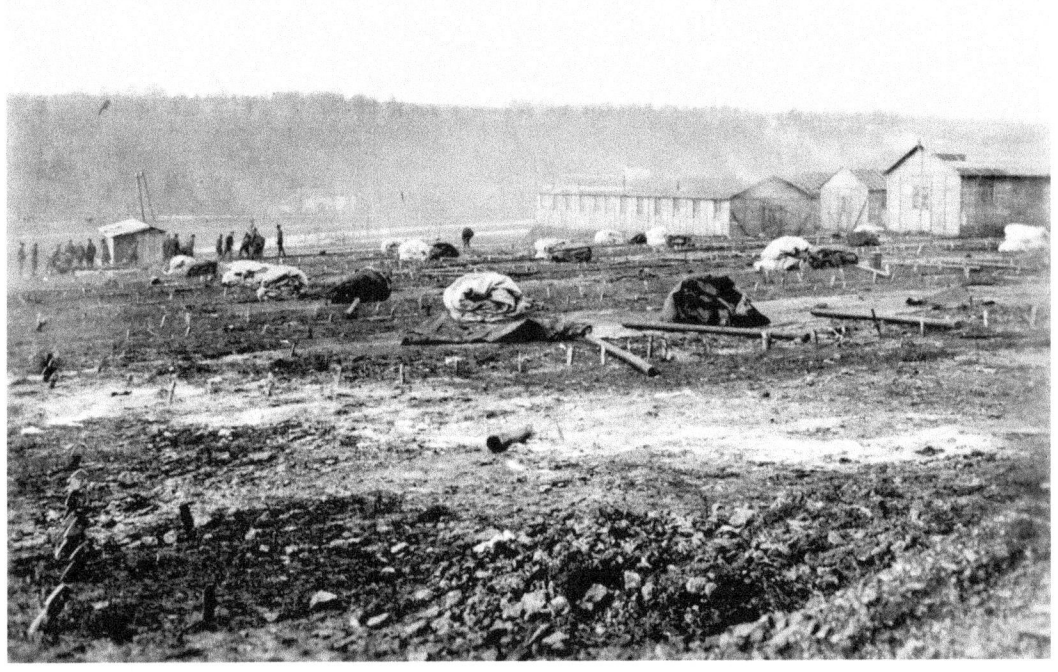

Breaking up the crisis expansion tentage at Base Hospital No. 116 which ceased operation on January 31, 1919 (author's collection).

groups in the Intermediate Section in central France. After November 11, Armistice Day, fewer patients were received. The First Army billeted in the areas surrounding Bazoilles-sur-Meuse and furnished a fair number of sick. In the last four months of its operation, the number of patients in Bazoilles Hospital Center was about 4,000.[30]

Discontinuation of Operation

On January 8, 1919, Evacuation Hospital No. 21 relieved Base Hospital No. 42. Base Hospital No. 18 turned over its patients and property to Provisional Base Hospital No. 1 on January 9.[31] Provisional Base Hospital No. 1 had been mobilized in the beginning of January 1919, when officers, nurses and enlisted personnel were transferred from various hospital units in the vicinity.[32] Base Hospital No. 46 evacuated all its patients to the other hospitals in the center on January 19.[33] Convalescent Camp No. 2 ceased to function on January 25. Base Hospital No. 116 ceased operation on January 31 and turned over its patients and plant including the neuropsychiatric department to Base Hospital No. 79. Base Hospitals Nos. 60 and 81 both ceased operation on March 31 and transferred their remaining patients to the other hospitals in the center. Evacuation Hospital No. 21 and Provisional Base Hospital No. 1 discontinued operation on April 22 and April 27, respectively, both

> # A COINCIDENCE
> While Fitting Out a Returned Soldier the Other Day It Developed that Frank A. Skofstad, Quartermasters' Depot of Base Hospital No. 79, at Bazoilles Sur Meuse, France, Had Outfitted the Same Soldier with Clothing Over There
>
> # OUR SERVICE
> Has Extended at Least two-thirds Around the World For it Has Gone West to Northern China and East as Far as Germany
>
> # SKOFSTADS
> # SELLING SYSTEM

Franklin A. Skofstad from Lawrence, Kansas, served as a private with the Quartermaster's Depot of Base Hospital No. 79. After the war he worked at the family-owned clothing service named Skofstads' Selling System. This June 1919 advertisement in *The Lawrence Daily Journal-World* refers to his overseas service at Bazoilles Hospital Center (A Coincidence. *The Lawrence Daily Journal-World*. June 17, 1919: 6).

transferring their patients to Base Hospital No. 79, the only hospital unit in operation until April 30. Bazoilles Hospital Center ceased operation on May 1. On that date, the 212 patients remaining in Base Hospital No. 79 were evacuated to Angers and Nantes. A large quantity of beds and bedding had already been shipped to Treves and the remaining property was shipped to Mars Hospital Center at Mars-sur-Allier. Bazoilles Hospital Center had been the first to start as an organized center and after ten months of operation was one of the last to close.[34]

From July 1, 1918, to April 30, 1919, 63,769 patients were treated at Bazoilles Hospital Center.[35] This indicates that 3 percent of the two million men and women that made up the American Expeditionary Forces[36] was admitted to Bazoilles Hospital Center at some point during their overseas service. The unit with the highest number of admissions was Base Hospital No. 116 where 12,119 patients were treated from July 1, 1918, to January 31, 1919. Among the principal hospital centers, only Toul Hospital Center, which was nearest to the front, listed more patients passing through with a number of 67,866 up to March 31, 1919.[37]

Two. Bazoilles Hospital Center in Operation

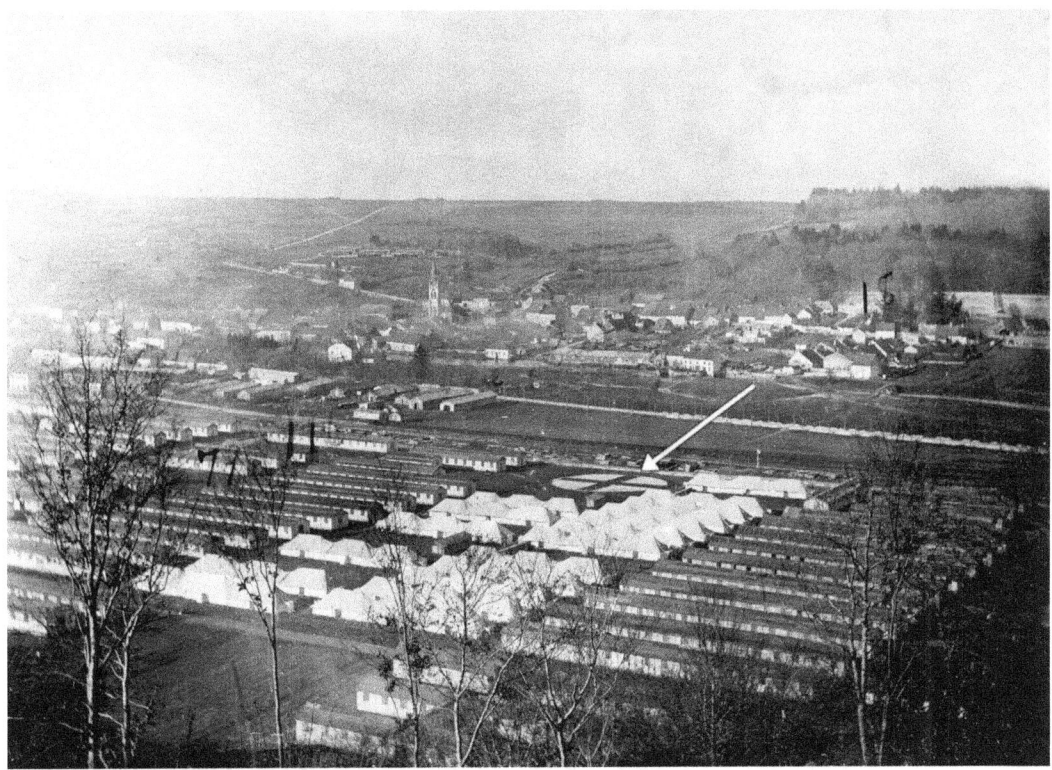

View towards Base Hospitals Nos. 42 and 79. The red cross sign next to the crisis expansion tentage clearly marks the location from the air as a hospital site. Three such signs were made in order to protect Bazoilles Hospital Center from air raids. The handwritten caption for this photograph reads: "Oct. 16, 1918 Bazoilles Sur Meuse France" (author's collection).

The Sound of the Siren

The air raid alarm sounded frequently at Bazoilles Hospital Center bringing about a sense of general discomfort and danger. Upon the shrill sound of the siren, all lights at the center were turned off. The medical personnel left their barracks and waited upon things to come while gazing toward the heaven above. Nurse Sarah Sand, Army Nurse Corps, described the routine of an air raid alarm in her war memoirs.

Air raid alarms occurred quite frequently at Bazoilles Hospital Center interfering with work in the wards as well as adding to the general discomfort of everyone.[1] There is conflicting information on whether or not the center has actually been bombed during air raids. In the book *Lamp for a Soldier: The Caring Story of a Nurse in World War I*, Nurse Sarah Sand from Bismarck, North Dakota, described the routine of an air raid alarm at Base Hospital No. 60 (her war memoirs were published in 1976 by the North Dakota State Nurses' Association on the occasion of the U.S. Bicentennial celebrations).

> Several evenings during October and up to November 11, the shrill siren sounded for air raids. We well understood its meaning. All lights vanished as if by magic [five winks of light were followed within seconds by blackness][2]; all French stoves were closed so there might not be a single glow. Each

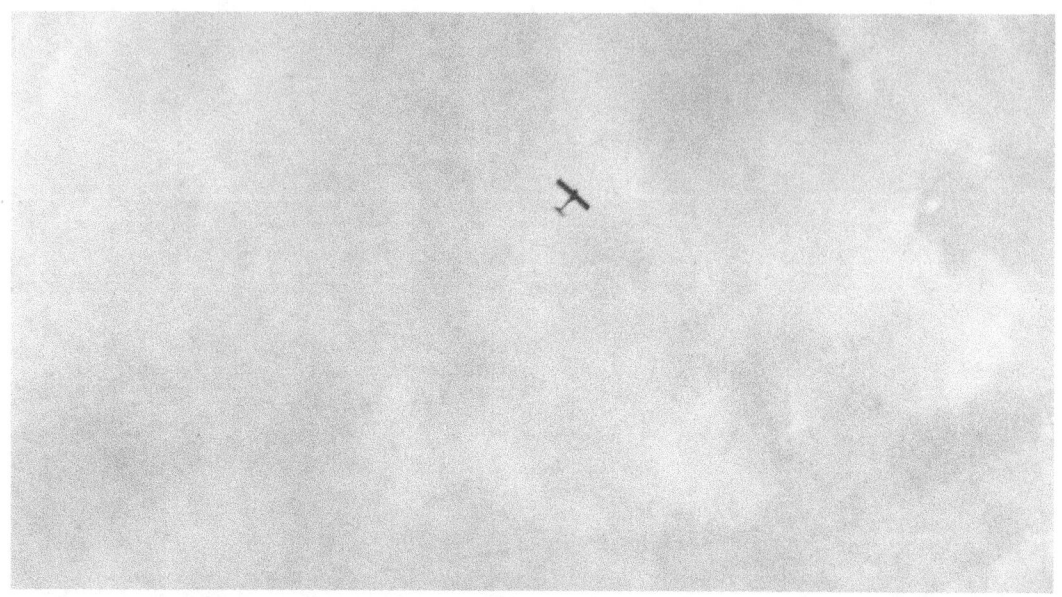

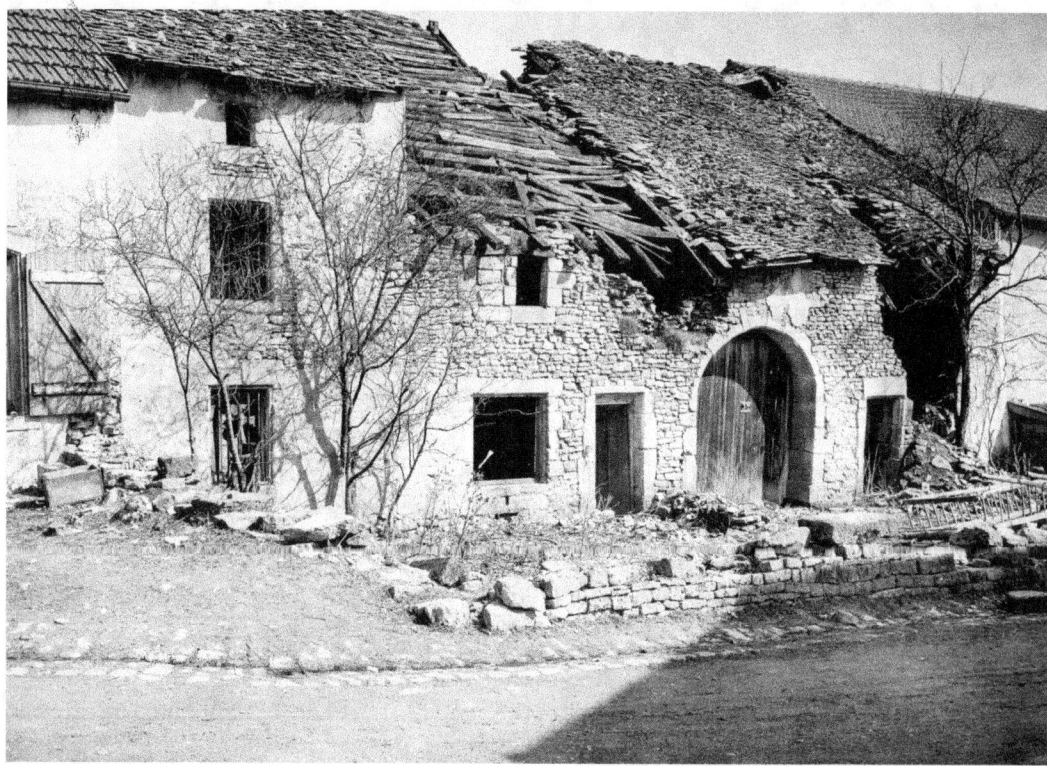

Top: An unidentified plane flies over Base Hospital 116 at Bazoilles Hospital Center (author's collection). *Bottom*: Sergeant Adolph C. Johnson from Prescott, Arizona, served with Base Hospital No. 79. His photograph album holds this picture with the handwritten caption: "Resident [residence] in Bazoilles-sur-Meuse hit by bomb." It remains unknown whether the damage was the result of a German air raid (courtesy Sharlot Hall Museum Library & Archives, Prescott, Arizona [Papers of A.C. Johnson: 1917–1973, Series 4: Photographs-DB 498A, Album #2]).

individual slid quietly out in front of his or her barracks where a guard was stationed and an officer appeared. There we would stand with our eyes gazing toward the heaven above. It seemed that these raids always took place on a beautiful moonlit night. The Germans would then decide to come out and do a little reconnoitering. One starry night we stood in front of our barracks shivering and gazing at the stars until 2:00 a.m. We were wondering just what would happen, when an officer kindly offered me his field glasses to look at two bright stars he indicated. They were not stars at all but two planes, one French, the other German. Their reflections gave the appearance of a star to the naked eye. To say my interest was increased is true, as they were directly over our camp and seemed to be merely watching each other. No harm was done on this occasion. It seemed during this time we never went to the Red Cross hut to enjoy a picture or a song but that the horrible notes of that shrill siren called us back to our barracks and brought to our minds thoughts of danger.[3]

There are conflicting reports on whether or not Bazoilles Hospital Center had actually been bombed. Nurse Alice Griffith Carr was attached to Base Hospital No. 18 which arrived at Bazoilles-sur-Meuse on July 26, 1917.[4] She described Bazoilles Hospital Center as a "never bombed 20,000 bed hospital" although "Germans flew over us constantly."[5] Base Hospital No. 46 arrived at Bazoillles-sur-Meuse on July 2, 1918, and its written history states that the frequent occurrence of air raid alarms caused great inconvenience but "nothing more serious than alarms ever occurred."[6] Private First Class Searle Fairfax Grove from Clear Ridge, Pennsylvania, arrived at Bazoilles Hospital Center with Base Hospital No. 60 on September 15, 1918. On December 16, he wrote to the folks back home that "our greatest danger was in the air but they were never able to do any damage to the hospitals here for as soon as a Bosche [Boche, German] plane would cross the lines the alarm would be sent back and the lights would be extinguished all over camp."[7] Yet, a newspaper item reporting the return of 29 nurses from Base Hospital No. 46 in Portland, Oregon, mentions that the hospital "was bombed by aircraft a number of times."[8] Similar information was provided upon the return from France of Lieutenant Colonel Edward Harry Schell from Harrisburg, Pennsylvania, who served with the Quartermaster Corps at Bazoilles Hospital Center from September 2, 1918, onwards.[9] He stated he "himself had numerous narrow escapes, of which he is reluctant to tell. He was present during ten German air raids over the hospitals at Bazoilles. One time he was sleeping 500 feet [approximately 150 meters] from one of the buildings which was hit direct by a high explosive shell, but escaped injury."[10] However, no official report on bombing of Bazoilles Hospital Center has been found.

Three

"With the Wounded"
Wound Care at Bazoilles Hospital Center

More than 26,000 soldiers were treated for injuries at Bazoilles Hospital Center, most of whom were brought in from the war zone by hospital trains. An important aspect of wound care at Bazoilles Hospital Center was prevention of wound infection. Therefore, prophylactic injections with anti-tetanus serum were administered to those patients who had not already received one in the evacuation chain. The so-called Carrel-Dakin method was keystone in the treatment of wounds at Bazoilles Hospital Center. After surgical removal of shell fragments, bullets and non-viable or infected tissue, the wound was irrigated with antiseptic Dakin's solution to kill bacteria. The wound was surgically closed once no bacteria could be detected in wound smears. Captain Charles R. Ball witnessed the different aspects of wound care at Bazoilles Hospital Center and wrote about his observations in the chapter "With the Wounded" of his war memoirs.

Admissions for Injury

In the ten-month period from July 1, 1918, to April 30, 1919, 63,769 patients were treated at Bazoilles Hospital Center, of which 26,604 (42 percent) were admitted for injuries.[1] By large, these injuries were sustained in the Second Battle of the Marne, the Battle of St. Mihiel and the Meuse-Argonne Offensive.[2] At Base Hospital No. 18, 4,486 patients were admitted because of gunshot wounds. The anatomic distribution of these wounds was as follows:

Fibula and tibia [lower leg bones]	15.0 percent
Femur [upper leg bone]	14.0 percent
Hands	9.0 percent
Radius and ulna [forearm bones]	9.0 percent
Head	6.1 percent
Metatarsus, tarsus and phalanges [foot bones]	6.0 percent
Humerus [upper arm bone]	5.0 percent
Chest	5.0 percent
Abdomen	4.0 percent
Buttocks	2.0 percent
Neck	2.0 percent
Penis and scrotum	0.4 percent[3]

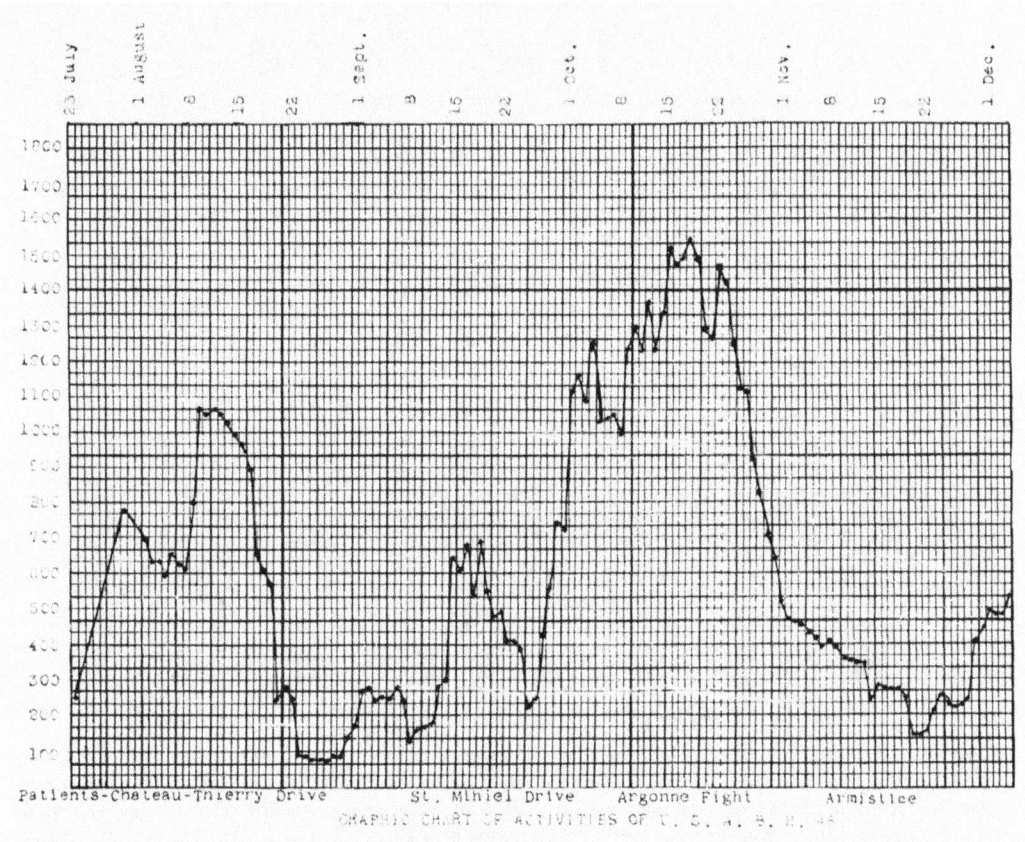

Chart showing the number of patients at Base Hospital No. 46 from July 23 to December 1, 1918. Patients were received from the Château-Thierry region (Second Battle of the Marne), the Battle of St. Mihiel and the Meuse-Argonne Offensive. On October 19, the maximum number of 1,544 patients was reached (*On Active Service with Base Hospital 46 U.S.A.* Portland, OR: Arcady Press; n.d.: 95).

Head and body injuries often proved fatal.[4] This explains the relatively large percentage of patients with gunshot wounds in the arms and legs admitted to Base Hospital No. 18. Patients with head and body injuries often did not live to reach Bazoilles Hospital Center.

The summary of sick and injured admitted to Bazoilles Hospital Center does not provide figures concerning wound infections, including often fatal tetanus and gas gangrene.[5] Yet, during the Meuse-Argonne Offensive, many wounded were received at Bazoilles Hospital Center with severe infections. Conditions in the advanced area were such that many battle casualties did not reach the center for four or five days after receiving their wounds, of which a fair proportion had not been operated on, with severe wound infections present.[6] Indeed, Corporal Joseph A. McGrath, Company D, 304th Engineers, 79th Division, died at Bazoilles Hospital Center on October 10, 1918, of "wounds infected with gas bacillus" (the bacterium referred to as "gas bacillus" is nowadays known as *Clostridium perfringens* and is the causative agent of gas gangrene), after being hit in the right leg near Nantillois on October 4 during the second phase of the Meuse-Argonne Offensive. He was buried on October 12 at the center's cemetery, known officially as United States Military Cemetery No. 6.[7] Corporal McGrath is listed among

```
                                                                              7
         McGrath,         Joseph A.          1,790,946      * White *Colored.
         (Surname)      (Christian name)   (Army serial number)

Residence:  4431   Mitchel St.        Philadelphia        PENNSYLVANIA
         (Street and house number)    (Town or city)    (County)    (State)

*Enlisted *R. A. *N. G. *E. R. C.*Inducted at Philadelphia Pa    on Oct 3, 19  17
Place of birth: Philadelphia Pa           Age or date of birth:  30  2/12 yrs
Organizations served in, with dates of assignments and transfers: Co D 304 Eng to death.


Grades, with date of appointment:  Pvt Oct 3/17; Pvt 1st cl Dec 7/17; Corp
                                   June 27/18.


Engagements:



Served overseas from July 9/18  to † death       , from †            to †
Died          Oct 10     , 19 18, of wounds received in action.
Other wounds or injuries received in action :                None
                                                      (If none, so state)
Person notified of death:  Thomas E. McGrath                 Father
                                  (Name)                (Degree of relationship)
          4431 Mitchell Street         Philadelphia            Pa
         (No. and street or rural route)   (City, town, or post office)  (State or country)
Remarks :
Form No. 724-7, A. G. O.   * Strike out words not applicable.   † Dates of departure from and arrival in the U. S.
    Nov. 22, 1919.                               3—7367
```

Service card of Corporal Joseph A. McGrath, Company D, 304th Engineers, 79th Division from Philadelphia, Pennsylvania, who died at Bazoilles Hospital Center on October 10, 1918, of gas gangrene after being hit in the right leg near Nantillois on October 4 (Ancestry. Pennsylvania, World War I Veterans Service and Compensation Files, 1917–1919, 1934–1948 for Joseph A. McGrath. https://www.ancestry.com; accessed February 10, 2017).

those who "died from wounds received in action."[8] It can, however, be argued that gas gangrene as cause of death could also have allowed for a listing among those who "died of disease."

"With the Wounded"

Charles Riggs Ball had been a civilian doctor before the war, working as a neurologist and psychiatrist in St. Paul, Minnesota.[9] In 1918, he enlisted in the U.S. Army Medical Corps in which he served as a captain.[10] He worked shortly at the Neuro-Psychiatric Board of a state-side base hospital examining the mental and nervous condition of drafted men,[11] but was soon assigned to Base Hospital No. 60, shortly before it went overseas.[12] Base Hospital No. 60 arrived at Bazoilles-sur-Meuse on September 15, 1918, as its fifth base hospital unit. However, by some logistic mistake, the hospital arrived without equipment and it did not began operation before October 4.[13] Captain Ball, therefore, spent his first days at Bazoilles Hospital Center watching the unloading of the wounded men from the hospital trains, their transferal by stretchers and ambulances to the hospitals and the wound care administered after admission.[14] He wrote about these observations in the chapter "With the Wounded" which was part of his war memoirs published in 1922 in *The Medical Pickwick*, "a monthly literary magazine of wit and wisdom."

At the time of arrival of Captain Ball at Bazoilles Hospital Center, hospital trains were coming in with wounded from the Battle of St. Mihiel (September 12–16, 1918).[15] "There were times when one hospital train was scarcely unloaded before another pulled in, each train bringing it [in] between 400 and 500 patients."[16] Upon arrival at Bazoilles Hospital Center, the patients were detrained by an unloading detail comprised of a quota of men from each base hospital in the center. Motor ambulances and trucks of the Motor Transport Corps were waiting at the station to transfer the newly arrived patients to the receiving wards of the base hospitals designated to admit them. At the receiving wards, patients were registered, undressed, examined, differentiated as to their underlying condition and as to the presence or absence of "cooties" (lice), deloused if necessary, assigned to a ward, bathed and clothed in fresh hospital garments.[17]

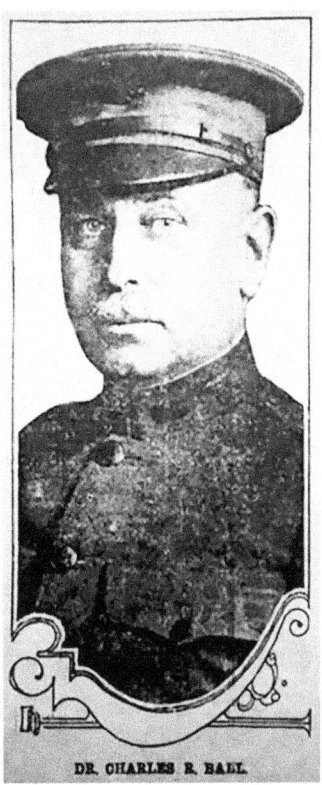

Right: Neuropsychiatrist Charles R. Ball served as a captain with the U.S. Army Medical Corps during World War I. He went overseas with Base Hospital No. 60 and arrived at Bazoilles Hospital Center on September 15, 1918, where he spent his first days watching the treatment of wounded men ("Looking at the Army from the Inside, or How Your Boy Was Treated in France." *The Saint Paul Pioneer Press.* September 14, 1919: 5).

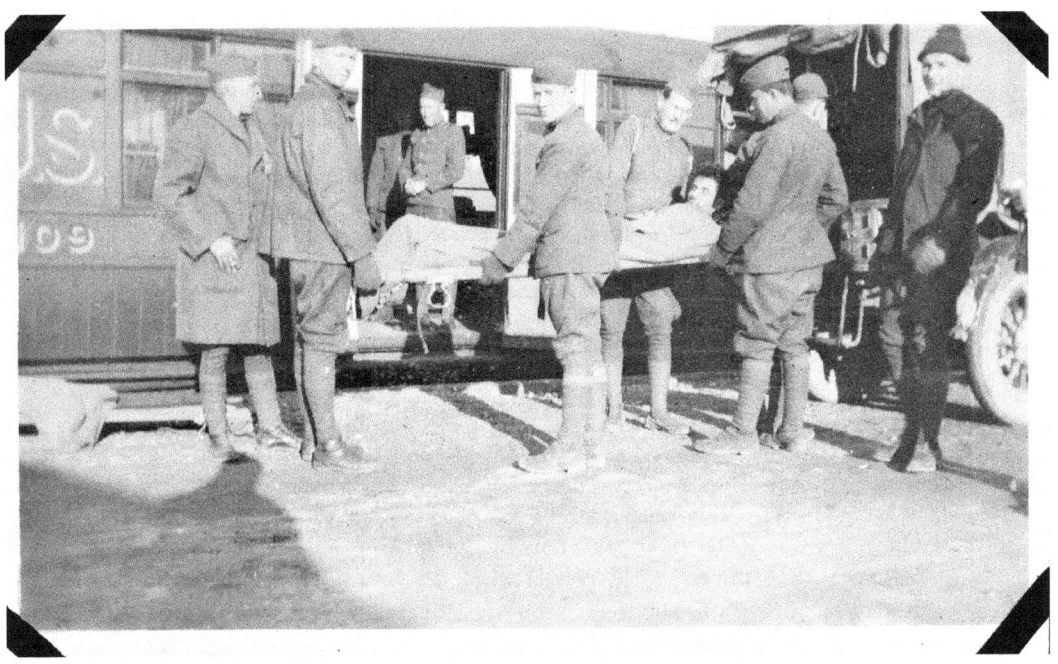

An unloading detail at Bazoilles Hospital Center lifts a patient from a hospital train to a motor ambulance or truck for transferal to the base hospital designated to admit him (author's collection).

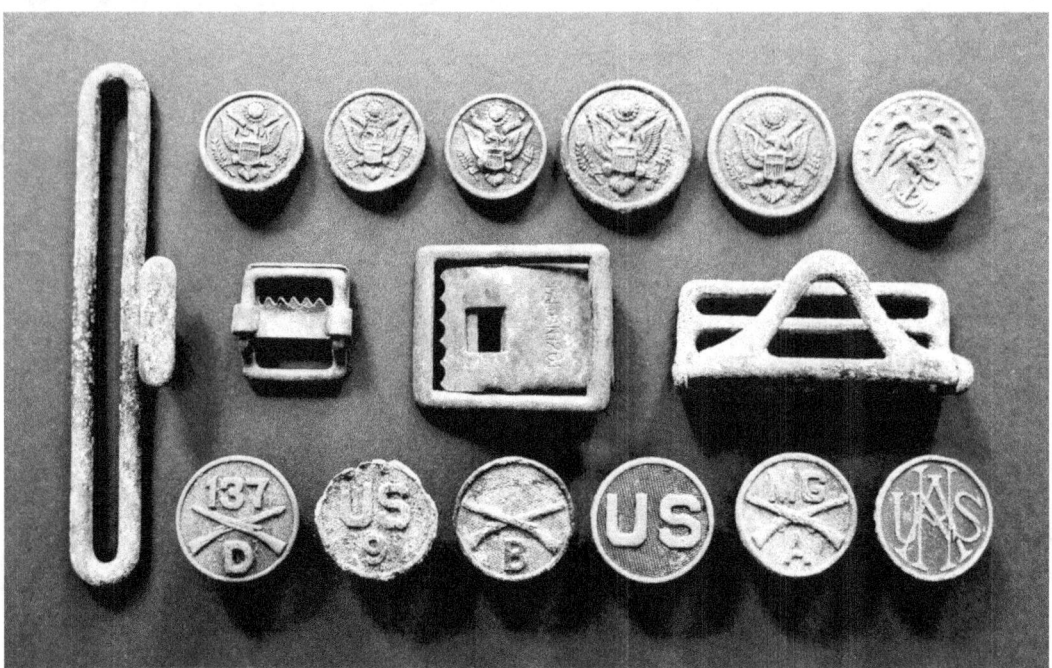

Service coat and trench coat buttons, collar disks and buckles recovered at the former site of Bazoilles Hospital Center illustrative of the removal of "blood-stained and dirt begrimed uniforms" from wounded U.S. Army soldiers after arrival in their designated base hospitals (courtesy Haye Wever [private collection] and author's collection).

The nurses carefully removed from the wounded the blood-stained and dirt begrimed uniforms, which in many instances had not been taken off for days. They bathed their feverish bodies which had not felt the soothing influence of a bath for weeks and then assisted them into a "spick and span" suit of pajamas which the Red Cross workers at home had sent across the seas for just that purpose.... All the wounded were tagged with what was called the field medical card, in the dressing stations or field hospitals where they were first taken care of. The field medical card had their name, rank, serial number [Army Service Number], organization to which they belonged, date and nature of their injury and the treatment recorded on it which they had received up to [that] date. As these cases were passed on from one hospital to another, additional data, pertinent to the case, was added by the different medical officers under whose charge they came.... The orders of the War Department were very strict in this regard. The continual changing of the patients from one hospital to another made the information furnished by this card very necessary in continuing the treatment of the case.[18]

Prophylactic Use of Anti-Tetanus Serum

Tetanus is an infectious disease of the nervous system which is often fatal without directed treatment. The disease is caused by the bacterium *Clostridium tetani* (known as *Bacillus tetani* at the time of World War I) which is commonly found in the intestinal tract of horses and other animals so that soil of cultivated lands, where manure has been used, is often highly infectious. Before World War I, tetanus was an uncommon disease in developed countries. However, immediately following the outbreak of World War I in 1914, an emergence of tetanus was observed among troops on both sides of the conflict. Among factors contributing to the emergence of tetanus during the first months of World

The front and back of a field medical card which was used to inform medical officers, under whose observation the patient successively came, of the specific treatment previously given (courtesy the National World War I Museum and Memorial, Kansas City, Missouri).

War I was the use of modern explosives. These caused deep tissue wounds in which dirt, originating from the richly manured soil on the fields of Belgium and Northern France, was driven inwards either directly or carried by penetrating objects. Furthermore, the contact between the soldier and the soil upon which he fought had never been more intimate than it was in the trenches and "no man's land." Men were literally "covered from

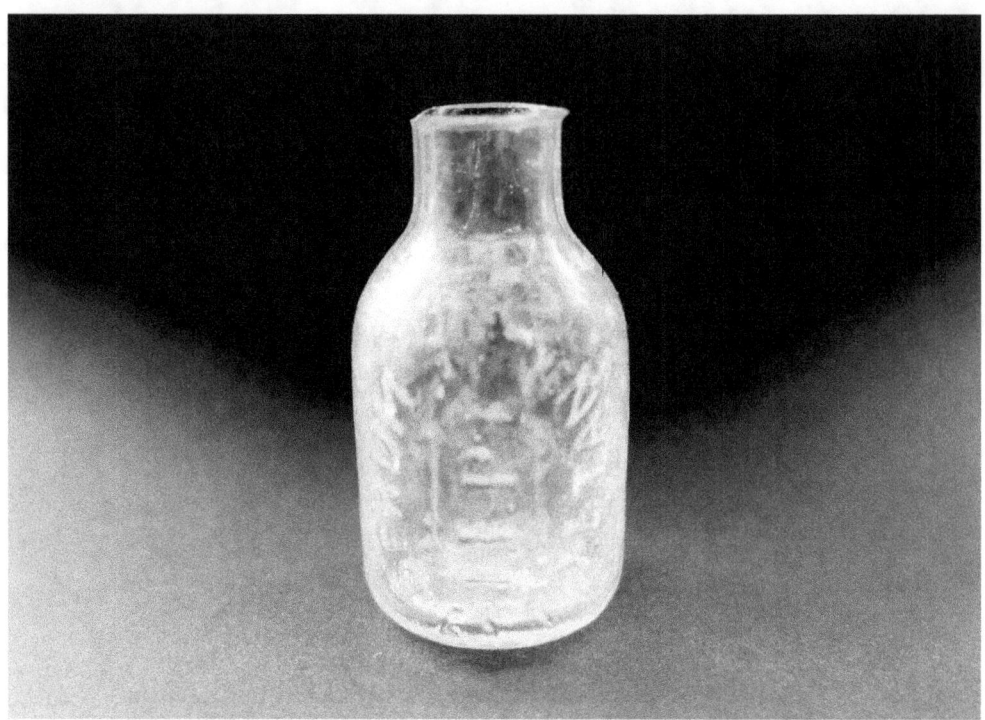

Glass vial with the inscription "SERUM ANTITETANIQUE" encircling the letters "IP" (acronym for "Institut Pasteur") recovered at the former site of Bazoilles Hospital Center. Apparently, the U.S. Army Medical Department used French supplies of anti-tetanus serum in France (author's collection).

head to foot with clay and earth and mud" and "this mud [was] largely manurial in origin." Therefore, from October 1914 onwards, routine prophylactic injections with anti-tetanus serum were given to wounded soldiers, which was followed by a steep fall in the incidence of tetanus in November 1914.[19]

In 1917, the U.S. Army Medical Department published the *Medical War Manual No. 1: Sanitation for Medical Officers* to "supply in a compact form that can be conveniently carried in the pocket of a uniform, such data as may be useful to medical officers as a guide for sanitary work."[20] Concerning the prevention of tetanus, the booklet stated that "all suspicious wounds, *i.e.*, all lacerated, contused, and punctured wounds inflicted under such circumstances that soil or dirt may have been introduced require prophylactic treatment.... a second dose ... is given when the patient arrives at the base hospital, if the wound is of any severity."[21] Indeed, also in Captain Ball's "With the Wounded" it is written that "every wounded soldier ... no matter how slight his wound, received at the Field Hospital or dressing station an injection of antitetanic serum."[22]

Thus, in theory, every wounded soldier that reached Bazoilles Hospital Center should have received a shot of anti-tetanus serum. However, in practice, this was not the case. The National Archives at Kansas City, Kansas City, Missouri, holds 12 reports of "failure to record administration of ATS" (anti-tetanus serum). These reports list wounded soldiers transferred "down the line" from different field hospitals and evacuation hospitals without a record of having received ATS. As a consequence, a prophylactic dose of ATS was administered at Bazoilles Hospital Center to each of the mentioned patients.

Base Hospital No. 116,
American E.F., APO 731,
September 23, 1918.

From :   Commanding Officer, Base Hospital 116, AEF.

To :   Chief Surgeon, AEF, (through the Director of General Surgery)

Subject :   Failure to record administration of ATS, per Cir., C.S.O. # 46, Par. 8 .

    1. The following cases were admitted to this hospital September 16, 1918, without record of having received ATS :

Hansen, J.C.,	Capt.	Co.B 356th Inf.	Passed	through	Evac.Hosp.# 1
Branson, Harold W.,	2nd.Lt.	185th Aero.Sqd.	"	"	Evac.Hosp.# 1
Ford, Olin H.,	2nd.Lt.	Co.A 23rd Inf.	"	"	Evac.Hosp.# 1
Gentile, Francis 120651	Cpl.	75th Co. 6 USMC	"	"	F.H.'s 15 and 23
Gotzen, Joseph 736062	Sgt.	Hdq. Co. 9th Inf.	"	"	F.H.'s 15 and 23
Gray, Jack 5431	Cpl.	Amb. Co. # 1 MD	"	"	Evac.Hosp.# 14
Hendrick, John 2222204	Pvt.	Co. I 23rd Inf.	"	"	Evac.Hosp.# 1
Ivins, Herbert H.1480328	Pvt.	Co. M 9th Inf.	"	"	Evac.Hosp.# 14
Jackson, Berry 1245015	Pvt.	Co. G 9th Inf.	"	"	Evac.Hosp.# 1
King, Vinton P. 200744	Chauf.	Co.E 406 Tel.Bn.	"	"	Evac.Hosp.# 3
Linn, Justin 162240	Pvt.	79th Co. 6 USMC	"	"	F.H.'s 15 and 23
McCormack, F., 2854296	Pvt.	Co. E 358 Inf.	"	"	Evac.Hosp.# 14
Walker, Francis 161139	Pvt.	16th Co. 6 USMC	"	"	Evac.Hosp.# 1
Weir, John 13499	Pvt.	Co. H 4 MGBn.	"	"	Evac.Hosp.# 1

German Prisoners :

Bruxner, Heindrich	Cpl.	7th Co. 163rd Inf.	"	"	Evac.Hosp.# 1
Frank, Alois	---	------ 59th F.A.	"	"	Evac.Hosp.# 14
Hoffman, Matthais	Pvt.	2nd Co. 332nd Inf.	"	"	Evac.Hosp.# 1
Jensch, Ernst	Sgt.	9th Co. 419th Inf.	"	"	Mobile Hosp.# 3
Jentsch, Richard	Pvt.	1st.Bn. 8th Gren.	"	"	Evac. Hosp.# 14
Kalz, Josef	Pvt.	MG.Bn. 419th Inf.	"	"	Evac.Hosp.# 1
Richard, Louis	Pvt.	5th Co. 6th Inf.	"	"	Evac.Hosp.# 14
Stelzner, Tony	Pvt.	6th Co. 257th Inf.	"	"	Evac.Hosp.# 14
Zaar, Hermann	Sgt.	9th Co. 332nd Inf.	"	"	Evac.Hosp.# 1

    2. A prophylactic dose of 1000 units was accordingly given to each of the above patients at this hospital .

HDQRS., HOSPITAL CENTER, A.P.O. 731
FORWARDED   30 SEP 1918

                                                          JOHN B. WALKER
                                                          Major , M.C.

A report dated September 23, 1918, mentioning wounded U.S. Army soldiers and German prisoners of war who were admitted to Base Hospital No. 116 without a record of having received anti-tetanus serum (ATS) (National Archives at Kansas City, Kansas City, Missouri [Record Group 120: Records of the American Expeditionary Forces (World War I), 1848–1942, Correspondence of the Hospital Center at Bazoilles, 1918–1919, National Archives Identifier 6636481, box 2 folder 705 Patients. Adm. of]).

Notably, these reports also list German prisoners of war who had not received ATS illustrating that they were given the same treatment as American soldiers.[23]

Fluoroscopic Examination of Wounds

The ability to localize foreign bodies (bullets, shrapnel, shell fragments) in the human body has been mentioned as perhaps one of the most important advances by the U.S. Army Medical Department during World War I. The method used was known as fluoroscopy. It had already been in use for some time before the war but it required large numbers of battle casualties to recognize its importance.[24] During World War I, fluoroscopes were used which consisted of a screen that had been coated on the inside with a layer of fluorescent chemicals. The screen was attached to a funnel-shaped cardboard eyeshade which excluded room light and could be worn with head straps. An X-ray tube placed under an operating table with a large central opening emitted X-rays through the patient's body. The fluorescent chemicals on the screen glowed when struck by X-rays. Hereby, an image of the patient's body appeared on the screen in which metal foreign bodies appeared dark. The use of such devices was accompanied by significant health hazards.[25]

Captain Ball's "With the Wounded" describes the application of fluoroscopy at Bazoilles Hospital Center.

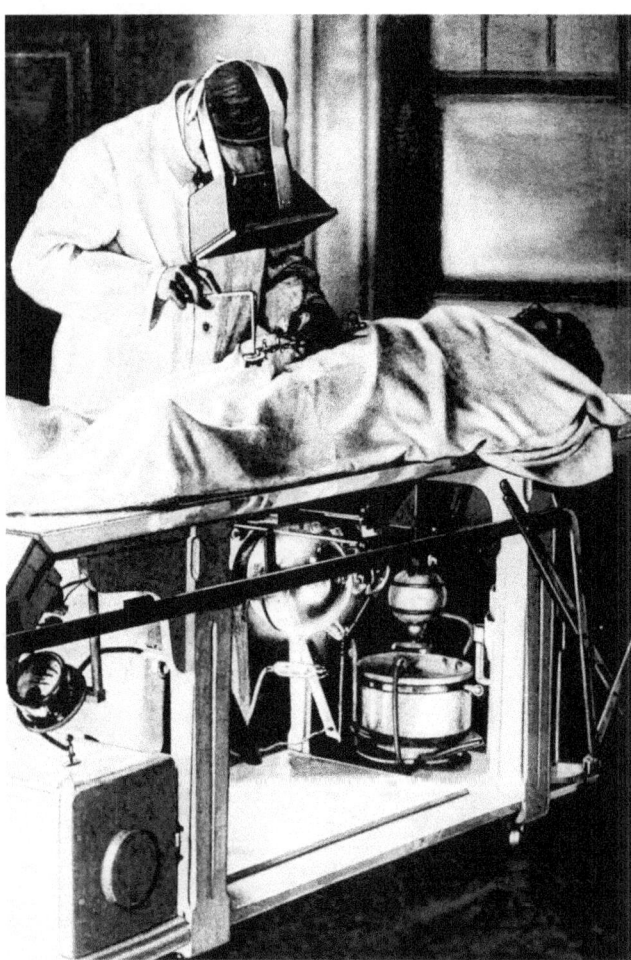

A 1917-dated image of a fluoroscope-assisted operation performed by a surgeon at the Roentgenographic Department of the American Ambulance Hospital at Neuilly, France. The X-ray tube is visible below the operating table. The surgeon is wearing a fluoroscope which is attached with head straps (Wikipedia. Surgical Operation during World War I Using a Fluoroscope to Find Embedded Bullets, accessed February 28, 2017).

> When the patients were first brought into the hospital, unless their field [medical] cards showed that it had already been done, one of the first things to do for them [the doctors] was to search with a fluoroscope all the wounds and their environment, for fragments of shell, machine gun bullets and spiculae of bone [needlelike bone fragments]. In enabling the medical

officer to locate foreign bodies of this nature, when embedded deeply in the tissues, the X-ray machine rendered the most valuable and efficient service. The X-ray equipment which the War Department furnished the hospitals everywhere, not only back in the S. O. S. [Services of Supply], but also in the zone of the advice [zone of the advance; Advance Section], was very complete. These machines were in constant use and practically every wound of any consequence had to be surveyed through the fluoroscope in order to make sure that it was free from foreign bodies. The method of making this search was unique. The wounded man was brought into an absolutely dark room, placed upon what was called an X-ray table, which was simply an operating table provided with a large oval opening in the center of it for the X-ray tube. When the rays were turned in on [on in] the tube fitted into this opening in the table all the operator had to do was to take his fluoroscope and move it up and down over the body, literally piercing the patient through and through with his gaze, the entire skeleton and any foreign body of greater density than the flesh being easily discernible in this manner.[26]

The Carrel-Dakin Method for Wound Treatment

During World War I, the allied armies adopted the so-called Carrel-Dakin method for wound treatment. The French surgeon Alexis Carrel had been awarded the Nobel Prize in Medicine in 1912 for work on suturing blood vessels and organ transplantation performed in the Rockefeller Institute for Medical Research in New York. He returned to France every year in the summer and was called to service as a major in the French Army at the outbreak of World War I. Supported by a Rockefeller Foundation grant of $ 20,000 he established a war research hospital in Compiègne, France. Along with the English biochemist Henry Dakin, he developed a method for treating wounds using a disinfectant solution known as Dakin's solution (0.5 percent weight per volume sodium hypochlorite).[27]

The Carrel-Dakin method included four distinct but occasionally overlapping phases. The first phase consisted of *débridement* (surgical removal) of infected surface tissues, in order to enable the necessary intimate contact between the Dakin's solution and invading bacteria. The second phase consisted of chemical sterilization by intermittent or continuous irrigation of all portions of the wound with Dakin's solution by means of insertion in the wound of small rubber tubes with perforated holes at half-inch intervals. To monitor the effect of healing and sterilization, daily clinical and bacteriological examinations were performed in the third stage. Once bacteriological wound smears failed to detect bacteria for three consecutive days, coincident with clinical improvement (good condition of the wound and regular temperature) the wound was surgically closed in the fourth stage (referred to as delayed primary closure).[28]

When the United States entered the war, the Rockefeller Foundation granted money to establish the War Demonstration Hospital on the grounds of the Rockefeller Institute in Manhattan, New York. The hospital served three principle functions: to make the Carrel-Dakin treatment available to civilian and military patients; to demonstrate and teach the Carrel-Dakin method to civil and military surgeons and nurses; and to test the feasibility of a portable military hospital unit. From July 1917 to March 1919, the hospital ran two-week courses in surgery, chemistry, laboratory work and special instruction with Alexis Carrel himself among the teachers.[29] A hundred so-called Carrel-Dakin apparatuses were part of the standard inventory of an overseas base hospital,[30] while four copies of the book *The Treatment of Infected Wounds*, co-authored by Alexis Carrel and Georges Dehelly and published in 1917, were among the standard inventory of its library unit.[31]

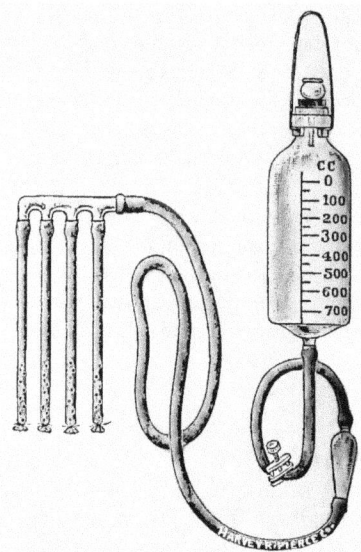 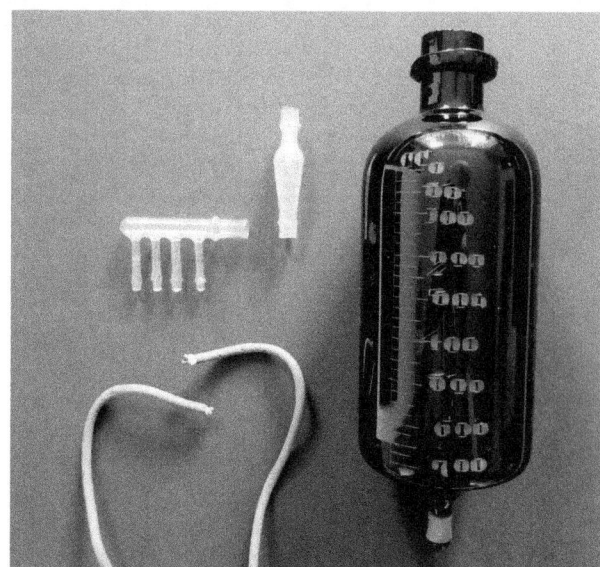

Left: Illustration of a Carrel-Dakin apparatus in which the different components are drawn out of proportion. A graduated reservoir is connected to a rubber tube with a clamp for flow control and a sight feed cup. The rubber tube is attached to a four-way glass distributor which connects to smaller rubber tubes with perforated holes at the end, which are inserted into a wound for irrigation with Dakin's solution (*List of Staple Medical and Surgical Supplies: Part I Surgical Instruments Selected to Meet War Conditions.* Washington, D.C.: Government Printing Office, 1918: 48). *Right:* Original components of a Carrel-Dakin apparatus left behind in France after World War I by the U.S. Army Medical Department. Shown are a graduated reservoir, a sight feed cup, a four-way glass distributor and rubber tubes with perforated holes at the end (author's collection).

Captain Ball's "With the Wounded" acknowledges that the Carrel-Dakin method for wound treatment "was in quite general use in the army" and describes its use at Bazoilles Hospital Center.

> The treatment of the wounds themselves was in general a simple matter. First, there was what was called the *debridement*, the French term for the cleaning up of the wound, the removal of any shell fragments and foreign bodies, together with a free incision, converting the narrow infected tract of the shell or bullet in the tissues into an open wound, triangular in shape, with the base of the triangle at the top and the apex at the bottom. This *debridement* was done to promote drainage and make all parts of the wound easily accessible. Before applying the dressings, perforated rubber tubes were put into the wounds, the ends of which stuck up outside of the dressings. It was through these tubes, coming up outside of the dressings that the Dakin's fluid was applied. Every two or three hours as per order, the nurse came along and with a small glass syringe squirted this Dakin's fluid into the tubes, thus keeping the interior of the wound continually bathed with it.... The Dakin's fluid may be briefly described as an anti-septic fluid, the chief object in its composition being to make it as potent as possible in destroying or retarding bacterial growth and at the same time as little injurious to the living tissues with which it came in contact.... The war wounds were practically all infected and their progress depended entirely on the number and variety of bacteria found in them.... For example, if the gas bacillus was found in the [wound] culture, a much more extensive dissection of the injured tissues was necessary than would otherwise be the case.... Practically all the wounds, because of the extensive debridement, had to be closed by sutures after the inflammation in the tissue had subsided and the germ growth had diminished.[32]

The application of the Carrel-Dakin treatment at Base Hospital No. 81 is mentioned in the war memoirs of Nurse Louise Kalkman. "I was assigned to a ward of fifty wounded

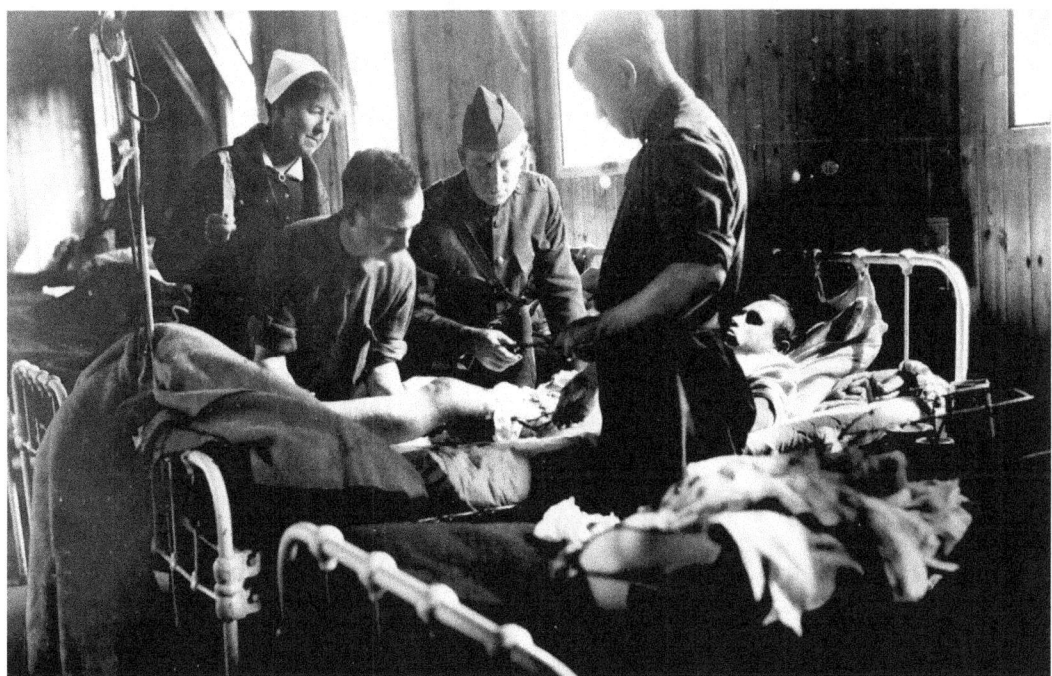

Installation of a Carrel-Dakin apparatus for irrigation of a wound above the right knee of a soldier admitted to Base Hospital No. 18. The man on the right side of the bed is holding several rubber tubes of which the ends are inserted into the patient's wound. A reservoir with Dakin's solution hangs from a pole attached to the foot end of the bed (National Archives at College Park, Maryland [Record Group 111: Records of the Office of the Chief Signal Officer, 1860–1985, Photographs of American Military Activities, ca. 1918–ca. 1981, National Archives Identifier 530707: photograph no. 111-SC-11889]).

soldiers, most of them had shrapnel wounds and suffered a great deal.... Many of the men had rubber drains in their wounds which were irrigated and cleaned daily."[33]

The Wound Bacteriology Division at the Center Laboratory

Although the various base hospitals at Bazoilles Hospital Center provided their own laboratory, a so-called center laboratory was set up for specific laboratory work. The center laboratory was first located in the greenhouse[34] of the *Château de Bazoilles-sur-Meuse*, which was occupied by Base Hospital No. 18 after its arrival in July 1917. The equipment of the central laboratory was moved on September 2, 1918, to a separate building next to the center's headquarters between Base Hospitals Nos. 60 and 79.[35] As the various hospital units arrived at Bazoilles-sur-Meuse, the laboratory personnel of each unit came under the control of the laboratory officer of the center, who was empowered to detail them to the center laboratory as needed. The work in the center laboratory of Bazoilles Hospital Center was organized in eight general divisions with one officer of the laboratory staff in charge of each of the divisions:

1. General bacteriology.
2. Typhoid-dysentery examination and water analysis.
3. Wound bacteriology.
4. Pneumococcus (a bacterium causing pneumonia) typing.
5. Serology.
6. Pathology, including all post-mortem examinations.
7. Preparation room.
8. Office and supplies.[36]

At the wound bacteriology division of the center laboratory, First Lieutenant Howard Osgood from Cambridge, Massachusetts, was in command. He had been granted his Doctor of Medicine degree from Harvard University on November 26, 1917, was commissioned First Lieutenant on December 6 and assigned to Base Hospital No. 116 on December 20. First Lieutenant Osgood had arrived at Bazoilles-sur-Meuse on April 10, 1918, and was sent to Dijon, France, in July for a course in wound bacteriology. After his return to Bazoilles-sur-Meuse, he assumed charge of the wound bacteriology division at the center laboratory.[37] In one of his letters home, First Lieutenant Osgood expressed his disappointment about the work in the wound bacteriology division.

> I have been rather discouraged over the work that we did in that department; it had seemed to me so merely barren & mechanical.... With the central laboratory so much detached from the clinical work, and with the center acting as a huge evacuation hospital center rather than a

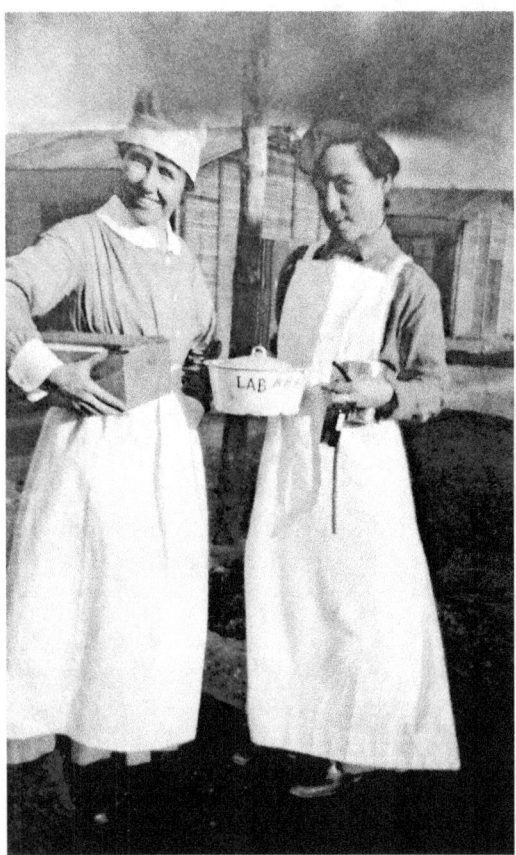

Two laboratory workers attached to Base Hospital No. 46 of which one is holding a cooking pan with the marking "LAB. B.H. 46." Presumably, these ladies were Vida L. Fatland and Agatha Holloway, who were both civilian employees working as laboratory technicians at Base Hospital No. 46 (courtesy Oregon Health & Science University, Portland, Oregon [Historical Collections & Archives, Grace Phelps Papers, Accession No. 20100-05, box 1 folder 5 Photographs]).

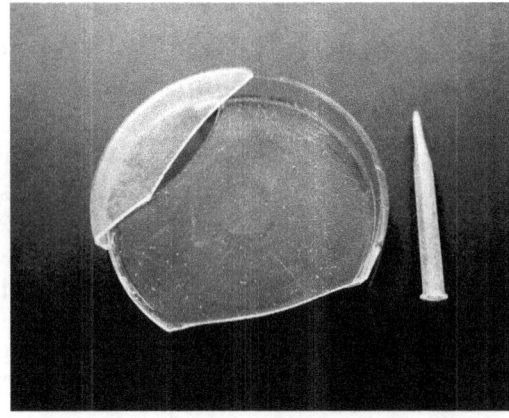

Culture dish (Petri dish) fragments and a dropping pipette (Pasteur pipette) recovered at the former site of Bazoilles Hospital Center (author's collection).

base [hospital], we were unable to get clinical data from cases as they passed through to go with the bacteriological data in our lab.

Clearly, many patients had moved on to hospitals further "down the line" before the results of their wound cultures became available and could be of use. On October 30, 1918, First Lieutenant Osgood penciled down his doubts on his contribution to the war effort in his diary.

> Very few wound cultures of any kind being sent in—am not sure of explanation [despite the fact that the Meuse-Argonne Offensive was still underway]. We have now myself & Capt. Harley [of Base Hospital No. 79] to work on them, while the actual work would only take one man half a day. With so much [clinical] work to be done, others working overtime on necessary & useful work, one feels unneeded & superfluous on a job like mine.

Still, upon analysis of wound cultures and surgical data for a general report on the subject, First Lieutenant Osgood came to the conclusion that "it seems we did as much if not more than most other similar hospitals in actual number of cultures."[38]

Changing of Wound Dressings

The changing of wound dressings (bandages) was a daily—and painful—routine at Bazoilles Hospital Center. At Base Hospital No. 60, Nurse Sarah Sand had been placed in charge of a surgical ward of fifty seriously wounded men nursed inside barracks and

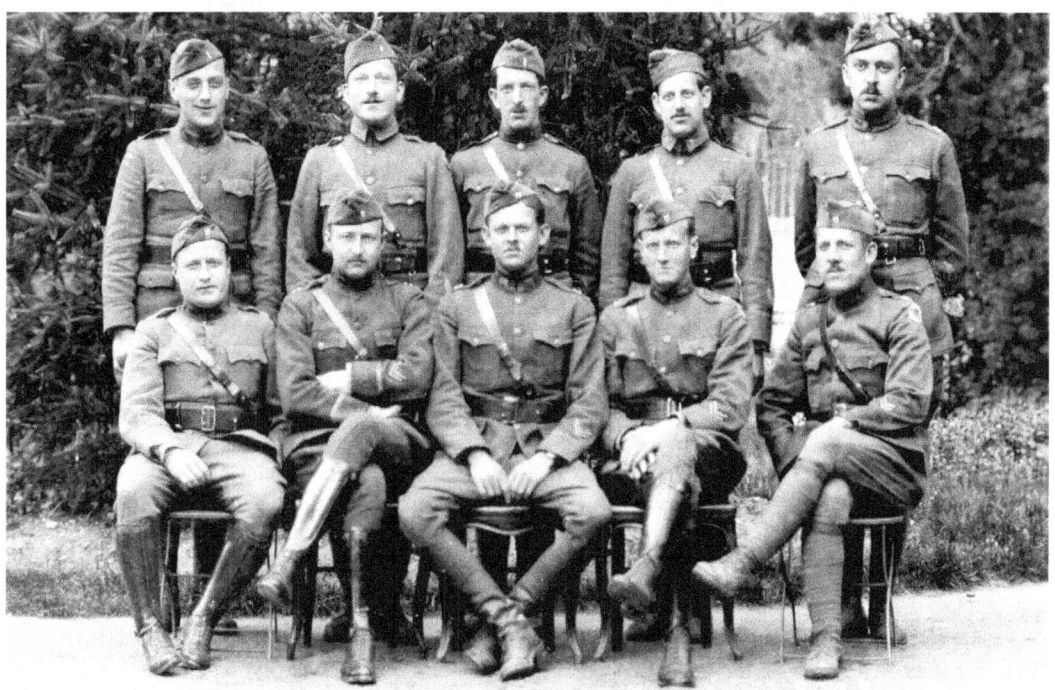

A photograph depicting several officers of Base Hospital No. 116. Seated second from the left is First Lieutenant Howard Osgood from Cambridge, Massachusetts, who was in charge of the wound bacteriology division at the center laboratory of Bazoilles Hospital Center (author's collection).

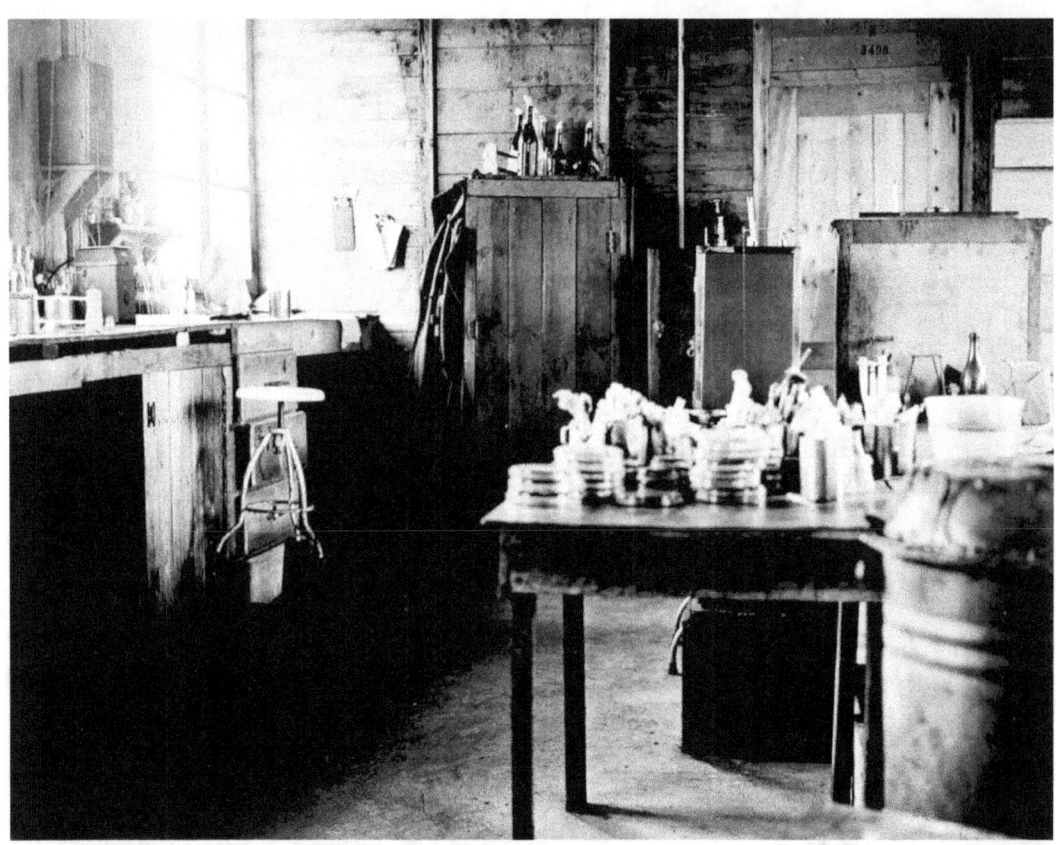

Laboratory benches at one of the bacteriology divisions at the center laboratory of Bazoilles Hospital Center. Several culture dishes can be seen on the bench at the right (U.S. National Library of Medicine. Digital Collections. http://resource.nlm.nih.gov/101399631; accessed February 18, 2017).

fifty less seriously wounded men located outside in a tent adjoining the barracks. She worked together with another nurse and two corpsmen. At the end of the ward was the dressing room which received a constant stream of men most of the day. There, bandages were cut off, wounds were irrigated and new sterile dressings were applied. She performed these duties for six weeks, dressing an average of 200 men in her ward each week. The work was supervised by the ward surgeon who dressed the most seriously wounded himself. Nurse Sand punctually noted the number of dressings performed during her shifts.

> Miss [Julia A.] Walton and I, during the day, dressed wounded soldiers as follows in [Surgical] Ward No. 13: October 18—dressed 60 wounded; October 19—dressed 15 wounded; October 20—dressed 40 wounded; October 21—dressed 33 wounded; October 22—dressed 30 wounded; October 23—dressed 18 wounded; October 24—dressed 18 wounded; October 25—dressed 23 wounded; and October 26—dressed 23 wounded.[39]

The extent of pain and agony suffered during the changing of the dressings at Bazoilles Hospital Center is described in Captain Ball's "With the Wounded."

> It was a trying experience to witness the changing of the dressings in the surgical wards after the arrival of a convoy train. During their trip of from 24 to 36 hours, sometimes longer, the dressings had become very dry and their removal was a tedious and painful procedure. Some of the most painful and extensive wounds which I saw were caused from burns of mustard gas. This gas affected

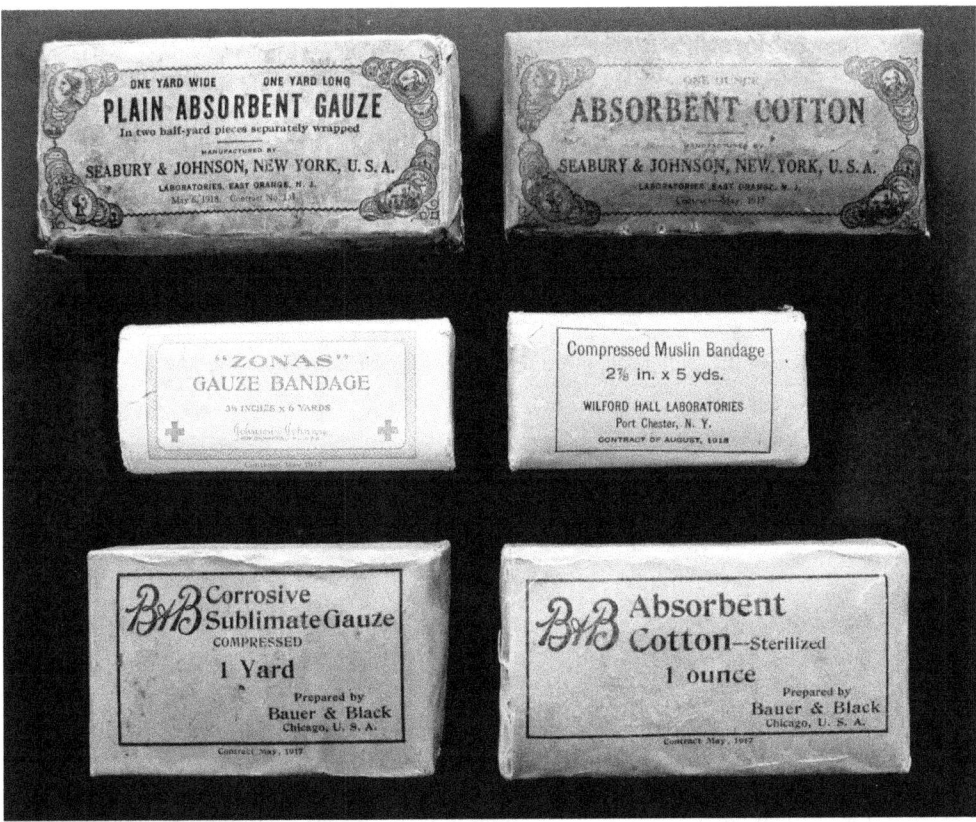

Different surgical dressings used by the U.S. Army Medical Department during World War I, all showing contract dates in 1917 and 1918. These dates indicate when a contract for the product was made between a U.S. Army contracting officer and the manufacturer (author's collection).

chiefly the portions of the body where moisture was present, such as the eyes, nose, genital organs and respiratory tract. The inflammation which this gas produced in the respiratory tract caused great suffering and was very often fatal.

The most horrible wounds, however, were those made by shell fragments. The laceration and destruction of the tissues by these fragments or eclats as the French called them was awful.

One afternoon, shortly after the arrival of a convoy train, I stood watching the dressing of a horrible wound of the thigh caused by shell fragments. The medical officer who was making the change in dressing was a great, big, red-faced fellow who in

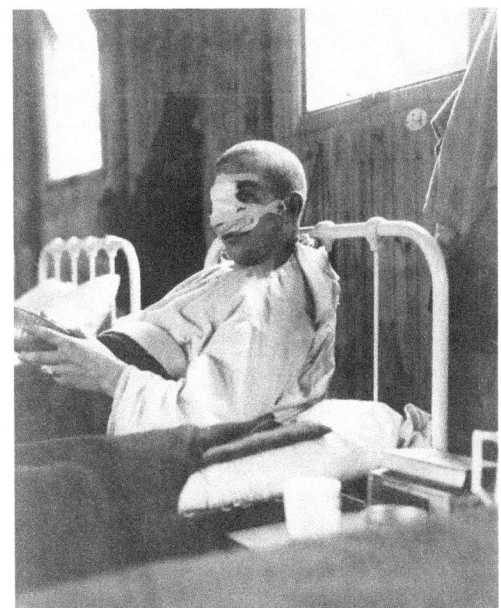

A soldier with a facial wound dressing admitted to Base Hospital No. 18 (National Archives at College Park, Maryland [Record Group 111: Records of the Office of the Chief Signal Officer, 1860–1985, Photographs of American Military Activities, ca. 1918– ca. 1981, National Archives Identifier 530707: photograph no. 111-SC-11895]).

his white apron somewhat resembled a butcher in his shop. The nurse was—well, she was just one of the trained nurses such as we see every day in the sick room at home. I think that this is the best compliment I can pay her. The dressings were so dry that every attempt to free them from the wound was agony to the patient. How slowly and carefully they went about this task although a whole wardful was awaiting their services. The ward orderly held the leg just so, and scarcely moved through the long, trying process, although I know his back must have felt like it was breaking long before the dressing was finished. The big doctor freed just a little surface at a time, and then only after the nurse had soaked it well with an anti-septic solution, giving the wounded man a rest whenever he asked for it and patiently waiting in the interval, until he had pulled himself together for another ordeal. It was not only a painful process for the patient but for everyone else concerned. When it was finished, my eyes were moist.... If the agonies of these poor wounded boys could only have been recorded on a monster phonographic record, so that future generations might hear their moans and cries of agony, I feel sure that this in itself would be a powerful appeal for the banishment of war forever.[40]

Gas! Gas! Treatment of Gas Cases

Medical care for gassed patients was purely symptomatic. Initial treatment was provided close to the front after which gas cases were transported back through the chain of evacuation. Several thousand gas casualties were treated at Bazoilles-sur-Meuse. The history of Base Hospital No. 46. describes the medical care provided after gas poisoning.

Initial treatment of gas poisoning was provided close to the front. While temporarily detached for clinical work from Base Hospital No. 116, First Lieutenant Howard Osgood wrote home from Bézu-le-Guéry about first care for gas patients at Field Hospital No. 1, 2nd Division.

> We get all kinds of cases from the front line, sick and gassed as well as wounded. On quiet days they trickle in in twos & threes, and on busy days they come with a rush.
> I think a note on our treatment of gas cases will get by the censor. When they arrive, their clothes which are more or less saturated with the stuff are taken away, and the men are thoroughly washed off—with warm water and soap. Then their eyes and throats are washed with [alkaline] bicarbonate solution & they are put to bed & given morphine if necessary. We only keep them a few hours until transportation is provided to evacuate them further back.[1]

Following a gas attack on May 27, 1918, Second Lieutenant Hugh Smith Thompson, Company L, 168th Infantry Regiment, 42nd Division, underwent first line treatment for phosgene gas poisoning at a U.S. Army hospital in Baccarat (possibly Evacuation Hospital No. 2). He vividly described his experiences in his war memoirs

> ... the [gassed] men who had been trapped in the cubbyhole shelters near the company dugout ... had been deposited in a receiving ward at Baccarat.... Strange people of both sexes, in gowns of rubber, had worked in a frenzy with oxygen tanks before [Private] Pierce had coughed his last. The rest of us ... had found ourselves in what seemed to be a basement room. Here, we had been stripped of all clothing, thoroughly fumigated [decontaminated], and had our heads shaved before we knew what it was all about.... Eyes had been treated, blood-pressure tests made amid rushing nurses and doctors.[2]

At Base Hospital No. 18, 1254 cases were treated for "absorption of deleterious gas."[3] In March 1918, before Bazoilles Hospital Center was in operation, around 250 badly

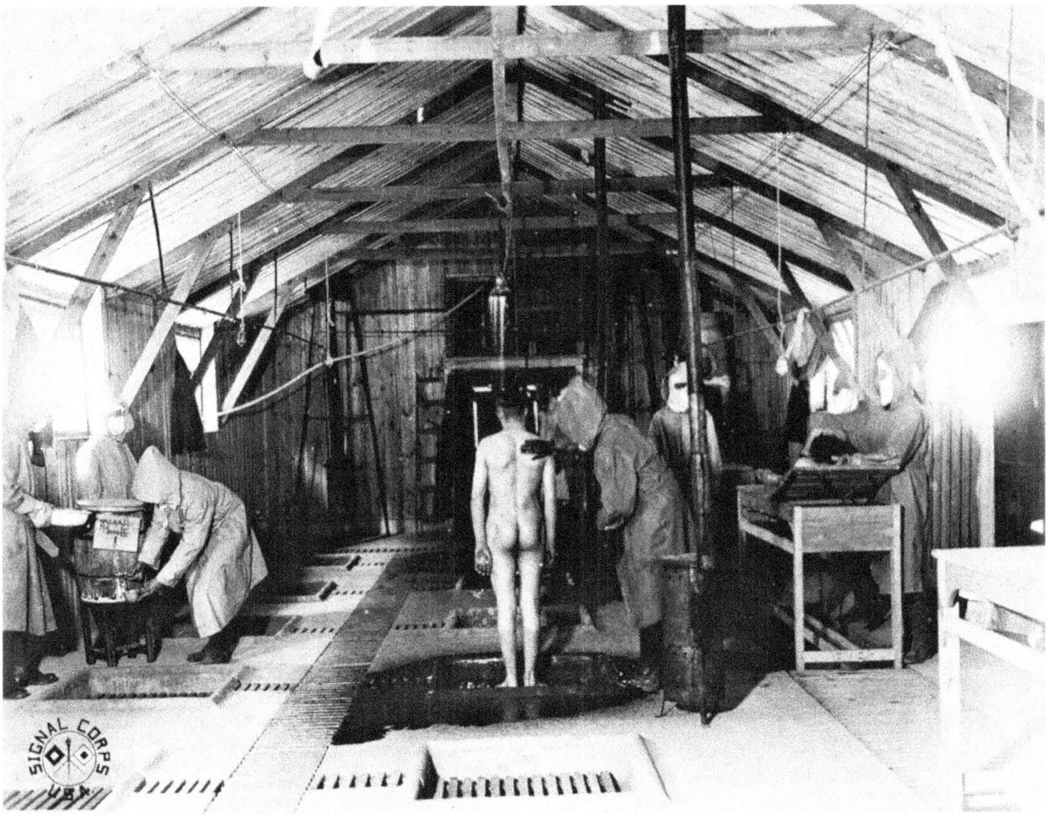

Interior view of the treatment room for gassed patients at Evacuation Hospital No. 2 in Baccarat, France. On the left side of the room, fluid is tapped from a reservoir marked "ALKALI Not for drinking" (U.S. National Library of Medicine. Digital Collections. http://resource.nlm.nih.gov/101399930; accessed March 21, 2017).

gassed cases from the 42nd Division came in by convoy, which was the largest number of gassed patients received at one time at that hospital.[4] Up to December 13, 1918, approximately 840 cases of gas poisoning were treated at Base Hospital No. 46, with mustard gas being the most common cause.[5] These figures indicate that in all several thousand gas casualties were treated at the different base hospitals constituting Bazoilles Hospital Center. The medical care for gassed patients is described in the history of Base Hospital No. 46.

> The first convoy on July 23 arrived not only before the hospital was adequately equipped, but also before there had been an opportunity to organize the staff. Coming from Chateau Thierry, it consisted mainly of patients gassed with Phosgene and to a lesser degree burned with the so-called

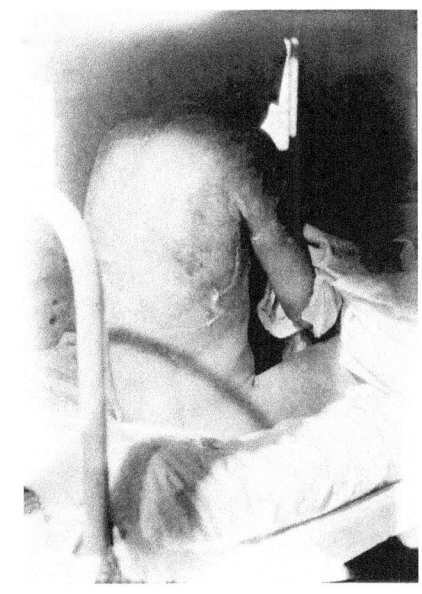

A patient at Base Hospital No. 116 with an extensive "mustard burn" on his back, shoulder and arm (author's collection).

"Mustard Gas." Up to August 1, there were 433 cases, practically all gas poisoning, being cared for in the medical wards. The treatment of these patients was purely symptomatic and on the whole far from satisfactory. Some developed secondary pneumonia, a complication which proved almost one hundred per cent fatal. While strictly speaking, mustard gas patients are to be classified as surgical [because of the blisters caused by chemical burning], the fact remains that a great many such were treated in medical wards. These included some of the most distressing cases with which the hospital had to deal. The pain and discomfort were intense; the weather very hot and the patients' sufferings were further augmented by great swarms of flies which infested the entire camp. Material with which to screen windows was unobtainable. About this time, one of the staff, Lieutenant Louis Mangan, impressed with the ineffectiveness of the method then in vogue for treating mustard burns, devised a scheme which consisted in merely injecting and re-injecting a simple alkaline solution into the blister. The result was truly remarkable and there can be no question that the suffering of many patients was not only reduced a hundred fold, but that lives were actually saved. It is to be regretted that the efforts of Lt. Col. W. R. Davis to have this method thoroughly investigated and tried out at various base and evacuation hospitals met with no success.[6]

After evacuation from the hospital in Baccarat, Second Lieutenant Thompson of the 42nd Division underwent further treatment at a U.S. Army hospital in Vittel (presumably at Vittel-Contrexéville Hospital Center), near Bazoilles-sur-Meuse.

A seemingly simple routine had followed our arrival at Vittel by hospital train—botanic acid in the eyes, no food for several days, liquid diet, and enforced rest for a week or ten days more. Later there had been a little exercise each day, between morning session choking and suffocating in the fumes of camphor steam. My inflamed eyes and a broken membrane in the mouth, evidently caused by zealous efforts to adjust my [gas mask] mouthpiece, had proved little more than temporary inconveniences. These were nothing to the first indescribable fears, when I had coughed, vomited, and wondered if the hemorrhages [bleedings] which had developed among some of those around me in those first hours at Baccarat were to be my fate, too.[7]

Four

Patients of Bazoilles Hospital Center
Three Soldiers Admitted Because of Battle Injuries

Bazoilles Hospital Center was in operation for 10 months from July 1, 1918, to April 30, 1919, during which period 26,604 patients were treated for injuries. This chapter describes three injured soldiers whose identification tags were recovered in 2016 at the former site of Bazoilles Hospital Center. All three men returned to the United States, but their wounds, resulting from gunfire, shell fire and (mustard) gas, had a lasting impact on their lives.

Private James L. Comfort, Army Service Number 2284154, Approximate Dates of Admission August 10 and/or October 14, 1918

James Lawrence Comfort was born on February 18, 1893, in Dalton, Georgia.[1] His mother and father passed away in 1903 and 1908 at the age of 37 and 61 years, respectively.[2] Together with his younger brother Quinlan, he was further raised in Lawrenceville, Georgia, by his widowed aunt Bessie L. Exum.[3] At the time of his registration for the World War I draft, on June 5, 1917, he listed Shamrock, Oklahoma, as home address, although he worked as a fruit packer at the Stewart Fruit Co. in San Bernardino, California.[4] In *The San Bernardino Daily Sun* of August 31, 1917, he was mentioned in the list of men certified for military duty.[5]

James Comfort entered the U.S. Army on September 19, 1917, at Redlands, California. He was assigned to the 364th Infantry Regiment, 91st Division, until February 26, 1918, after which he was transferred to Company G, 47th Infantry Regiment, 4th Division.[6] On May 10, his regiment sailed for Brest, France, where the troops disembarked on May 25.[7] The name of Private James L. Comfort from Lawrenceville subsequently appeared in a casualty list in *The Atlanta Constitution* of September 18, 1918, in which he was reported as missing in action.[8] The next day, *The Atlanta Constitution* printed a correction stating that James L. Comfort had been reported by the War Department as missing in action since August 10, 1918, while his aunt Bessie was in receipt of a letter from him dated August 13. This letter stated that he was in a hospital after being gassed with mustard gas.[9] On August 10, 1918, the 47th Infantry Regiment was located south of Bazoches-sur-Vesles near the Vesle River in the *département* Aisne, Northern-France. The written history of the 47th Infantry Regiment reads: "The heaviest barrage which the enemy had so far attempted occurred between midnight August 10th and six o'clock on the morning of the following day. Gas shells were thrown first, followed by shrapnel and high explosive."[10] The list of "Casualties among enlisted men" in the written history of the 47th Infantry Regiment mentioned Private James L. Comfort of Company G as being gassed ("G").[11] In the *Official U.S. Bulletin* of November 21, 1918, James L. Comfort is mentioned among those previously reported missing in action but now reported wounded of undetermined degree.[12]

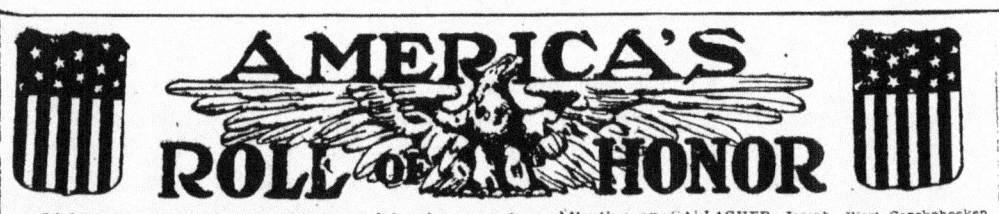

The Roll of Honor published in *The Atlanta Constitution* of September 18, 1918, mentions Private James L. Comfort from Lawrenceville, Georgia, as missing in action (America's Roll of Honor. *The Atlanta Constitution*. September 18, 1918: 6).

REPORTED AS MISSING, GEORGIAN IS GASSED

Lawrenceville, Ga., September 18.—(Special.)—James L. Comfort, reported by the war department as missing in action since August 10, was a prominent young man of Lawrenceville. He was reared by his aunt, Mrs. Bessie L. Exum, of this city, who is in receipt of a letter from him dated August 13, stating that he was in a hospital, having been gassed with mustard gas. Mr. Comfort went west some years ago, and was drafted from California in company G, 47th infantry.

In *The Atlanta Constitution* of September 19, 1918, a correction is printed stating that James L. Comfort, reported as missing in action, has in fact been hospitalized after being gassed with mustard gas (Reported as Missing, Georgian Is Gassed. *The Atlanta Constitution*. September 19, 1918: 7).

On August 28, after discharge from hospital, Private Comfort was transferred to the 148th Infantry Regiment, 37th Division. He was gassed a second time on October 14 when his division occupied the Pannes Sector in Lorraine, France.[13] In the *Official U.S. Bulletin* of February 26, 1919, James L. Comfort is, therefore, mentioned again but this time among the slightly wounded.[14] On March 29, he returned in the United States and was honorably discharged from the U.S. Army in good physical condition at Camp Gordon, Georgia, on April 30, 1919.[15]

James Comfort died at the age of 34 years on August 7, 1927.

Four. Patients of Bazoilles Hospital Center

K—Killed. W—Wounded. G—Gassed. D—Died. TD—To Duty. M—Missing.

Cavett, DeWitt, Mechanic D, W TD
Cawley, Joseph J., Pvt C, K
Cecchi, Colombo, Pvt E, K
Celani, Paul, Pvt H, W TD
Celetti, August, Pvt MG, W
Cerio, Joseph, Pvt B, W
Cermak, Charley J., Pvt G, G

Coll, Daniel B., Cpl Hdq, G
Colley, Harley E., Pvt 1-Cl E, W
Colley, Warren, Cpl E, K
Collings, Hayes, Pvt H, W TD
Collins, Rhodifer, Pvt M, W
Colombo, Alfred, Pvt C, W
Comfort, James L., Pvt G, G

The list of "Casualties among enlisted men" in the written history of the 47th Infantry Regiment mentions Private James L. Comfort of Company G as being gassed ("G"). He did not return to duty ("TD") with this regiment as he was transferred to the 148th Infantry Regiment, 37th Division (*The Forty-Seventh Infantry: A History, 1917–1918 1919*. Saginaw, MI: Press of Seemann & Peters, 1919: 136).

He is buried at Old Shadowlawn Cemetery in Lawrenceville, next to his father and mother.[16] Buried at the same plot is his brother Quinlan who died at the age of 45 years.[17] Notably, the cover plate of his grave reads "JAMES LAWRENCE COMFORT DIED OF INJURIES RECEIVED IN THE WORLD WAR."[18] The certificate of death of James Comfort lists that he had worked as a linotype operator and was of single marital status. He died in U.S. Veterans' Hospital No. 62 in Augusta, Georgia. The cause of his death was myeloid leukemia complicated by acute fibrinous pleurisy.[19] His leukemia might have been caused by exposure to mutagenic mustard gas during World War I while his lungs might also have been badly damaged as a result of this exposure.

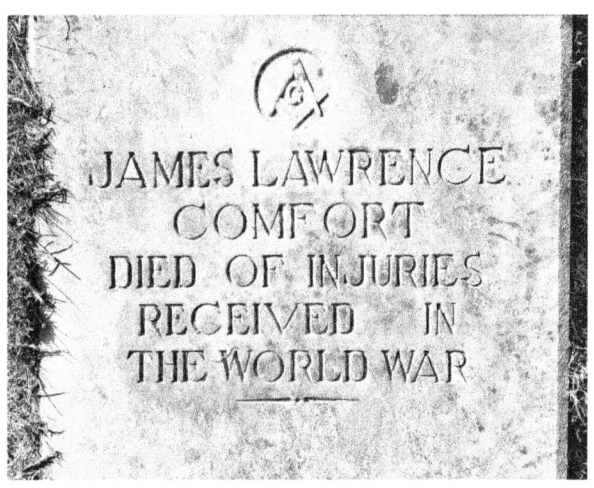

James L. Comfort is buried at Old Shadowlawn Cemetery, Lawrenceville, Georgia. The cover plate of his grave reads "JAMES LAWRENCE COMFORT DIED OF INJURIES RECEIVED IN THE WORLD WAR" (photograph by author).

In August 2016, an identification tag was recovered at the former site of Bazoilles Hospital Center inscribed, although barely readable, on one side with "COMFORT JAMES L" "U S A" and on both sides with Army Service Number "2284154." The combination of name and Army Service Number provides certainty that this identification tag had belonged to Private James. L. Comfort described above. The identification tag is heavily corroded which might be due to the effect of mustard gas on aluminum or the result of burning of military gear of gassed soldiers.

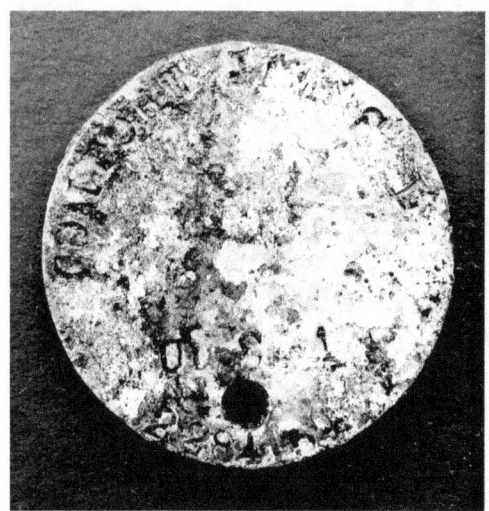 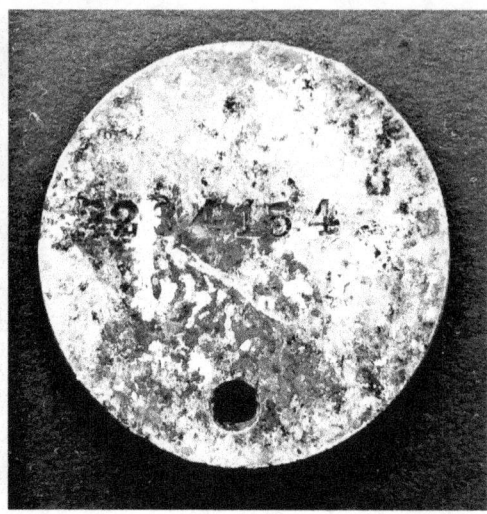

The heavily corroded identification tag of James L. Comfort recovered at the former site of Bazoilles Hospital Center in August 2016. It is inscribed on one side with "COMFORT JAMES L" "U S A" and on both sides with Army Service Number "2284154" (author's collection).

Sergeant Fred Smith, Army Service Number 737107, Approximate Date of Admission September 12, 1918

Fred Smith was born on October 1, 1884, in Spring Valley, Ohio. In 1911, at the age of 27 years, he entered the U.S. Army. He was sent to the Philippines during the Moro Rebellion and participated in the Mexican Expedition in 1916–1917.[20] From April 24, 1918, to September 8, 1919, he served with the American Expeditionary Forces as sergeant in Company M, 11th Infantry Regiment, 5th Division.[21]

Early in the morning of September 12, 1918, the first day of the Battle of St. Mihiel, Fred Smith was gassed and shot through the shoulder near Viéville. He refused to return to a first aid station for treatment and continued to lead his platoon throughout the day.[22] The actions of the 11th Infantry Regiment near Viéville on September 12, 1918, are described in the written history of the 5th Division in World War I: "The Eleventh Infantry descended on Viéville, protected by its belt of wire and strong machine-gun nests. They took the town while the barrage was leaving it. The men in steel gray [the color of German uniforms] came out of their cellars and deep dugouts to find the olive-drab [the color of American uniforms] waiting to receive them. There was resistance only from the isolated machine gunners."[23]

Fred Smith was wounded severely. After a month of hospitalization, he returned to his unit to participate in the Meuse-Argonne Offensive. As the oldest man in his company, he was usually asked to lead patrols as "the kids looked up to him to bring them back."[24] In 1919, Fred Smith was awarded the Distinguished Service Cross, the second highest military award in the U.S. Army, for his actions on September 12, 1918.[25]

After the war, Fred Smith remained in service but eventually thought he "wouldn't live long enough in the Army." He left the service in 1923 and went into railroading as an employee of the Erie Railroad. On December 12, 1969, at the age of 85 years, Fred

Four. Patients of Bazoilles Hospital Center

The Cincinnati Enquirer of March 12, 1919, mentions Sergeant Fred Smith among those announced by the War Department as having been awarded the Distinguished Service Cross for acts of extraordinary heroism (Honored for Heroism. *The Cincinnati Enquirer.* March 12, 1919: 2).

HONORED FOR HEROISM.
SPECIAL DISPATCH TO THE ENQUIRER.

Washington, March 11.—Included in lists of members of the American expeditionary forces, announced yesterday by the War Department as having been awarded the Distinguished Service Cross for acts of extraordinary heroism, are the following Ohio Valley men: Sergeant Fred Smith, Dayton, Ohio; Private Joseph Thornton, Glencoe, Ohio; Sergeant Samuel Clarkston, Druprock, Ky.; Sergeant Corbett Meeks, Lee City, Ky.; Sergeant George Berkley, Golden Pond, Ky., and Sergeant Fred M. Marlowe, Greensburg, Ind.

SMITH, FRED (737107)............ | Sergeant, Company M, 11th Infantry, 5th Division.
Near Vieville, France, Sept. 12, 1918. | After being gassed and shot through the shoulder early in the morning, he continued to lead his platoon throughout the day, refusing to return to the first-aid station for treatment.
R—Dayton, Ohio.
B—Spring Valley, Ohio.
G. O. No. 37, W. D., 1919.

The citation for the Distinguished Service Cross of Fred Smith, Army Service Number 737107, awarded for his actions near Viéville, France, on September 12, 1918 (*American Decorations: A List of Awards of the Congressional Medal of Honor, the Distinguished-Service Cross and the Distinguished-Service Medal Awarded under Authority of the Congress of the United States, 1862–1926.* Washington, D.C.: Government Printing Office, 1927: 567).

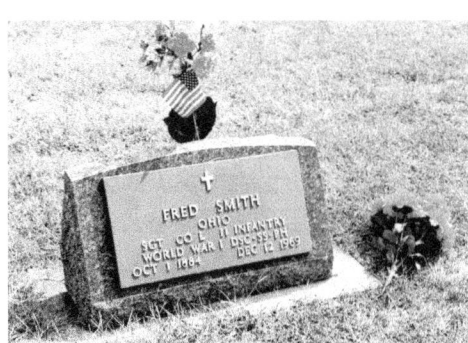
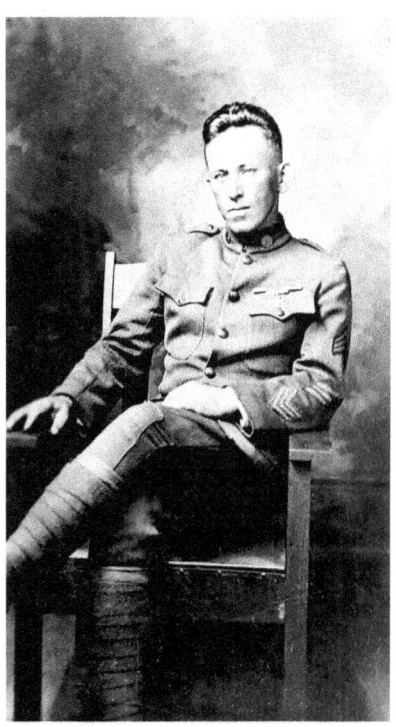

Above: Headstone of the grave of Fred Smith at Enon Cemetery in Enon, Ohio. The headstone honors him as a veteran of World War I awarded with the Distinguished Service Cross, Silver Star and Purple Heart. Incorrectly, the inscription mentions that Fred Smith served with Company L instead of Company M, 11th Infantry Regiment (courtesy John L. Poling, Dayton, Ohio). *Right:* This studio photograph shows Fred Smith after World War I wearing a custom made uniform decorated with a sharpshooter badge. The left sleeve of his uniform shows his sergeant's insignia, his three service stripes each indicating three years of service and his three War Service Chevrons ("overseas stripes") each indicating a six month period of service in the Zone of the Advance (courtesy John L. Poling, Dayton, Ohio).

Smith died in the Veterans Administration Hospital in Dayton, Ohio. He is buried at Enon Cemetery in Enon, Ohio.[26]

In August 2016, an identification tag was recovered at the former site of Bazoilles Hospital Center inscribed on one side with "F. SMITH" "CO. M" "(??). INF." "U. S. A." and on the other side with Army Service Number "737107." The combination of name and Army Service Number provides certainty that this identification tag had belonged to Sergeant Fred Smith described above. The identification tag is heavily corroded which might be due to the effect of gas on aluminum or the result of burning of military gear of gassed soldiers.

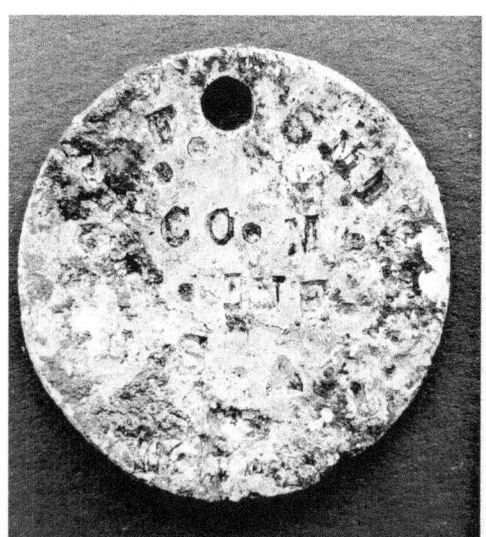 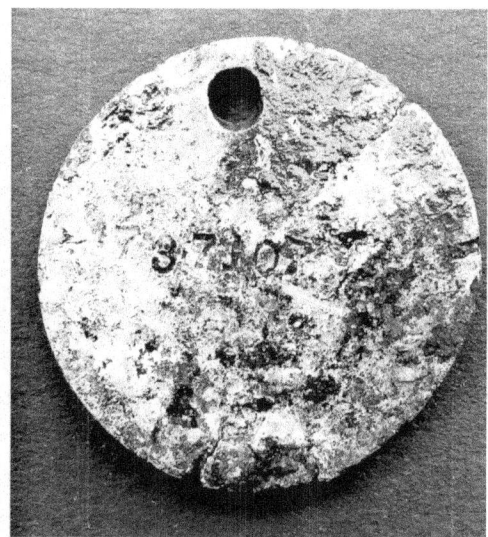

The heavily corroded identification tag of Fred Smith recovered at the former site of Bazoilles Hospital Center in August 2016. It is inscribed on one side with "F. SMITH" "CO. M" "(??). INF." "U. S. A." and on the other side with Army Service Number "737107" (author's collection).

Private Michael J. O'Connor, Army Service Number 1907027, Approximate Date of Admission October 9, 1918

Michael Joseph O'Connor was born on November 1, 1894, in Worcester, Massachusetts, from parents who had emigrated to the United States from Ireland. At the time of his registration for the World War I draft, on June 5, 1917, he was imprisoned at the House of Correction at Worcester, where he was put to work caning chairs.[27] He was inducted in the U.S. Army at Worcester on September 20, 1917. Training was received in 2nd Company, 151st Depot Brigade at Camp Devens, Ayer, Massachusetts. On October 26, he was transferred to Company G, 327th Infantry Regiment, 82nd Division. Promotion to the rank of corporal was made on December 12. He sailed for Europe on board the *RMS* (Royal Mail Ship) *Baltic* leaving on April 25, 1918, arriving at Liverpool on May 7. That

Four. Patients of Bazoilles Hospital Center

Service card of Private Michael J. O'Connor who was severely wounded on October 9, 1918, near Cornay during the second phase of the Meuse-Argonne Offensive (courtesy the Archives-Museum Branch, the Adjutant General's Office of Massachusetts, Concord).

same day his unit proceeded to Southampton from where it sailed to Le Havre, France, which was arrived on May 11. For unknown reason, Michael O'Connor was demoted to the rank of private on May 18.[28]

The 327th Infantry Regiment participated in the Battle of St. Mihiel and the Meuse-Argonne Offensive. In the morning of October 9, during the second phase of the Meuse-Argonne Offensive, units of the 327th Infantry Regiment advanced through the small village of Cornay meeting fierce resistance. A German counterattack in which Cornay was recaptured forced the American troops to surrender or withdraw to Hill 180, east of Cornay.[29] It was during the events on this day that Michael O'Connor was severely wounded by shell fire.[30] His injuries led to the loss of his left leg.[31] While under medical treatment he was repatriated to the U.S. where he arrived on February 12, 1919. Discharge from hospital followed on June 9 after which he was transferred to 2nd Company, Convalescent Center at Camp Devens. There, he was honorably discharged on June 13, while reported 60 percent disabled.[32]

Michael O'Connor returned to Worcester as a disabled war veteran.[33] In 1930, he lived there together with his parents and a younger brother and was without employment.[34] He died at the age of 72 years on December 18, 1966, and was buried in a family grave at St. John's Cemetery in Worcester.[35]

In October 2016, an identification tag was recovered at the former site of Bazoilles Hospital Center inscribed on one side with "MICHAEL J. O'CONNOR" "U. S. A." and

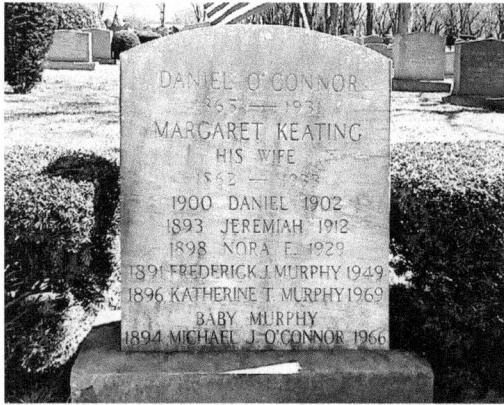

The front and back of the 1942 World War II draft registration card of Michael J. O'Connor indicate that he was a disabled veteran without employment who had lost his left leg during World War I (Ancestry. U.S., World War II Draft Registration Cards, 1942, for Michael Joseph O'Connor. https://www.ancestry.com; accessed December 13, 2016).

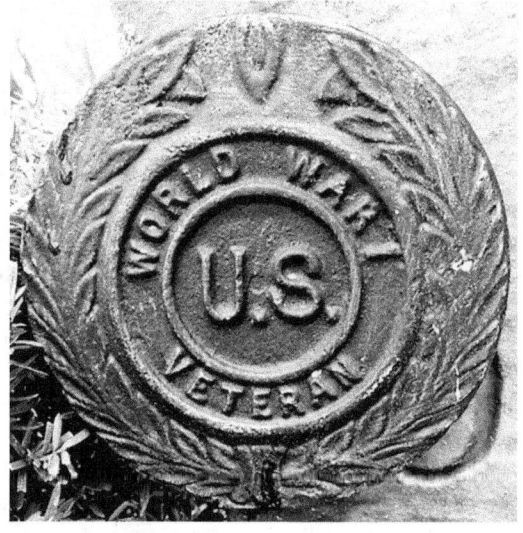

Above: Michael J. O'Connor is buried together with his father and mother in a family grave at St. John's Cemetery in Worcester, Massachusetts (BillionGraves. Grave Information for Michael J O'Connor. https://billiongraves.com/grave/Michael-J-OConnor/7479731#/; accessed December 14, 2016). *Right:* Next to the family grave where Michael J. O'Connor is buried, stands a marker honoring him as a World War I U.S. veteran (courtesy Jim Shetler, Minneapolis, Minnesota).

on the other side with Army Service Number "1907027." Notably, on the front side of the identification tag, several inscriptions have been made illegible. Presumably, these inscriptions had mentioned the unit of Michael J. O'Connor. They were made unreadable so as not to provide information on his unit would he be captured by German forces. The combination of name and Army

Service Number provides certainty that this identification tag had belonged to Private Michael J. O'Connor described above.

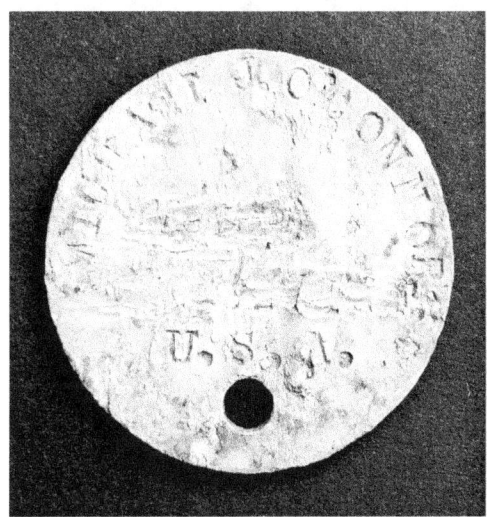 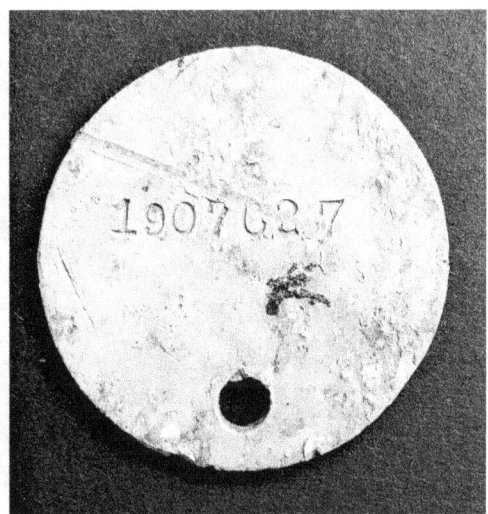

The identification tag of Michael J. O'Connor recovered at the former site of Bazoilles Hospital Center in October 2016. It is inscribed on one side with "MICHAEL J. O'CONNOR" "U. S. A." and on the other side with Army Service Number "1907027." On the front side of the identification tag, several inscriptions have been made illegible. Presumably, these inscriptions had mentioned the unit of Michael J. O'Connor. They were made unreadable so as not to provide information on his unit would he be captured by German forces (author's collection).

Treatment of Wounded German Prisoners of War

At Bazoilles Hospital Center, medical care was provided not only to U.S. Army soldiers but also to French soldiers and German prisoners of war. In principle, the German wounded were treated alike American soldiers, although they were at times harassed. Nurse Sarah Sand, Army Nurse Corps, recollected of the treatment of German prisoners of war in her war memoirs.

Both American and German wounded were transported collectively to Bazoilles Hospital Center by hospital train.[1] Illustratively, during its period of operation, 215 German prisoners of war and 41 French soldiers were treated at Base Hospital No. 46.[2] In the book *Lamp for a Soldier: The Caring Story of a Nurse in World War I*, Nurse Sarah Sand described the medical care provided to German prisoners of war at Base Hospital No. 60.

> It was during this time that thirteen German prisoners were brought into our ward. Several of them were seriously wounded but none died. Our ward was carefully marked off with a large white line where the prisoners were to remain and one of our guards stood at the end of the barracks continually. There was no talking allowed back and forth with our wounded soldiers but the German prisoners were allowed to talk to each other and they did this in German. They were always wondering what had happened to the Crown Prince's troops but, to my knowledge, no one enlightened them.
> We always fed our own soldiers first and we always dressed their wounds first but otherwise we

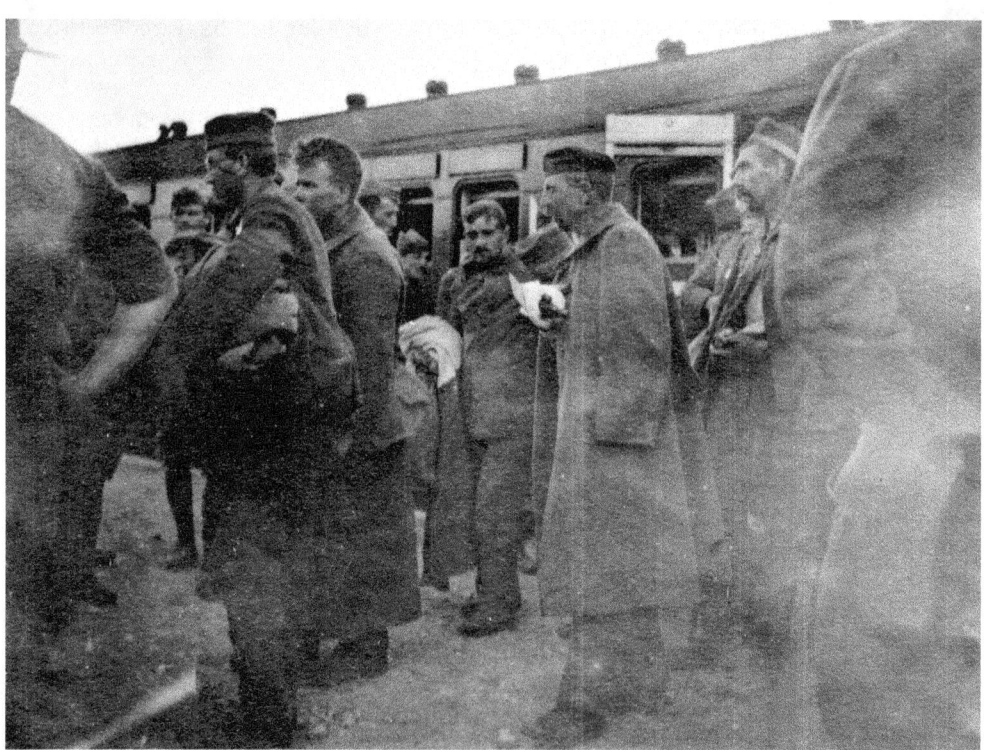

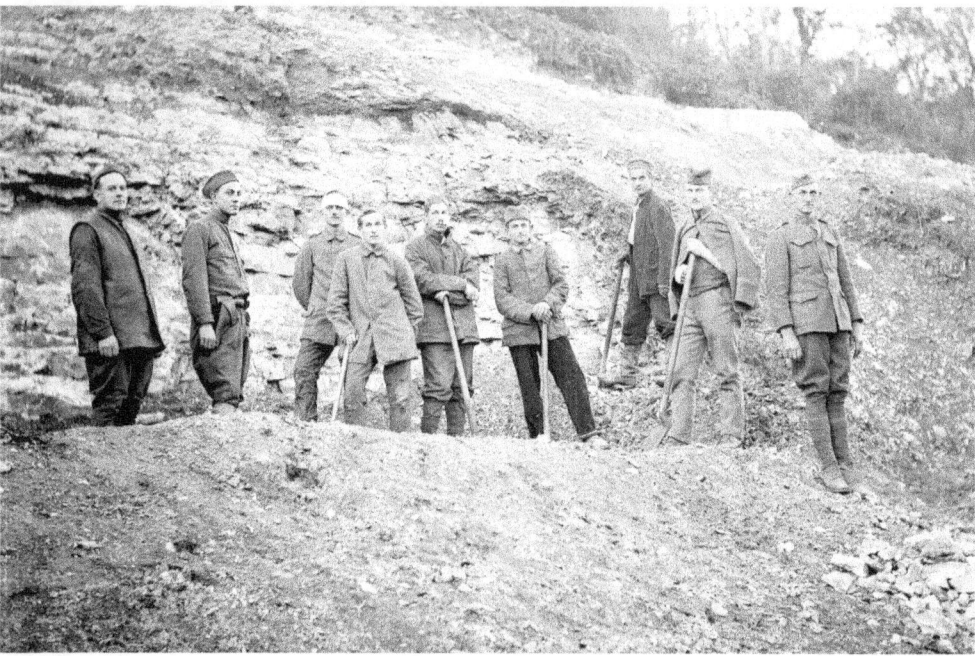

Top: Wounded prisoners of war have just been unloaded from a hospital train at Bazoilles Hospital Center (author's collection). *Bottom:* Six German prisoners of war and three American guards in the gravel pit near Bazoilles Hospital Center (courtesy Oregon Health & Science University, Portland, Oregon [Historical Collections & Archives, Otis B. Wight Base Hospital 46: Glass Plate Negative Collection, Accession No. 20060-12, box 1]).

Four. Patients of Bazoilles Hospital Center

treated the German prisoners the same as our own. The prisoners were a great help to us. I could talk a few German words and could show them how to make dressings and those not seriously ill or wounded used to make them for us almost all the time. Each morning I would cut up the gauze and they would diligently fold it for me. In this way they not only helped themselves but our wounded too. The nurses had precious little time to fold gauze and our home supply was running low. One day, before our ward was closed up, some of our prisoners were allowed to go outside the barracks for an airing. I heard great merry-making and upon investigation found our boys busy cutting the buttons of the Germans' coats for souvenirs. I requested them not to do this as it was still cold weather; they never said a word but stopped at once [in one of his diary entries, First Lieutenant Howard Osgood from Base Hospital No. 116 also mentions American soldiers laughing and joking with "Boche prisoners" who came in by train in a convoy of sick].[3]

One or our German prisoner's name was William. He was a fine looking, well mannered man, a student from the Berlin University. He spoke English fluently and served as an interpreter for the others. Their wounds were of the same nature as our own soldiers! One had a steel injury of his eye and it was causing him to go blind in the other eye. A young captain from Alsace-Lorraine had a serious abdominal and hip wound; another, a leg injury and so on; they rarely complained of pain.[4]

Five

Spanish Flu
*The Toll of Influenza
and Secondary Pneumonia*

The period during which Bazoilles Hospital Center was in operation coincided with the highly fatal second and third waves of the Spanish flu epidemic in 1918 and 1919. Yet, the summary of sick and injured admitted to Bazoilles Hospital Center does not specifically mention influenza cases. This chapter sets out to show not only the toll of influenza and secondary pneumonia among admitted patients, but also the impact of Spanish flu on medical care at the center, making adequate staffing and treatment almost impossible.

Summary of Sick and Injured

Bazoilles Hospital Center was in operation for 10 months from July 1, 1918, to April 30, 1919. During this period, 63,769 patients were treated at the center, of which 26,604 (42 percent) were admitted for injuries and 37,165 (58 percent) because of disease.[1] It seems plausible that soon after November 11, 1918, Armistice Day, the number of admissions because of injuries decreased, explaining to some extent the relatively high proportion of admissions because of disease. Indeed, the surgical ward of Base Hospital No. 60 was closed in the latter part of November 1918.[2] Yet, in war, disease had long been responsible for more loss of life than gunfire. Illustratively, of the six million occasions on which British doctors treated soldiers in World War I, three-and-a-half million were for illness rather than injury.[3]

The overall mortality rate at Bazoilles Hospital Center was low (1.3 percent; 850 deaths) with a slightly higher mortality rate for disease (1.5 percent; 564 deaths) compared to injuries (1.1 percent; 286 deaths).[4] With this low mortality rate, the valley in which Bazoilles Hospital Center was situated hardly deserved the name "Death Valley," as it was reportedly sometimes referred to.[5] On the other hand, the number of deaths at the center exceeded the number of inhabitants of Bazoilles-sur-Meuse, namely 412,[6] by a proportion of two to one. Overall, infectious diseases (pneumonia, dysentery, venereal diseases, (para)typhoid, measles, cerebrospinal meningitis and scarlet fever) accounted for at least 85 percent of disease-related mortality with the cause of the remaining 86 disease-related deaths remaining unspecified.[7]

Summary of sick and injured admitted to hospital center, Bazoilles-sur-Meuse, France, July 1, 1918, to April 30, 1919

Cases of sickness	Total					Pneumonia	Dysentery	Malaria	Venereal	Paratyphoid	Typhoid	Measles	Cerebrospinal meningitis	Scarlet fever	All other diseases
	Hospital	Quarters	Total	Disease	Injury										
Remaining [a]	1,248	0	1,248	447	801	5	0	0	24	20	0	0	0	2	416
Admitted	62,521	0	62,521	36,718	25,803	1,450	85	18	1,481	45	280	111	80	72	33,096
Total treated	63,769	0	63,769	37,165	26,604	1,455	85	18	1,505	45	280	111	80	74	33,512
Died	850	0	850	564	286	414	2	0	1	2	28	1	28	2	86
Transferred to organization	15,908	0	15,908	11,254	4,654	324	42	5	576	10	43	33	6	24	10,191
Otherwise disposed of [b]	46,799	0	46,799	25,135	21,664	705	41	12	828	33	209	67	43	48	23,149
Remaining sick [c]	212	0	212	212	0	12	0	1	100	0	0	10	3	0	86

[a] The remaining 1,248 cases comprises total number of patients in Base Hospitals Nos. 18 and 116 on July 1, 1918, the date the hospital center was established.
[b] Sent to other hospitals, replacement depots, regulating stations, etc.
[c] In Base Hospital No. 79, the only hospital operating April 30, 1919.

Summary of sick and injured admitted to Bazoilles Hospital Center from July 1, 1918, to April 30, 1919 (Ford, J.H. *The Medical Department of the United States Army in the World War, Volume II: Administration American Expeditionary Forces.* Washington, D.C.: Government Printing Office, 1927: 545).

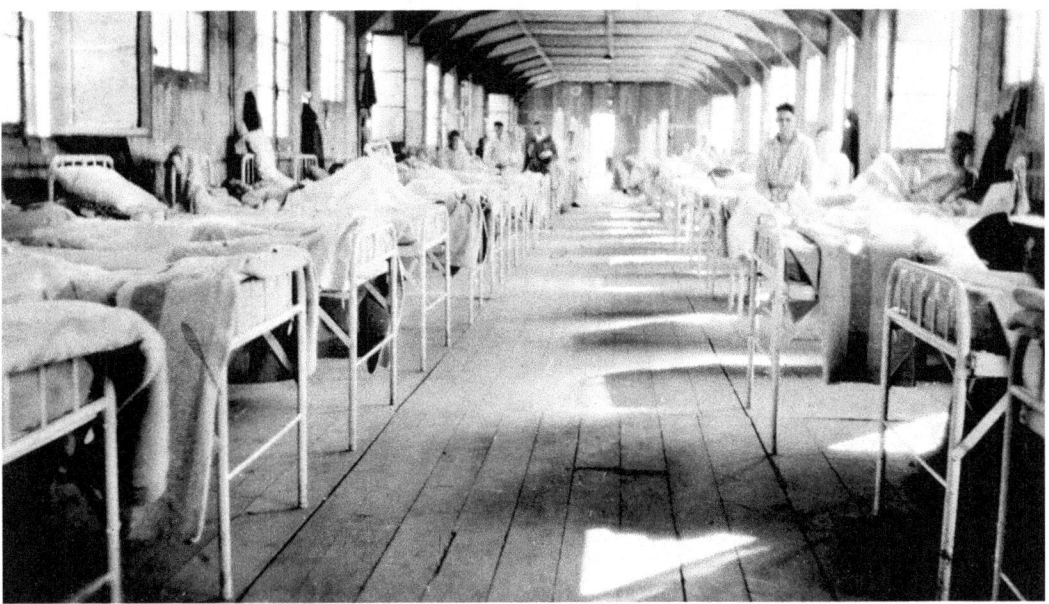

Ward No. 7 of Base Hospital No. 116 at Bazoilles Hospital Center. Wards like these were used as pneumonia wards during the Spanish flu epidemic (author's collection).

Fatal Cases of Spanish Flu and Secondary Pneumonia at Bazoilles Hospital Center

By far the most important cause of death at Bazoilles Hospital Center was pneumonia (414 deaths), accounting for 49 percent of all-cause mortality and 73 percent of disease-related mortality. Among the reported 1,455 cases of pneumonia, the mortality rate was

28 percent illustrating the high case-fatality rate.[8] Secondary pneumonia was a feared complication of the Spanish flu (influenza), which ran its deadly course in 1918 and 1919. A notable characteristic of the Spanish flu epidemic is that it occurred in waves of varying lethality. The first wave, which took place in the spring of 1918, was relatively mild and caused few deaths. After a period of calm in the beginning of the summer, the virus reemerged in an extremely virulent fashion during the second wave in the 1918 autumn months and caused tens of millions of deaths throughout the world. A third wave, also responsible for considerable mortality, occurred during the initial months of 1919, while a final fourth wave, although not always acknowledged as such, spread during the first months of 1920. Notably, Spanish flu was caused by an at that time unknown agent (the virus influenza A subtype H1N1) for which there was no specific treatment, while the often fatal secondary pneumonia was caused by respiratory bacteria.[9]

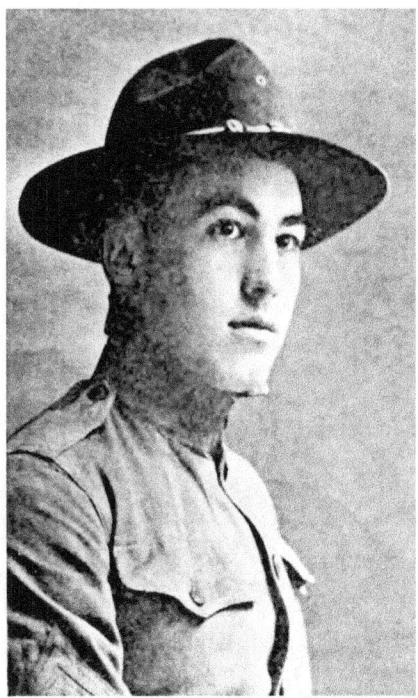 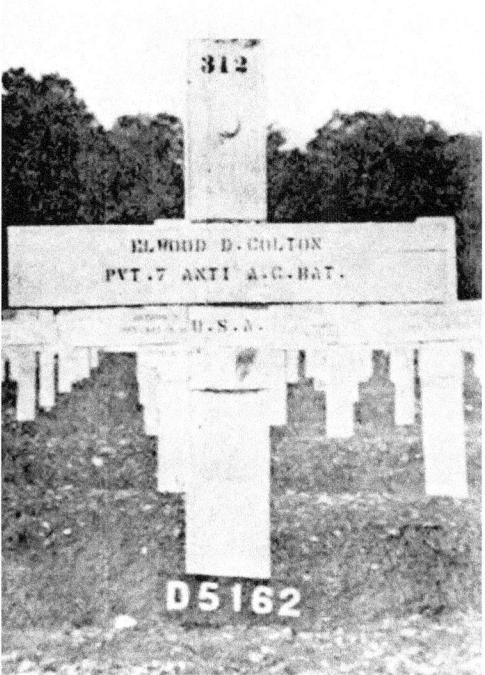

Left: **Private Elwood D. Colton from Evansville, Indiana, served as a medical attendant with the 7th Anti-Aircraft Battery, Coast Artillery Corps. He died on October 24, 1918, at Base Hospital No. 18 of Spanish flu complicated by broncho-pneumonia** (Blatt, H. *Sons of Men: Evansville's War Record.* Evansville, IN: Abe P. Madison, 1920: 45). *Right:* **The grave marker of Private Elwood D. Colton at U.S. Military Cemetery No. 6 at Bazoilles Hospital Center where he was buried in grave No. 312** (Blatt, H. *Sons of Men: Evansville's War Record.* Evansville, IN: Abe P. Madison, 1920: 46).

Privates Elwood Digby Colton and Cleveland Hicks were both residents of Evansville, Indiana.[10] Elwood Colton served as a medical attendant with the 7th Anti-Aircraft Battery, Coast Artillery Corps. While en route to Verdun, he unselfishly ministered to the needs of his comrades suffering from Spanish flu. Later, he himself was brought to Base Hospital No. 18 as a flu victim. His disease was complicated by broncho-pneumonia which was treated in vain with oxygen for the last two days. He died October 24, 1918, and was buried in grave No. 312 of U.S. Military Cemetery No. 6 at Bazoilles Hospital Center. His body was later repatriated to the U.S. where he rests at Oak Hill Cemetery in Evansville.[11] Cleveland Hicks was assigned to Company B, 333rd Infantry Regiment, 84th Division. In France, he contracted Spanish flu which developed into broncho-pneumonia. He was admitted to Base Hospital No. 42 where he died on November 4, 1918, after a few days of illness. Following his death, his mother received a letter written by a representative of the Red Cross Home Communication Service.

> You have no doubt received a cable telling you about the death of your son in hospital here. I know that many questions will arise during these dark days and I want to answer a few of them. Your boy came to us suffering from a bad attack of the influenza. It soon developed into pneumonia and in spite of all the tender care of nurses and doctors, he passed away at 6:40 a. m., Nov. 4. It is hard to have loved ones pass away when they are so far from home. One keeps thinking and wondering about his care and those who comforted him. It certainly is a comfort to me to be able to assure you that no boy ever had more skillful attention in his own home. And the nurses and doctors as well as all the rest of us love these boys and give them all that is possible and well for them to have.
>
> Your son had a military burial [at U.S. Military Cemetery No. 6 at Bazoilles Hospital Center; he was later reburied at the Meuse-Argonne American Cemetery in Romagne-sous-Montfaucon in Plot C, Row 38, Grave 34].[12] The casket was covered with the flag he loved and died for. Six of his comrades carried him out. At the grave the Chaplain, who had comforted him when he was ill, conducted the service while all the soldiers stood at attention about the grave. Then we lowered the casket and the bugler sounded taps [bugle call played at military funerals]. A little cross with his name and number was raised and then we left him to sleep with his comrades all about. There is no more fitting place for a soldier to sleep than in this friendly French valley with those who fought with him for freedom.
>
> The cemetery is on the sunny slope of a quiet hill. Above the slope is a forest of trees turning brown and gold in the autumn crispness. Below are green meadows dotted with herds tended by little children. These little children love our brave boys too, and stand at attention with their little caps in their hands when we pass them with our soldiers who have paid the price of their lives. And then lower down is the river [Meuse] winding along among the trees. Even yet the wild flowers linger in the sheltered places—falming, red poppies and yellow mustard.[13]

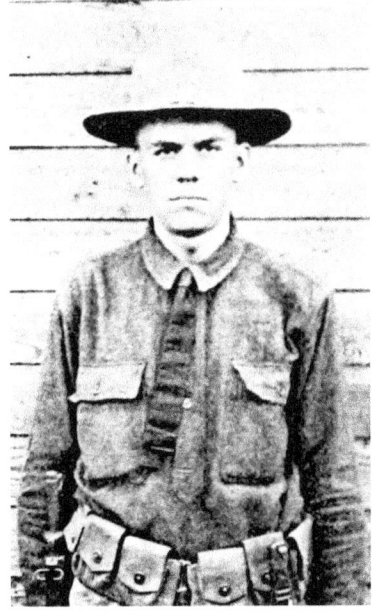
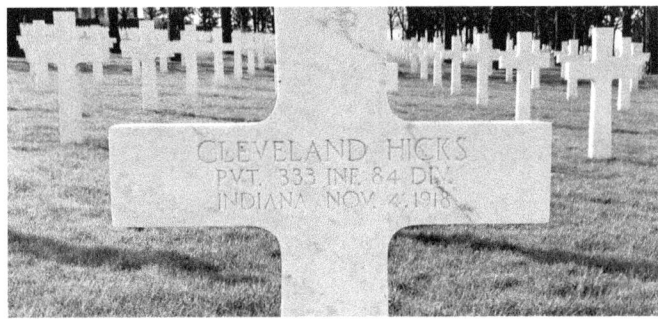

Left: Private Cleveland Hicks from Evansville, Indiana, was assigned to Company B, 333rd Infantry Regiment, 84th Division. He was admitted to Base Hospital No. 42 where he died on November 4, 1918, of Spanish flu which had developed into broncho-pneumonia (Blatt, H. *Sons of Men: Evansville's War Record*. Evansville, IN: Abe P. Madison, 1920: 85). *Above:* Headstone of the grave of Private Cleveland Hicks at the Meuse-Argonne American Cemetery in Romagne-sous-Montfaucon (courtesy American Battle Monuments Commission [Overseas Operations Office, Paris, France; photograph by author]).

The Appendix lists 36 other American servicemen and women who died or were buried at Bazoilles Hospital Center because of fatal influenza and/or pneumonia. Notably, these pneumonia cases occurred during either the second or third waves of the Spanish flu epidemic, suggesting that the pneumonia was secondary to influenza. The number of deaths because of influenza and/or pneumonia at Bazoilles Hospital Center seems to peak in the seven-day period from 22 to October 28, 1918 (the number of deaths due to any cause in the center seems highest on October 24). Moreover, the Appendix shows that influenza and pneumonia patients were admitted to the various base hospitals at Bazoilles Hospital Center, despite the fact that Base Hospital No. 18 had been designated to receive all contagious disease cases coming to the center.[14] Many of these soldiers, and presumably most, if not all, of them, were initially buried at U.S. Military Cemetery No. 6 at Bazoilles Hospital Center. They were later exhumed and transported to the U.S. or to the Meuse-Argonne American Cemetery at Romagne-sous-Montfaucon.[15]

German prisoners of war at Bazoilles Hospital Center also succumbed to influenza and/or pneumonia during the Spanish flu epidemic. Illustratively, *Soldat* Emil Steglich, serving with *1. Kompanie, Königlich Sächsisches 13. Infanterie-Regiment Nr. 178, 123. Infanterie-Division*, was admitted to Base Hospital No. 46 on October 18, 1918, and died of broncho-pneumonia on November 6.[16]

Report of death of *Soldat* Emil Steglich who served with *1. Kompanie, Königlich Sächsisches 13. Infanterie-Regiment Nr. 178, 123. Infanterie-Division*. Steglich died of broncho-pneumonia during the Spanish flu epidemic, on November 6, 1918, as a German prisoner of war admitted to Base Hospital No. 46 (National Archives at Kansas City, Kansas City, Missouri [Record Group 120: Records of the American Expeditionary Forces (World War I), 1848–1942, Correspondence of the Hospital Center at Bazoilles, 1918–1919, National Archives Identifier 6636481: box 2 folder 383.6 Enemy Prisoners of War]).

The Toll of Influenza and Secondary Pneumonia Among the Fighting Forces

While the summary of sick and injured admitted to Bazoilles Hospital Center does not specifically mention influenza figures,[17] the written histories of the various base hospitals indicate that numerous influenza cases were present among the 33,512 unspecified disease cases. In fact, while Spanish flu struck all the armies, the highest morbidity rate was found among the Americans as the disease sickened over one million men, 26 percent of the U.S. Army, in both training camps in the U.S. and in Europe. Overall, Spanish flu killed around 45,000 U.S. Army soldiers. In comparison, this number by far exceeds the 26,000 American deaths during the Meuse-Argonne Offensive, which is still considered "America's deadliest battle." It has even been stated that more Americans were buried in France because of Spanish flu than of enemy fire.[18]

Up to December 13, 1918, the Medical Service of Base Hospital No. 46 received 1,158 cases of influenza (almost 14 percent of the total number of admissions at this base hospital).[19] Early in September 1918, the prevalence of influenza at Base Hospital No. 46 took a sharp rise,[20] coinciding with the arrival of the second wave of Spanish flu on the Western Front roughly around September 15, 1918.[21] As the epidemic progressed, cases became complicated more frequently by broncho-pneumonia.[22] There were 142 broncho-pneumonia cases, besides 43 cases of lobar pneumonia, with eight cases of subsequent empyema.[23] A double ward, No. 22, was designated for the exclusive management of broncho-pneumonia at Base Hospital No. 46. During September and October 1918, 119 cases were admitted to this ward of which 71 were fatal. The mortality rate of 59 percent at Ward No. 22 exceeded all others of the hospital combined. Many cases received by convoy died within 48 hours of admission. The disease was reportedly "absolutely atypical, both as to its clinical features and its associate bacteriology."[24] Illustratively, on September 29, 1918, an otherwise unknown doctor described in a letter the rapid clinical course of fatal influenza with secondary pneumonia at Camp Devens, a U.S. Army training camp in Massachusetts.

> These men start with what appears to be an ordinary attack of LaGrippe or Influenza, and when brought to the Hosp. they very rapidly develop the most viscious [vicious] type of Pneumonia that has ever been seen. Two hours after admission they have the Mahogony [Mahogany] spots over the cheek bones, and a few hours later you can begin to see the Cyanosis [blue or purple coloration of the skin or mucous membranes] extending from their ears and spreading all over the face, until it is hard to distinguish the colored men from the white. It is only a matter of a few hours then until death comes, and it is simply a struggle for air until they suffocate. It is horrible. One can stand it to see one, two or twenty men die, but to see these poor devils dropping out like flies sort of gets on your nerves. We have been averaging about 100 deaths per day, and still keeping it up. There is no doubt in my mind that there is a new mixed infection here, but what I don't know. My total time is taken up hunting Rales [breath sounds which can be heard in the lungs of patients with pneumonia using a stethoscope], rales dry or moist, sibilant or crepitant or any other of the hundred things that one may find in the chest, they all mean but one thing here—Pneumonia—and that means in about all cases death.[25]

At Base Hospital No. 18, 52 percent of the 2,014 cases of infectious and epidemic diseases were cases of influenza (over 6 percent of the total number of admissions at this base hospital, which began operation 11 months before the organization of Bazoilles Hospital Center).[26] Broncho-pneumonia was responsible for 31 percent of deaths at Base Hospital No. 18 exceeding the number of deaths due to wounds incurred in battle.[27]

The disease burden of non-fatal Spanish flu is well illustrated by the diary entries of Private Charles L. Wells, a cook with Battery F, 115th Field Artillery, 30th Division, who was admitted with influenza at Bazoilles Hospital Center for almost a month during the second wave of the epidemic.

> November 21: I have a high fever and am feeling very tough.
> November 22: I am barely able to sit up.
> November 23: I am forced to take my bed on the floor of the little shack we built out of some salvaged lumber.
> November 24: The medical man says I have influenza. The ambulance is taking me to the hospital at Commercy.
> November 28. For the last four days I have been delirious and unable to write. Today is Thanksgiving and Turkey is being served for dinner but too bad, I am too sick to eat any.
> November 30: My Twenty-Fifth birthday.
> December 1: I was transferred to Base Hospital. Ward number 60, at Bazoilles near Newfchatear [Neufchâteau]. I was taken in an ambulance. On my way I passed through the town of Dorami [Domrémy-la-Pucelle], the home of Joan De Arc and saw the church where she worshipped and the hill where she saw her vision. ...
> December 15: Was transferred to duty ward.
> December 25: A fine Christmas dinner, the first real meal I have had since I left the states.
> December 26: Left Bazoilles for my organization, landing at Toul the same day and going into a replacement camp.
> December 28: Was fully equipped again.

Significantly, Private Wells writes on February 12, 1919, that his outfit was "quarantined for the influenza" indicating the arrival of the third wave of the Spanish flu epidemic.[28]

Treatment options for Spanish flu and secondary pneumonia were limited. At the pneumonia ward of Base Hospital No. 60, Nurse Sarah Sand made rounds with hypodermics (medication injected under the skin) and bags of oxygen. This was supplied from large oxygen tanks and given to each patient who was cyanotic.[29]

The Impact of Spanish Flu on Medical Care at Bazoilles Hospital Center

Although the medical services of the American Expeditionary Forces were equipped to handle wounds as well as disease, the magnitude of the Spanish flu epidemic overwhelmed the system. The impact of Spanish flu was felt throughout the complex network of medical stations and transportation lines. For a time, it even appeared as though the ravages of influenza would seriously affect military operations during the Meuse-Argonne Offensive by overwhelming the sanitary formation. Moreover, Spanish flu could also put medical personnel out of commission at the very time they were needed most.[30] Indeed, doctors, nurses and orderlies fell ill from influenza, making adequate staffing and treatment almost impossible.[31] Illustratively, on September 23, 1918, a request was made that nurses on temporary duty at Base Hospital No. 66 in Neufchâteau were returned to Base Hospital No. 46 at Bazoilles-sur-Meuse. It was stated that "on account of sickness among the members of the Nurses Corps of this hospital, the services of above nurses are badly needed."[32]

First Lieutenant Howard Osgood from Base Hospital No. 116, who was responsible for wound cultures at the center laboratory of Bazoilles Hospital Center, experienced a chilliness in the evening of October 30, which made him fear for the "grippe." The next morning, he "felt rotten" suffering from "malaise, pains, headache, etc." On November 1, he was admitted to an officers' ward where he stayed for one week. It was November 10 that he was "feeling much better" after being ill for ten days.[33]

The Appendix lists six names of medical professionals and a social worker who died of fatal influenza and/or pneumonia and had worked or been admitted to Bazoilles Hospital Center. The death of Nurse Ima Ledford from Base Hospital No. 116 on October 7, 1918, has been described in the war memoirs of fellow Nurse Louise Kalkman.

> One of our nurses, Miss Ledford, a pretty dark-eyed girl from Washington, developed pneumonia and passed away. She was only ill three days and everyone felt very badly as she was loved by all. The boys made a coffin of rough boards and she was laid away in her uniform with autumn leaves as flowers. As the taps blew that morning, we all bowed our heads with tears in our eyes, and said a prayer for our little sister who had been so brave.[34]

Nurse Jeannette Bellman from Base Hospital No. 18 was taken ill on November 2, 1918. After a short and severe illness, she died on November 12.[35] The *Dayton Daily News* published the news of her death on November 30:

> Miss Jeanette Belleman [Bellman], 36, a Red Cross nurse who formerly lived in and near Dayton, died this week in France, a victim of bro[n]cho-pneumonia. Word of her death was received in a dispatch sent by Adjutant General Harris, of Washington, to her brother, Ira Belleman, R. F. D. [Rural Free Delivery] No. 3. Just the day before the sad message was delivered Mr. Belleman had received a cheerful letter from his sister, in which she said that she was enjoying excellent health, though working so hard that she did not have time to change her wet clothes when it rained and that she found it necessary to go to bed in order to get warm and dry. Miss Belleman had been working among the soldiers for two years and six months. She first entered the Red Cross service during the Mexican trouble and remained at Ft. Sam Houston, Texas for a year. Very soon after America entered the war she was sent overseas.[36]

In her war memoirs, Nurse Sarah Sand of Base Hospital No. 60 described her grief over the death of a stretcher bearer due to pneumonia at Bazoilles Hospital Center. "My heart went out to one stretcher-bearer of this hospital train. He fell over while carrying in a wounded patient and was brought to our [pneumonia] ward. He had worked day and night in the cold and wet until he completely collapsed with pneumonia. In his delirium he thought I was his mother and he kept repeating over and over that nobody thought of the stretcher-carriers. A few hours after being brought in he made the supreme sacrifice for his country."[37]

Died of Disease.
LIEUTENANT.
DURGIN, Robert G. Frank H. Durgin, Exeter Street, New Market, N. H.
NURSES.
BELLMAN, Jeannette. Ira Bellman, R. F. D. 3, Dayton, Ohio.
HOFFMAN, Katherine. Sam Hoffman, R. F. D. 2, Queen City, Mo.

Nurse Jeannette Bellman of Base Hospital No. 18 is listed in the *Official U.S. Bulletin* of December 5, 1918, among those who died of disease (Casualties Reported by Gen. Pershing. *Official U.S. Bulletin*. December 5, 1918: 22).

Synopsis

At least 2,200 cases of influenza have been admitted to Base Hospitals Nos. 18 and 46 (cases admitted to Base Hospital No. 46 after December 13, 1918, not included).[38] The fatal cases of influenza and/or pneumonia listed in the Appendix indicate, however, that patients with these conditions were also admitted to Base Hospitals Nos. 42, 66, 79 and 116 and Evacuation Hospital No. 21. Furthermore, Base Hospital No. 60 had its own pneumonia ward.[39] This suggests that the total number of Spanish flu patients admitted to the different hospitals of Bazoilles Hospital Center might well exceed 6,000, thereby nearing 10 percent of the total number of cases treated at the center. Accounting for 414 deaths among both the fighting forces and medical personnel, pneumonia—a feared complication of Spanish flu—was by far the most important cause of death at Bazoilles Hospital Center. In the written history of Base Hospital No. 18, it was stated that "the death statistics … point out that a soldier not mortally wounded in battle has an excellent chance for eventual recovery, if he can be afforded proper treatment, and that the Army has more to fear from the virulent respiratory diseases than the shells of the enemy."[40]

Convalescent Camp No. 2

On November 12, 1918, the day after Armistice Day, the number of patients in overseas U.S. Army hospitals totaled 193,026, distributed in 153 base hospitals, 66 camp hospitals and 12 convalescent camps.[1] Convalescent camps were part of large hospital centers or situated in their vicinity. Patients whose medical or surgical treatment had been completed,

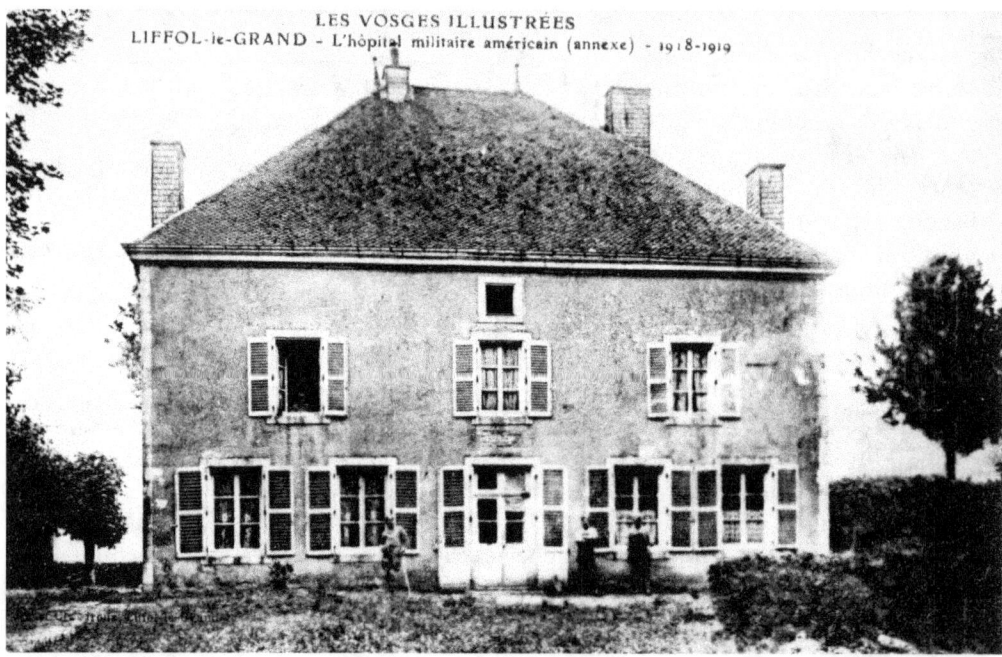

A postcard showing the (annex to the) 1918–1919 American military hospital in Liffol-le-Grand. Another postcard (not shown) refers to this same building as *Le Château* (Castle). This indicates that this building was part of Convalescent Camp No. 2 which "contained a number of small structures and a 14-room château" (author's collection).

Five. Spanish Flu

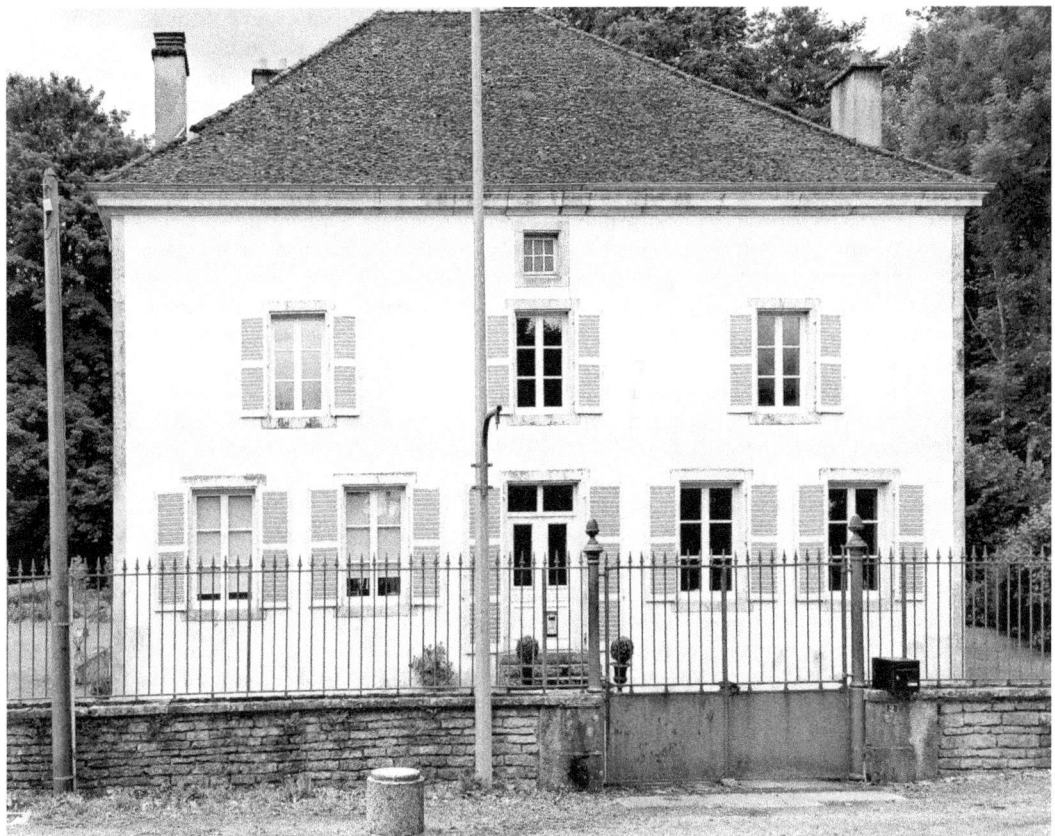

Present-day view of the building in Liffol-le-Grand that was part of Convalescent Camp No. 2 from July 13, 1918, to January 25, 1919 (photograph by author).

but whose physical condition was such that their attending doctors did not consider them fit for duty, could be sent to convalescent camps. Thereby, base hospital beds were cleared of patients allowing for the reception of new patients from the front. This was particularly important for those base hospitals nearest to the front.[2]

The convalescent camp connected to Bazoilles Hospital Center was situated in nearby Liffol-le-Grand and designated Convalescent Camp No. 2. It started operation on July 13, 1918, and ceased to function on January 25, 1919. Its operation is described in Volume II of the commemorative series *The Medical Department of the United States Army in the World War*.

> The chief surgeon in a letter of June 21, 1918, ordered that a convalescent camp be operated in connection with the center. The proportion of beds was fixed at one convalescent bed to five of the base hospital capacity of the center, all crisis expansion accommodations being excluded. For this purpose, the number of active beds in buildings was assumed to be 7,000, thus fixing the bed capacity of the camp at 1,400. The site for the camp was selected at Liffol-le-Grand, a village 4 miles west of Bazoilles. This site had been used at one time as a camp hospital and contained a number of small structures and a 14-room château. The personnel of Convalescent Camp No. 2, consisting of 10 officers and 90 enlisted men, arrived on June 10, 1918.
>
> The preparation of buildings and grounds with provision of new barrack buildings, water supply, and roads was begun at once. A satisfactory water supply was not obtained until November, 1918.

The medical organization of the camp was quite simple. On admission after the bath, the patient was weighed, stripped. He was outfitted with essential clothing and assigned to a bed in the barracks. At once a physical examination was made, and he joined in the class work the following day. This class work consisted of physical exercise in the morning, followed by a short period of squad drill. After dinner and after an hour's complete relaxation in bed, he was sent on a mile march. On returning, he took part in various games according to his ability. After supper, varying amusements, held in the Y. M. C. A. hut, were available. At the discretion of the medical officer, he was promoted to Company 2, with its increased physical demands, and then to Company 3, where the work consisted of 40-minute setting-up exercises, an hour's squad drill, and a 5-mile march in the afternoon. By the time the patient had successfully passed the physical examination in this company and could successfully perform the strenuous exercises, he was discharged to duty.... It is worthy of comment that these tests were of much greater value as a basis for classification than those heretofore employed; that is, the stethoscope, physician's opinion of patient's statement. Great emphasis was laid on the necessity for military discipline; and although on a patient's status, all convalescents were treated as soldiers training for the front line. Great difficulty was experienced in the lack of standardization of the type of patients received. Thus, one convoy would comprise a case of pneumonia out of bed one day, a mumps patient convalescent three weeks, a patient with flat-foot, gas cases of varying degrees of severity, and superficial gunshot wounds. An oc[c]asional [cardiac] valve lesion was discovered, a few cases of pulmonary tuberculosis were found, and not infrequently patients were sent directly from the admitting office to the camp hospital suffering from acute infections, such as bronchopneumonia, influenza, and tonsillitis. Another interesting feature is the fact that promotions were made daily instead of at weekly intervals. This increased markedly the capacity of the camp, and cut down the stay in camp of those physically fit on admission to the remarkably short period of 72 hours. It was this factor that allowed 2,431 admissions and 998 discharges in October, when the camp was in full working order.

A follow-up system was instituted, and the final proof of the success of the camp as measured by the ability of members of the outgoing drafts to perform front-line duty was supplied by the medical officers of units to which the patients were returned.

The constant support and assistance afforded by the American Red Cross carried the camp far beyond the standards obtainable under purely military control. Games and other equipment for the amusement of the patients were all supplied through this organization. A regular representative of that society did not arrive for some weeks after the camp was opened because of the lack of such officers, but thereafter it engaged in numerous activities for the promotion of morale.[3]

Six

"Dear Mother"
Letters from Bazoilles Hospital Center

Tens of thousands of letters from hospitalized soldiers and medical personnel to worried mothers back home must have been written at Bazoilles Hospital Center. Some letters provided comfort, but in other cases, they bore bad news. Three of these letters—written by a Medical Department soldier, a chief nurse and a hospitalized soldier—are reproduced in full below.

Private Henry A. Ladd, Base Hospital No. 46, to Mrs. Mary L. Ladd, Portland, Oregon

July 30, 1918.

Well, at least, mother dear, I am writing.... Shortly after I wrote my last letter (days and dates mean nothing to me now—I had to ask three boys the date before I found it) we moved our own hospital site to another near by, which, I believe, is more desirable-nearer the little village and will be slightly more protected from winter winds [Base Hospital No. 46 was shortly situated on the east bank of the river Meuse before moving, presumably around 18 July,[1] to its final location on the west side of the river]. In less than three days, long before we were really settled, came orders to receive patients [Base Hospital No. 46 began operation on 23 July[2]; the first convoy of patients was received on that date and consisted mainly of gassed patients from the Battle of Château-Thierry, which was fought on July 18].[3] From then on my heart has increased in vigor. I have been a different boy, indeed. I have put all I had each day into work and the work has taken all I had, but has given me, oh, so much satisfaction! For about three or four days I worked in a supply building, handling boxes and checking, checking, checking supplies of one nature or another from 7 in the morning until often 9:30 or later at night. That work was hard, but very important just then. Soon a larger convoi [convoy] of patients came and I was put in a ward. Late hours continued. My patients were mostly gassed. The first night I spent up all night with one nurse. We worked incessantly. I had sleep the next day, that is, some, and then I was on regular day duty. After a couple of days I was shifted to a surgical ward just being filled by patients of which I have had charge as ward master ever since. The nurse over me is a woman of about thirty-four or five, and the ward surgeon, Lieutenant McCrown [First Lieutenant Arthur C. McCown] is a corker. He is a man I like and am eager to assist at dressings though my duties give me little time for the latter. But here I must pause, the call to Quarters has blown and I'm at the Red Cross building. Good night, more tomorrow.

Here is the second night on this letter. I have had quite a confining day with seemingly lots to do and little to show for the doing. Besides one of the men who has been mending rapidly, has tonight taken a turn for the worse and I have a sort of depressed feeling over his condition, for he is one of the most lovable boys in the ward. My hours end at seven p. m. but tonight, as usual, I didn't finish until a few minutes ago (about 8 o'clock), so I just sat down here in the ward kitchen to write.

It has been a lovely day and I should have liked to have had it alone in some woody region. The evenings grow rather chilly after the sun sets, but the atmosphere is wonderfully clear and delightfully fresh this evening.

Well, last night I believe I was talking about changing wards, and being put here under Lieutenant McCown, and a fine head nurse, when I had to stop. I suppose that means little to you, but you see that a ward master's job can be made "hell," or "pleasant hell," by the gods directly in charge of said personage, and just now I'm having a very interesting bit of "pleasant hell," as it were. Furthermore, the boy who happened to be assigned here with me as chore man, is a mighty good chap. I had not known him before, but I have grown to like him more and more as we work together. …

And now my work again. Besides my regular duties of tending to the care of the ward, etc., I have been able to see most of the more serious dressings, and of course have tended to the patients somewhat. I honestly enjoy all that work and I try to get into all the surgical bits of it that I can, for experience in assistance there means, of course, a chance for a surgical team and the front–sometime–which is quite my present aspiration, but the realization of which I fear is somewhat in the distant future. It is marvelous, mother, how some of the boys pull through and what wonders nature does of its own accord with good nursing. …

A heart of love again.[4]

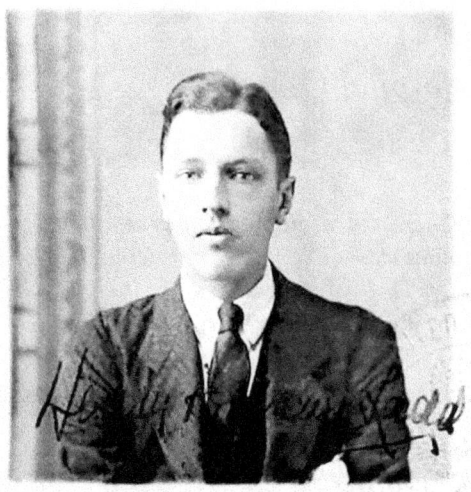

This photograph of Henry A. Ladd was attached to his emergency passport application dated May 15, 1919, which was submitted to the American Passport Bureau in Paris. Henry Ladd had been transported to France without having ever owned a passport (Ancestry. U.S. Passport Applications, 1795–1925 for Henry A Ladd. https://www.ancestry.com; accessed November 13, 2016).

Author's note: later in life, Henry Andrews Ladd became an art critic, author and professor.[5] He died, aged 46, as a resident of Kent, Connecticut, and a teacher at Sarah Lawrence College, Bronxville, New York, of a sudden heart attack on June 27, 1941.[6]

Chief Nurse Grace Phelps, Base Hospital No. 46, to Mrs. Sarah A. Royer, Snoqualmie Falls, Washington

Base Hospital No. 46
A. P. O. #731
September 18, 1918

Mrs. Sarah Agnes Royer,
Snoqualmie Falls,
Washington

My dear Mrs. Royer:

You will find enclosed your letters to Norene, which were received, but which she never read.

I wish I had some way of telling you without bluntly writing that your dear child was taken very sick with pneumonia on the 10th of this month and died at 2:1t [2.15] a. m. on the 17th of September.

You doubtless have received an official notice telling of the death of Norene by this time. A telegram was sent to your son [Master Engineer Ed. Royer, Headquarters Company, 35th Engineers stationed at La Rochelle, France] when she became so ill and we wired him again just as soon as she had passed away yesterday morning. Everything possible that the doctors and nurses could do was done for her. She made a brave fight to live, but her God has called her and she has gone to Him.

Father Dinan [Chaplain Thomas A. Dinan of Base Hospital No. 46], the Priest here was with her and gave her the last Sacraments. She seemed to know that she was going as she said when she was first taken sick that she did not believe she would get well. Miss [Anna C.] Berg who has been her very good friend was with her as one of her special nurses and of course, will write to you very soon.

Norene was laid away at 9:30 this morning in the cemetery with our brave men who have died in the service. Some of them she has taken care of. She was given all military honors. The six senior officers, majors and captains of our unit were the honorary pall bearers; six first-class sergeants were in attendance as active pall bearers. Most of the officers, nurses and enlisted men of the unit attended.

Certificate of identity issued by the War Department to Chief Nurse Grace Phelps of Base Hospital No. 46 (courtesy Oregon Health & Science University, Portland, Oregon [Historical Collections & Archives, Grace Phelps Papers, Accession No. 20100-05, box 2 folder 4]).

I wish I could tell you how beautiful she looked in her Red Cross uniform, white—white shoes and her Red Cross cap with the unit flag draped around her casket and a beautiful silk flag, which is the particular pride of the nurses of the unit, placed over her as a covering.

We will all miss her so much; the men because she was nice to them and such a good nurse, doing the thing to be done in a sisterly way and the nurses because she was one of them and they loved her. She roomed next door to me and I will miss her songs, for she was always singing and seemed very happy.

The cemetery is just back of the nurses' quarters and where we can look right over and see where she is at rest. Enclosed is a poem [*In Flanders Field* by John McCrae], which you may have seen before. It means much to us. The poppies will grow on Norene's grave as they do everywhere here. The Officers went to the nearest town and bought some beautiful flowers, but what they got were no more beautiful than the boquet [bouquet] of red, white and blue flowers we gathered from the field— the red poppies, the blue corn flowers and the white asters.

Within the next few days, we will have her things ready to return to you, all with the exception of a few things supplied by the Red Cross, which are supposed to be returned to them.

It is impossible for us to know the extent of your grief, but we do wish you to know that we send all the sympathy in the world. We hope to get in touch with your son, although we have not heard from him yet.

Father Dinan was perfectly splendid; came to see her often and was so nice to arrange for the service, which was held in the quaint and historic cathedral in the village near where we are stationed. There was High Mass and the service was beautiful.

We will be very glad indeed to hear from you. It likely will be sometime before you will receive Norene's things. They will be sent thru the regular military channels.

Again assuring you of my great sympathy and the sympathy of the entire unit, I am,

Very sincerely yours,
Chief Nurse

> GP JLD
> Grace Phelps, Chief Nurse
> Base Hospital No. 46,
> A. P. O. #731,
> Amer. E. F.[7]

Chief Nurse Grace Phelps kept a notebook with details on the service of the nurses of Base Hospital No. 46. These pages show her entries on and a picture of Nurse Norene M. Royer and mention her death of pneumonia (courtesy Oregon Health & Science University, Portland, Oregon [Historical Collections & Archives, Grace Phelps Papers, Accession No. 20100-05, box 3]).

Author's note: the body of Nurse Norene Mary Royer was exhumed from U.S. Military Cemetery No. 6 at Bazoilles Hospital Center in 1921. She was included in a group of 5,212 war dead transported to the army pier in Hoboken, New Jersey, on the United States Transport *Wheaton*, which docked on May 18.[8] Her body arrived in Portland, Oregon, on June 2, from where she was transported to Spokane, Washington.[9] There, she was reburied in the legion plot at the Riverside Park Cemetery. She received a full military funeral service in the presence of twenty Red Cross nurses in full uniform.[10]

Six. "Dear Mother"

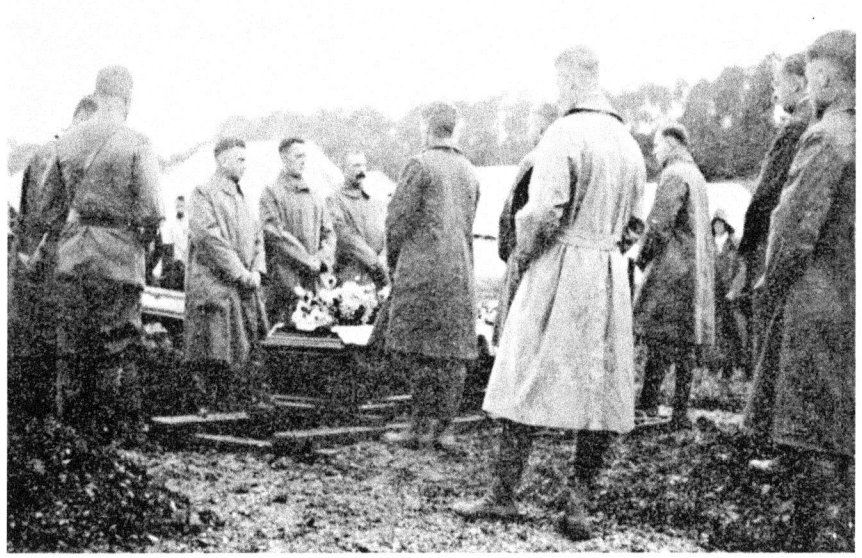

Love Tragedy of World War Related by Veteran

Claude M. Bristol, Portland Legionnaire, who is now in Paris covering the American Legion for The Telegram, today tells an unusual and touching reminiscence of the great struggle. Many brave lads have marched away to war and many a girl left behind has mourned their passing, but in the story today, the monster War, claims both the man and his beloved.

By Claude M. Bristol.

PARIS, Sept. 28.—(Special.)—Just a dream of yesterday, though it seems we are living it now as we pound the old Underwood which has been with us all these years.

We have only to close our eyes and we hear the tramp of countless feet and the clank of artillery harness. The hushed hum of "There's a Long, Long Trail a Winding" reaches our ears through the darkness, sounding the spirit of the troops, their soul released to the night.

We were driving an auto, intuitively, for lights on this march would bring quick death from overhead. We could hear the droning but intermittent throbbing of a Boche plane circling in the vicinity. Suddenly, right before us loomed men—coming like apparitions out of the inky night and we were forced to hit the ditch to avoid running them down. A tire blew with a sharp crack, attracting passing troops to our aid. Quickly we were hoisted back upon the road and then the soldiers, cannon and horses go on into the night, moving, always moving toward the front. We limp along being then on the rim, seeking a place for repair.

LOVE IN WAR ZONE.

Then we spotted a tiny glow, which seemed to beckon us to adventure as irresistibly as a great lighthouse beckons ships to safety. It was the glow of a cigaret. We knew that the man with nerve enough to defy the military police would have nerve enough to get us help. He did, and shortly we were being questioned by a captain in an old barn while his men were putting on a new tire for us.

The gleam of a candle revealed that the captain's face was not so much the face of a man seamed with the cares of war, but rather that of a man uncomfortable with an affair of the heart. Almost in the core of the maddened, battle torn maelstrom was romance. He wrote a short note to a girl at base hospital 46, which was at Neufchateau, and asked us if we would not deliver it as we went by there.

TRAGEDY.

We delivered it the very next day. She was a beautiful girl, too, and we could see, brief as was the message, that it meant vastly more to her than just news. Again we had encountered love where you would least expect to find it.

And then, seemingly as a terrible indication that war is death to everything that is good and fine, came news that the girl had contracted the flu and died. Later we learned that while the disease was claiming her, her captain "went west" in the St. Mihiel scrap. That's war.

This little tale will probably be more interesting to Portland folk when we tell them that the woman in charge of the nurses at base hospital 46 and who directed us to the captain's girl was Miss Phelps, who is now head of the Doernbecher hospital in the Rose City.

There isn't a man or woman who was with base 46 who doesn't know the girl of whom we speak, but few know the part we played in delivering the message from the captain. He had been with some sanitary train and had stopped a few hours at base 46. There he had met the girl.

Now we are in France and it's our hope, though we make no promises, to drift into Neufchateau and down to Bazoilles (Americans call it Bazuillie) the site of base 46, just four or five kilometers from the original first army headquarters. The incident above, left an impression and we're going back just to see whether it was a dream.

Above: Burial of Nurse Norene Royer at U.S. Military Cemetery No. 6 at Bazoilles Hospital Center on September 18, 1918. Her coffin is decorated with flowers. Tents of Base Hospital No. 46 can be seen in the background (*On Active Service with Base Hospital 46 U.S.A.* Portland, OR: Arcady Press; n.d.: 9). *Left:* More tragedy was added to the story of Nurse Norene Royer's death when a newspaper item from 1927 suggested that there had been a romantic fling between her and a U.S. Army captain. This otherwise unknown captain served with a sanitary train and was killed during the Battle of St. Mihiel (September 12-14, 1918), while Nurse Norene Royer was vainly fighting pneumonia (courtesy Oregon Health & Science University, Portland, Oregon [Historical Collections & Archives, Grace Phelps Papers, Accession No. 20100-05, box 2 folder 4]).

Private James V. Lewis, Base Hospital No. 81, to Mrs. Clara E. Lewis, Stockton, California

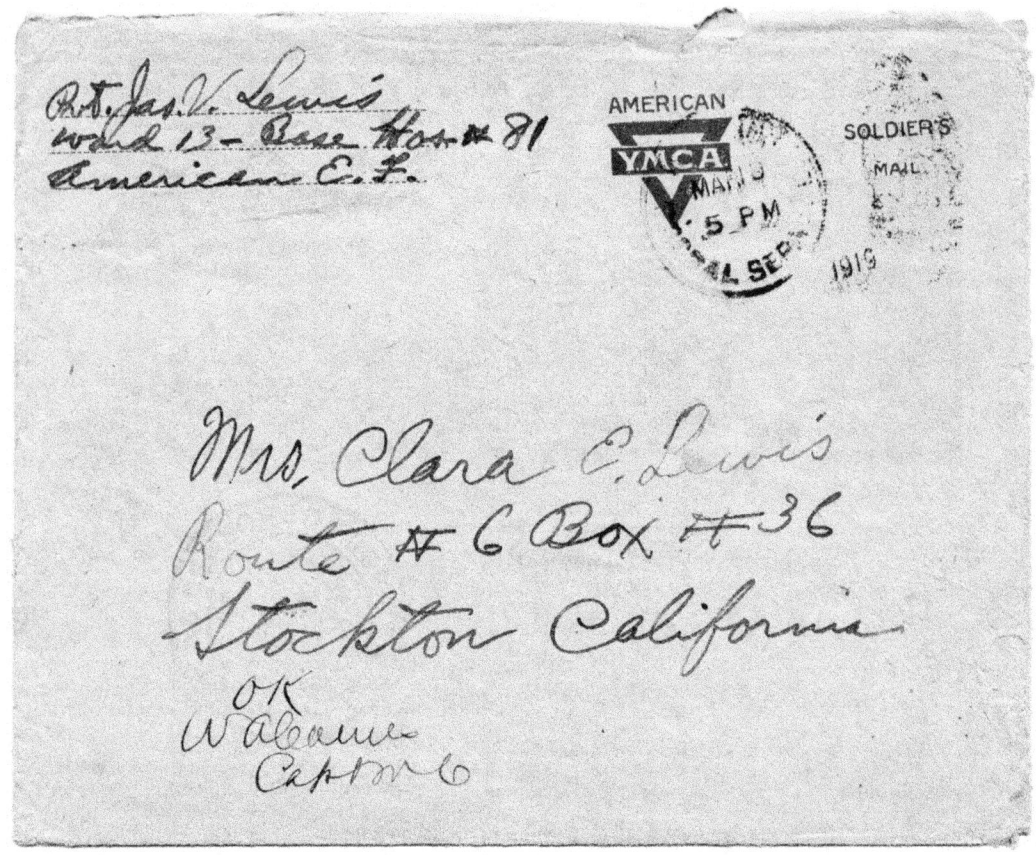

Envelope for the letter sent from Base Hospital No. 81 by Private James V. Lewis to his mother in Stockton, California, on March 18, 1919 (author's collection).

> Base Hospital # 81
> ward # 13 —
> Mar–18 1919

Dear Mother —

I'm in the hospital yet. I feel much better than I did when I landed here. I guess it is because I've had a chance to rest up a bit. The doctor has decided to operate on me here. You may write to me here at the address I gave you in my other letter. The operation will not be very serious but I will be here for several days. Probably a month or more.

I guess the company is at Le Mans now. They were supposed to leave for there last Saturday. I wrote to them Sunday to send my mail to me here.

I have just finished my dinner. It is real class to have my meals served to me at my bed. But I guess it won't seem so classy when I have to stay in bed for a couple of weeks. That is the only thing I dread about being operated on. Two of the patients were operated on yesterday for the apendicitus [appendicitis]. Their beds are right next to mine and it was rather amusing to hear them talk as they came out of the anesthetic. The doctor told me yesterday that I would not have to take an anesthetic if I didn't want it. So I decided I would do without it.

I guess I've been transfered out of my outfit all right. They will probably be on their way to the states before I get out of here. So I'll be a casual when I start home if I'm not put into some other outfit.

I'll close for this time. Love to all, your affectionate son

> Pvt. James V. Lewis
> ward # 13   Base Hospital # 81
> American Ex F.

(ps. send my mail to this address.)
(ps. p.s.) Everything is lovely and theres no need for you to worry. Don't do it!— Jim[11]

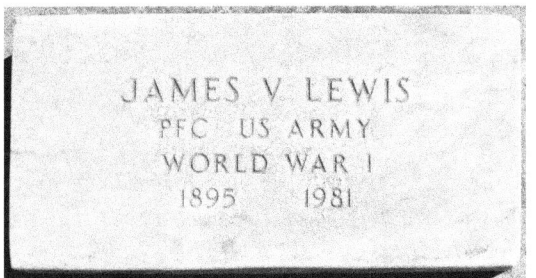

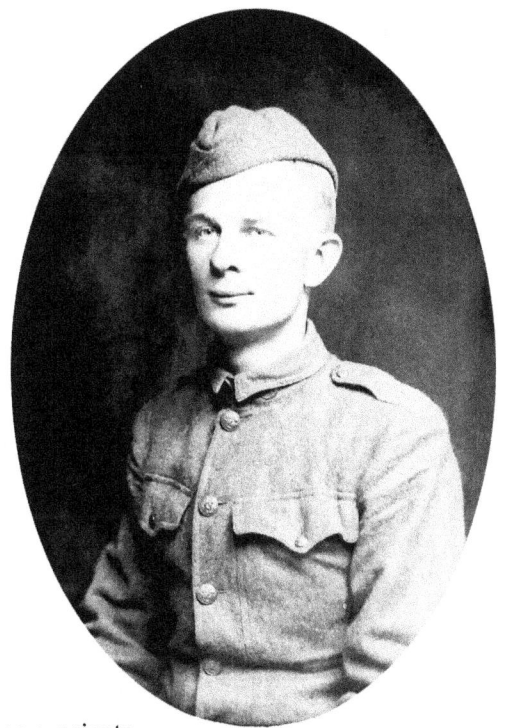

Above: Headstone of the grave of James V. Lewis at Oakdale Citizens Cemetery in Oakdale, California. The headstone honors him as a veteran of World War I in which he served as a private first class (Find a Grave. James Varus Lewis. https://www.findagrave.com/memorial/54809418; accessed November 8, 2017 (courtesy Wes Keat). *Right:* A studio photograph of Private First Class James V. Lewis. The handwritten caption reads: "1st cl.p James V. Lewis 22d Engineers-co. a-A. E. F. [American Expeditionary Forces] France" (Ancestry. California, World War I Soldier Photographs, 1917–1918 for James V Lewis. https://www.ancestry.com; accessed April 26, 2017).

Author's note: James Varus Lewis served as a private with Squad No. 19, Company A, 22nd Engineers,[12] which was a light railway construction regiment made up of army troops. In France, the regiment served with the First Army from September to November 1918.[13] After his operation, James Lewis returned to the United States, as a private first class, with Detachment No. 283 on board the USS (United States Ship) *Great Northern* among a contingent of "walking cases requiring no dressing class "B."" He sailed from Brest, France on May 23, 1919, and arrived in Hoboken on May 30.[14] He was discharged from service on August 9, 1919.[15] After the war, he returned to his work at the Southern Pacific Railroad.[16] He died, aged 86, on May 23, 1981.[17] The headstone of his grave at Oakdale Citizens Cemetery in Oakdale, California, honors him as a veteran of World War I.[18]

Seven

The Ministering Angels of Base Hospital No. 60
The Spanish Flu Outbreak on Board the USS Leviathan

On their way to Bazoilles-sur-Meuse, the nurses of Base Hospital No. 60 travelled overseas on the USS Leviathan *during its ninth overseas trip as a troop transport carrier. Their trip turned for the worst because of the Spanish flu outbreak on board with over 2,000 cases and 99 deaths. As the nurse corps of the* Leviathan *numbered only nine navy nurses, the 191 nurses of Base Hospitals Nos. 60 and 62 were also assigned to take care of patients in various sick quarters on the ship. They worked day and night and were described as "ministering angels." About 30 nurses fell ill themselves and two died the day after arrival in France at Kerhuon Hospital Center. Nurse Eileen L. Forrest of Base Hospital No. 60 is still honored today at the Forrest-Gunderson-Klevgard American Legion Post 264 in her hometown Gilmanton, Wisconsin.*

The USS Leviathan

Considered the "queen of the troop transport fleet," the USS *Leviathan* carried to Europe, during a period of almost 11 months, over 100,000 troops, approximately one-twentieth of the entire American Expeditionary Forces.[1] The *Leviathan* was originally built at Cuxhaven, Germany, as the *Vaterland* for the Hamburg-American Line. It was launched in the early part of 1914 and was Germany's largest passenger ship. When World War I broke out, the *Vaterland* was at her pier in Hoboken, New Jersey, ready to sail on August 1, 1914. However, all German ships in Hoboken were ordered by the German Admiralty not to sail for fear of the British Navy. The *Vaterland* stayed in port at Hoboken until it was seized—together with 90 other German ships in different American ports—by armed forces on April 5, 1917, the day before the U.S. Congress declared war on Germany.[2] In the months thereafter, the ship was converted from a luxurious passenger ship to a troop transport ship with a crew of 68 officers and 2,240 men. On September 6, the name of the *Vaterland* was changed by order of the Secretary of the Navy to the USS *Leviathan*, meaning "monster of the deep." When the ship was reported ready for sea, a trial trip to Cuba was made, leaving port on November 17, 1917.[3] On December 15, the *Leviathan* left harbor for the first of 19 transatlantic trips as a troop transport carrier.[4]

Seven. The Ministering Angels of Base Hospital No. 60

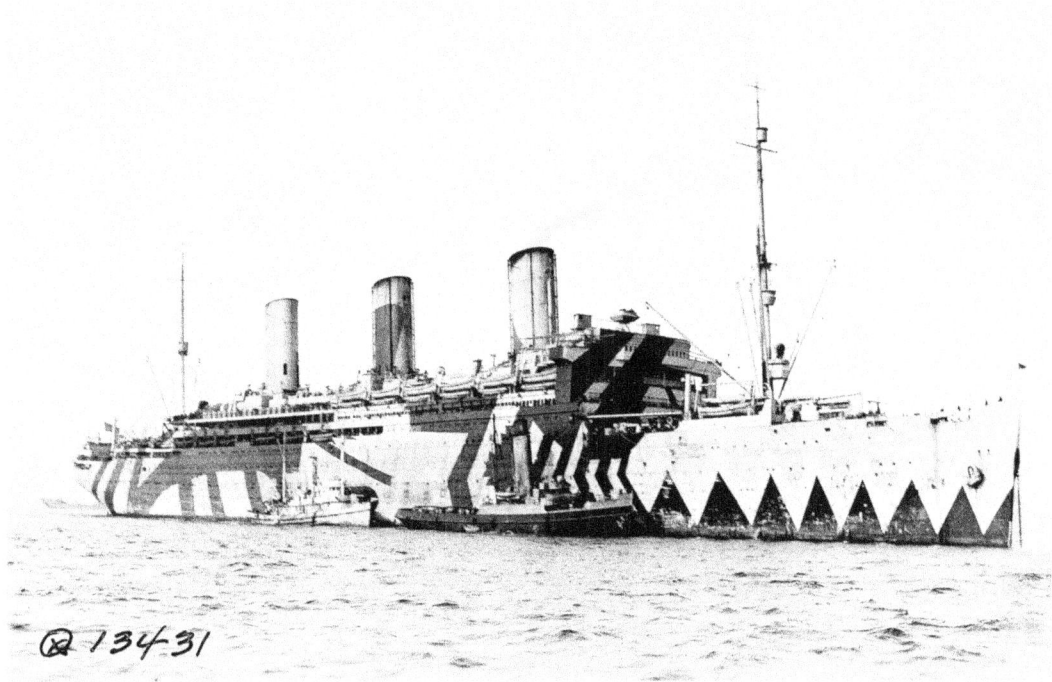

The troop transport carrier USS *Leviathan* at Brest, France, on May 2, 1918, painted in so-called dazzle camouflage (National Archives at College Park, Maryland [Record Group 111: Records of the Office of the Chief Signal Officer, 1860–1985, Photographs of American Military Activities, ca. 1918–ca. 1981, National Archives Identifier 530707: photograph no. 111-SC-13431]).

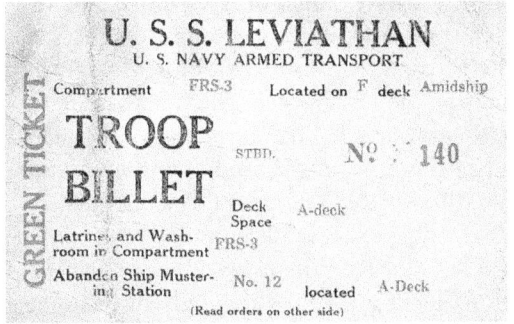

The front and back of a troop billet ticket for the USS *Leviathan*. After checking an individual's name upon the passenger lists, the person was supplied with this ticket showing among others his or her compartment, deck space, bunk number and abandon ship station, etc. (courtesy Naval History & Heritage Command, Washington, D.C. [catalog numbers NH 104240-KN and NH 104240-A-KN]).

The Ninth Overseas Trip

On September 29, 1918, the *Leviathan* left its pier at Hoboken for the ninth overseas trip. On board were 9,366 troops from several units including the 57th Pioneer Infantry, the 323rd Field Signal Battalion, Medical Replacement Unit No. 73 and 191 nurses of Base Hospitals Nos. 60 and 62.[5] The nurses of Base Hospital No. 60 were on their way to

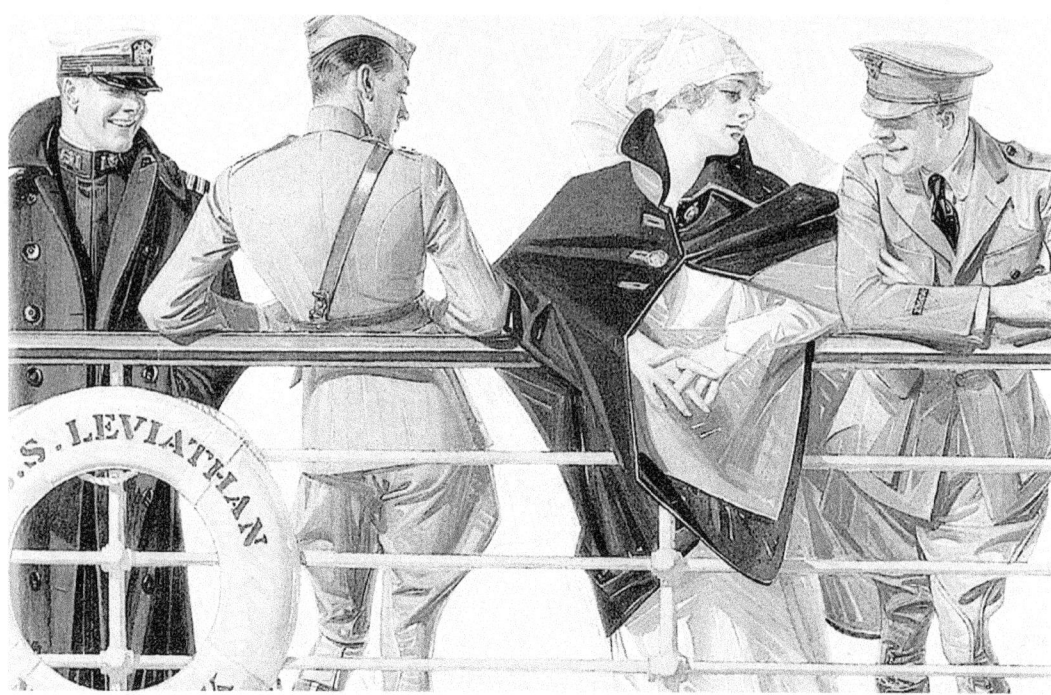

A romanticized illustration of army and navy personnel on board the USS *Leviathan* drawn by the popular artist J.C. Leyendecker for a 1918 advertisement of The House of Kuppenheimer, a men's clothing and retail operation (Daily Art Fixx. J. C. Leyendecker: 1874–1951. http://www.dailyartfixx.com/2016/03/23/j-c-leyendecker-1874-1951/; accessed May 6, 2017).

Bazoilles Hospital Center.[6] Their trip turned for the worst because of the Spanish flu outbreak on board.[7] A main factor responsible for the outbreak was the widespread infection among several units before embarking and their assignment to many different parts of the ship.[8] Already on their march from the camp to the ferry which would take them to the *Leviathan*,[9] a number of men had fallen by the wayside. On the pier, some of the men dropped helpless on the dock. Before casting of the lines of the ship, many men and several nurses were obliged to leave the ship.[10] All available bunks in the sick bay were filled before the morning of September 30.[11] That day, the second day out, the first death, a sailor who did duty in the Hospital Corps, was recorded.[12] It was estimated that 700 Spanish flu cases had developed by the night of September 30. By the night of October 3, additional room for the sick was created on E-deck capable of bunking 878 men. The navy medical officers confined their efforts mostly to those in the sick bay, while the sick quarters below were turned over to army medical officers. Besides, there were many ill men in various troop spaces in other parts of the ship.[13] In total, the number of Spanish flu cases on board exceeded 2,000,[14] while the daily number of deaths steadily increased each day reaching 31 deaths on October 7, the day of arrival.[15]

The Ministering Angels of Base Hospital No. 60

The *Leviathan* provided in its own medical department consisting for the greater part of the time of nine medical officers, pharmacy staff, about 130 navy hospital corpsmen

Seven. The Ministering Angels of Base Hospital No. 60

and nine navy nurses including a chief nurse. The normal bed capacity of the sick bay was 182 with 132 beds in Medical and Surgical Wards, 40 beds in the Isolation Ward and ten beds in the Sick Officers' Quarters.[16] It has been considered "the one bit of luck on the voyage" that almost 200 army nurses were on board during the Spanish flu outbreak on the *Leviathan*.[17] The army nurses of Base Hospitals Nos. 60 and 62 were assigned to take care of the improvised sick quarters below, of pneumonia cases in the Isolation Ward, sick officers in the Sick Officer's Quarters and sick nurses and officers in the ship's staterooms. About 30 nurses had fallen ill themselves and required the constant attention of healthy nurses and an army medical officer.[18] With the Spanish flu causing nasal hemorrhages (nosebleeds) among one fifth of the sick, pools of blood were scattered throughout the troop compartments. Furthermore, seasickness caused vomiting among the sick and the healthy. On October 2, because of fear for the pestilence below, army personnel refused to provide cleaning details for the troop compartments and bring up any man who was found sick or dead. Instead, despite tradition and standing orders, the nurses and navy hospital corpsmen made a valiant effort to clean up. The voyage turned into a nightmare of weariness and anxiety for the nurses, medical officers and hospital corpsmen. No one thought of bed and all hands worked day and night.[19]

Not all of the sick could be cleared from the *Leviathan* on the day of arrival in Brest on October 7. About 200 patients remained on board during the night. These were taken off the ship by army personnel the next day, but not before 14 more deaths had occurred. The nurses remained on board until the last sick man was taken off.[20] When they left the *Leviathan*, the army nurses wept and bade its sailors an affectionate goodbye. The army nurses on board the *Leviathan* have been described as "ministering angels during that dreadful scourge ... [with] unwearying patience and generous self-denial." "They were brave American girls who had left home and comfort in order to undergo peril and sacrifice abroad. Surely they have earned a place in Heaven."[21]

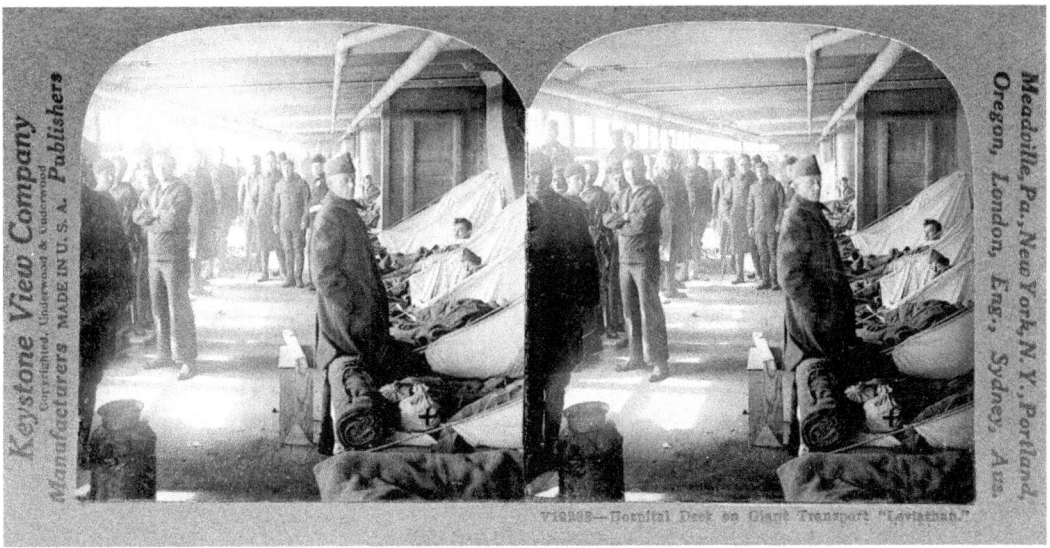

World War I era stereocard view of the sick bay of the USS *Leviathan* (author's collection).

The Ordeal of Nurse Sarah Sand

In April 1917, when the U.S. Congress declared war upon the German Empire, Sarah Sand was Director of Nurses at the Bismarck Evangelical Hospital in Bismarck, North Dakota. Shortly after, she volunteered her services to her country signing up with an Emergency Surgical Unit. As she was never called to report, she subsequently signed up with Base Hospital No. 60. On April 29, 1918, she took the oath of allegiance to the United States as a member of the Army Nurse Corps. After basic training at Camp Jackson, South Carolina, the nurses of Base Hospital No. 60 left for New York and embarked onto the *Leviathan* for its ninth overseas trip.[22]

A few days into the trip, Nurse Sand became ill with Spanish flu during a lifeboat drill. An officer next to her in the lifeboat ordered her back to her stateroom and instructed her to disregard any emergency calls. Her condition worsened as she developed bleedings from nose, ears and throat and purple discoloration of her skin. When a friend, Nurse Margaret L. Brown of Base Hospital No. 60, came in to see her and noted her serious condition, she said in a sad tone: "Have you any message to send back to your people? I fear you are about to die. I will deliver it if I return alive." But Nurse Sand responded that people knew that her trip would be an uncertain journey. Instead, she asked for Major Haig, a sanitary inspector, to come and help her. When Major Haig came, he shook his head and muttered that if he only had adrenalin, he could save her life. Instead, he gave her a hypodermic injection (medication injected under the skin) and ordered her to take some pills. During the night, however, the raging sea tossed everything to the floor including the pills. At some point during this hardship, a seemingly dead soldier with full pack rolled into the stateroom door. He was pushed up along the hall by a guard to prevent blockage of the passageway until a stretcher bearer carried him away.[23] Nurse Sand herself was so near death that a nurse who peeped into her stateroom actually thought she had succumbed.[24] She tried hard not to sleep as her mouth and throat filled with choking blood, but when awake was constantly nauseated from the foul-smelling odors on the ship. To make matters worse, as the *Leviathan* was nearing Brest, all the water was turned off, making Nurse Sand and the other sick suffer terrible thirst. Yet, Nurse Sand, although still ill, was able to leave the boat walking when the ship reached port in Brest.[25]

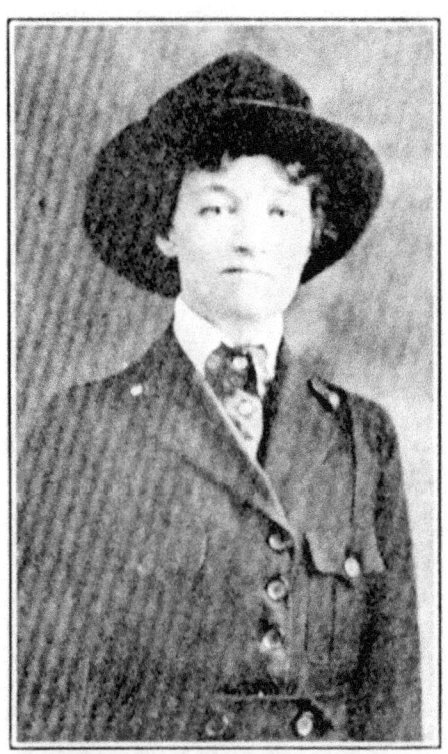

Army Nurse Sarah Sand was Director of Nurses at the Bismarck Evangelical Hospital in Bismarck, North Dakota, before signing up with Base Hospital No. 60 in 1918. Nurse Sand was among those who became severely ill with Spanish flu during the ninth overseas trip of the USS *Leviathan* (North Dakota Nurses Association. Sarah Sand Stevenson [Sixth President]. http://www.ndna.org/Main-Menu/About/NDNA-History-Library/Stevenson.pdf; accessed May 6, 2017).

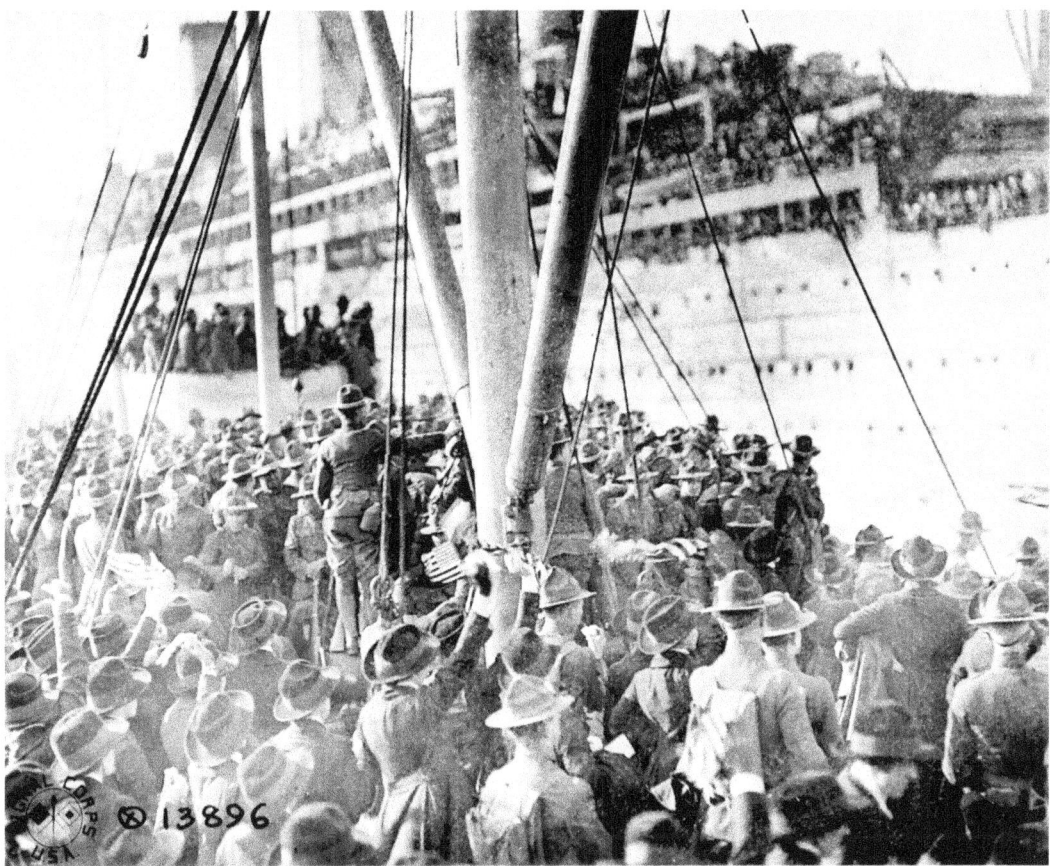

Soldiers and nurses leaving the USS *Leviathan* at Brest, France, in 1918 (National Archives at College Park, Maryland [Record Group 111: Records of the Office of the Chief Signal Officer, 1860–1985, Photographs of American Military Activities, ca. 1918–ca. 1981, National Archives Identifier 530707: photograph no. 111-SC-13896]).

Tragedy After Disembarking

Upon arrival in Brest on October 7, the *Leviathan* carried 99 deaths, 96 soldiers and three sailors. As the *Leviathan* transported 9,366 troops, the mortality rate among soldiers exceeded 1 percent. As over two thousand cases of influenza and pneumonia were counted, the onboard case-fatality rate approximated 5 percent. Yet, it is assumed that probably hundreds of men that had disembarked the *Leviathan* died in the next few days. Of the 57th Pioneer Infantry alone, 123 men died at Kerhuon Hospital Center, 40 at Base Hospital No. 23 and several at Naval Hospital No. 5 and the hospital at Landernau. Almost 200 Spanish flu victims of the 57th Pioneer Infantry were buried in the American cemetery at Lambézellec. It seems likely that the other units which had disembarked the *Leviathan* fared no better.[26]

Twenty sick nurses went ashore from the *Leviathan* of which seven were on stretchers and the others escorted by army men. On the lower decks, they had to step around stretchers and climb over the sick and dying, who were obstructing the gangways. The nurses were taken to barracks at "Camp Kerihou" (Base Hospital No. 65 at Kerhuon

> **DIED OF DISEASE**
> Corp. Arthur E. Wallin, Grantsburg.
> Nurse Eileen L. Forrest, Gilmanton.
> Pvt. Earl E. Faaberg, Bruce.
> Pvt. Oscar Hansen, Lake Mills
> Pvt. Otto E. Knutson, Colfax.
> Pvt. Julius Dove, Galesville.
> Pvt. Herbert S. Higby, Sheboygan.
> Pvt. James Ruzicka, Germantown.

A clipping from the "Day's Casualty List" published in *The Capital Times* on December 5, 1918, lists Nurse Eileen L. Forrest from Base Hospital No. 60 among those from Wisconsin who died of disease. She died of Spanish flu one day after disembarking the USS *Leviathan* at Brest, France (Day's Casualty List. *The Capital Times*. December 5, 1918: 5).

Hospital Center),[27] a few miles outside of Brest. While nurse Sarah Sand was still shivering violently with chills, she witnessed Nurse Eileen Louisa Forrest of Base Hospital No. 60 trying to get out of bed and screaming in her delirium that she would take care of the wounded. A sick nurse from another unit (presumably Nurse Nellie G. Galliher of Base Hospital No. 62)[28] chewed her tongue until the blood oozed from her mouth. In the morning of October 8, both were quietly carried out of the barracks and died shortly afterwards.[29] Nurse Forrest succumbed from Spanish flu at age 27 and was buried at the American cemetery at Lambézellec. Her par-

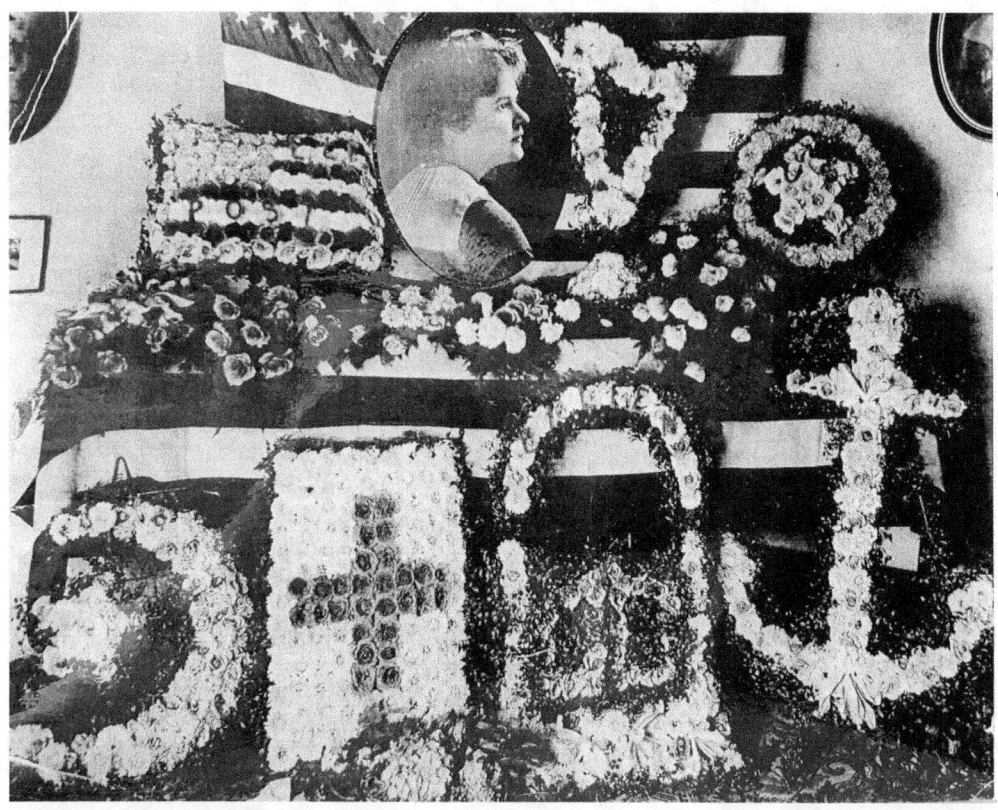

The flag-draped coffin of Nurse Eileen L. Forrest with flower arrangements and memorial sprays at the memorial service in her hometown Gilmanton, Wisconsin (courtesy Forrest-Gunderson-Klevgard American Legion Post 264, Gilmanton, Wisconsin).

ents were notified in mid–November that their daughter had passed away. No letter to Eileen's mother was sadder than the one written from France by First Lieutenant Albert T. DeBaun, Jr of the 306th Engineers, 81st Division: "I realize that nothing I can say can make the burden any easier for you and your family. Your burden I don't believe is heavier than mine, because if Eileen had lived we would have been married next month when I would have had my seven days leave, instead I will spend my leave visiting where she is buried and making arrangements to have her body returned to you." On August 3, 1920, 22 months after her death, Nurse Forrest was laid to rest in the cemetery of her hometown Gilmanton, Wisconsin. Speaking on the occasion, the Reverend Pinkney of Gilmanton urged the citizens of the village "to keep green the memory of her unselfish spirit and patriotic service." A few days earlier, on August 1, the application for an American Legion Post at Gilmanton had been granted, which was named the Eileen L. Forrest American Legion Post 264.[30] In 1922, on the occasion of Armistice Day, 161 names were made public of "gold star women." Eileen Forrest is named on this list of service women of the American Expeditionary Forces who gave their lives in the world war.[31] Notably, the last entry in her journal had been:

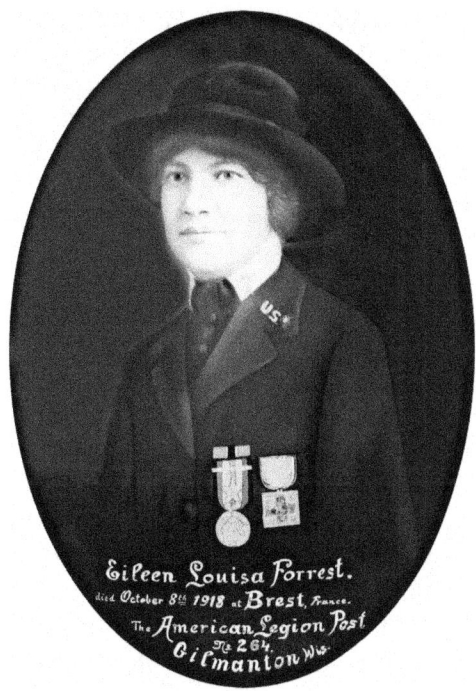

Oil painting of Nurse Eileen L. Forrest which hangs in the Forrest-Gunderson-Klevgard American Legion Post 264 in Gilmanton, Wisconsin. The painting is one of ten images of service men and women of the Gilmanton area that died in World War I (4), World War II (5) and the Korean War (1) (courtesy Forrest-Gunderson-Klevgard American Legion Post 264, Gilmanton, Wisconsin).

> You ask of me poetic skill
> The task seems hard for me to fill.
> And now a task I ask of thee
> "T'is simply this—remember me."[32]

Aftermath

Nurse Sarah Sand, together with other ill nurses, remained hospitalized at Kerhuon Hospital Center for several days. On October 9, it was ordered that 94 nurses and one dietitian of Base Hospital No. 60 would proceed to Bazoilles-sur-Meuse, as soon as transportation could be arranged. Before leaving, the nurses were to be equipped with gas masks and helmets and instructed in their use. On one of the following days, Chief Nurse Jessie P. Allan notified the sick nurses that those who wanted to go to the front should get ready for gas mask drill. All but four arose and started to dress. Some of the nurses were, however, still too sick to go in the gas chamber. The lieutenant in charge of the drill demanded to know who had sent pneumonia patients out but his question remained unanswered. The nurses left Kerhuon Hospital Center the next day. For five days and four nights, the nurses travelled across France by train. Bazoilles-sur-Meuse was reached on a dark and rainy night. The next day, the nurses entered upon their duties. Nurse Sand was placed in charge of Ward No. 13, a surgical ward. Her notebook mentioned that on October 18, less than two weeks after near death from influenza, Nurse Sand, together with Nurse Julia A. Walton, dressed the wounds of 60 men.[33]

The *Leviathan* remained for three days in Brest and left for its westward return trip in the evening of October 9. It carried the bodies of 40 deaths of which 33 were brought back to the United States. The morning after its departure, following a prayer at sunrise by the chaplain, the flag was half-masted, taps were sounded, the volleys were fired and seven bodies were given a burial at sea. The *Leviathan* returned in New York in the morning of October 16.[34] Around that time, by mid–October 1918, it was recommended that only troops from U.S. Army camps which had passed through the influenza epidemic were selected for shipment overseas. Soldiers from such camps who had actually had Spanish flu could be transported with safety while those who had not suffered from the disease were assumed to have been exposed to it and might be considered immune.[35] Indeed, recent analysis of repeated illness data among seasoned troops in five U.S. Army training camps, indicated that the first wave of Spanish flu provided 49–94 percent protection against clinical illness during the second wave and 56–89 percent protection against death.[36] In December 1918, the official newspaper of the American Expeditionary Forces, *The Stars and Stripes*, stated that 1,180 American soldiers had died at sea in September and October and 2,336 within five days after landing in France. These numbers omit the hundreds who died in Halifax, Canada, the last possible stopping place in North America to put men ashore, and the unknown number who died within five days after landing in Britain. Therefore, it has been stated that probably no less than 4,000 American soldiers died in transit from the United States to Europe in the last two months of World War I. Yet, also in February 1919, American soldiers would die on board of the *Leviathan*, presumably as a result of the third wave of Spanish flu, but this time on their way back to the United States.[37]

War Is Over

On November 11, 1918, Armistice Day, hostilities came to an end. The news of the Armistice was received with relief and joy throughout the world. At Bazoilles Hospital Center, enlisted men started parading arm in arm, singing and pounding on tin pans. Nurse Sarah Sand recollected of the festivities at Bazoilles Hospital Center in her war memoirs, while First Lieutenant Howard Osgood from Base Hospital No. 116 described the expressions of joy in his diary. Their writings are printed below in their entirety.

In the book *Lamp for a Soldier: The Caring Story of a Nurse in World War I*, Nurse Sarah Sand of Base Hospital No. 60 described her initial disbelief and subsequent joy when hostilities finally ended on November 11, 1918.

> In the afternoon one of the older officers came to our ward and said. "Well nurse, they have signed the Armistice!" I fairly shouted, "What do you mean?" "Why, the war is over! Come in to Neufchateau and take dinner with me and we will celebrate this occasion!" I said, "No, captain, you can

ARMISTICE SIGNED, END OF THE WAR! BERLIN SEIZED BY REVOLUTIONISTS; NEW CHANCELLOR BEGS FOR ORDER; OUSTED KAISER FLEES TO HOLLAND

Front page headlines of the *New York Times* on November 11, 1918, Armistice Day (Armistice Signed. *New York Times*. November 11, 1918: 1).

fool me only once. You said last week it was over and now I simply cannot believe it." But soon I heard the church bells ringing without ceasing and in a few moments our soldiers were marching arm in arm, up and down the road in front of our camp, pounding tin pans and playing and singing all at once, without interruption. We than realized it was true. All guards were called off duty and everyone celebrated. Several of us nurses decided we would go out and look around. We walked up the road in front of our camp where everyone we met insisted we go to town with them and have dinner but this we did not do because it was a most hilarious occasion. Instead we stood in the shadow of a large tree in the moonlight, watching the stream of people come and go, shouting out the deepest secrets of their hearts. One dignified officer came down the road telling aloud how he had eloped with his wife, eluding her parents and marrying her, and now he was wild with joy, not that the war was over, but that he could again go home to his wife! So it seemed each one thought of his or her loved ones at home. We realized that this awful death-dealing, property-destroying war was at last at an end. We finally returned to our barracks to rejoice in our own way and we began at once to plan to go home.[1]

The diary entry for November 11, 1918, of First Lieutenant Howard Osgood from Base Hospital No. 116, who was responsible for wound cultures at the center laboratory of Bazoilles Hospital Center, describes the same high-spirited atmosphere.

Monday Nov 11

Papers this morning (yesterday) confirmed abdication of Kaiser & renunciation of rights by Crown Prince; report is that they have fled to Holland.

At noon. Lt. Col. Walker read telegrams announcing signing of armistice at 5 A.M. today, with cessation of hostilities at 11 A.M.

All the morning & early afternoon an American division—the 82nd—has been marching along the road southward under full equipment footsore but happy, coming from front.

Officers who went to N- [Neufchâteau] said news was received there about noon; town immed. blossomed out in flags; swarmed c [with] poilus [French infantrymen] delerious c joy. [Lieutenant] Youland said poilus saluted U.S. officers c enthusiams.

Just after dark heard fanfare & shouting across valley in village—probably French troops passing through.

Officers & nurses messed together in celebration; Lt. Col. Walker read bulletin giving terms of armistice—simply crushing but the only way of absolutely preventing any possibility of fighting again—to remain in effect for 30 days when peace negotiations will be under way. Enlisted men had parade c tin pans & bugles until dispersed. We do not feel much elation, will take day or so to realise fully.[2]

Eight

A Medical Officer's Photo Album
Pictures of Daily Life

    Major Theodore J. Abbott from New York City was Chief of Medical Service at Base Hospital No. 116.[1] He compiled a photo album containing over 200 pictures illustrating daily life and medical care at Bazoilles Hospital Center.[2] At some point, the album came into possession of a historian from Hudson Valley, New York. After his death, it was bought by an antiquarian bookseller from Garrison, New York.[3] The author bought the album in 2016. Here, photographs from this album are reproduced to show what daily life at Bazoilles Hospital Center looked like.

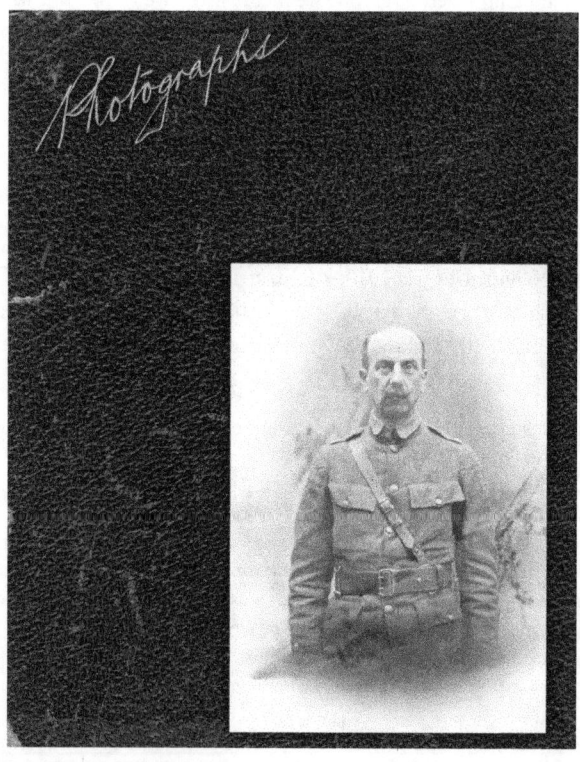

Cover of the photograph album of Major Theodore J. Abbott, who was Chief of Medical Service at Base Hospital No. 116. The inset shows the photograph of Major Abbott that is attached to the first endpaper of the album (author's collection).

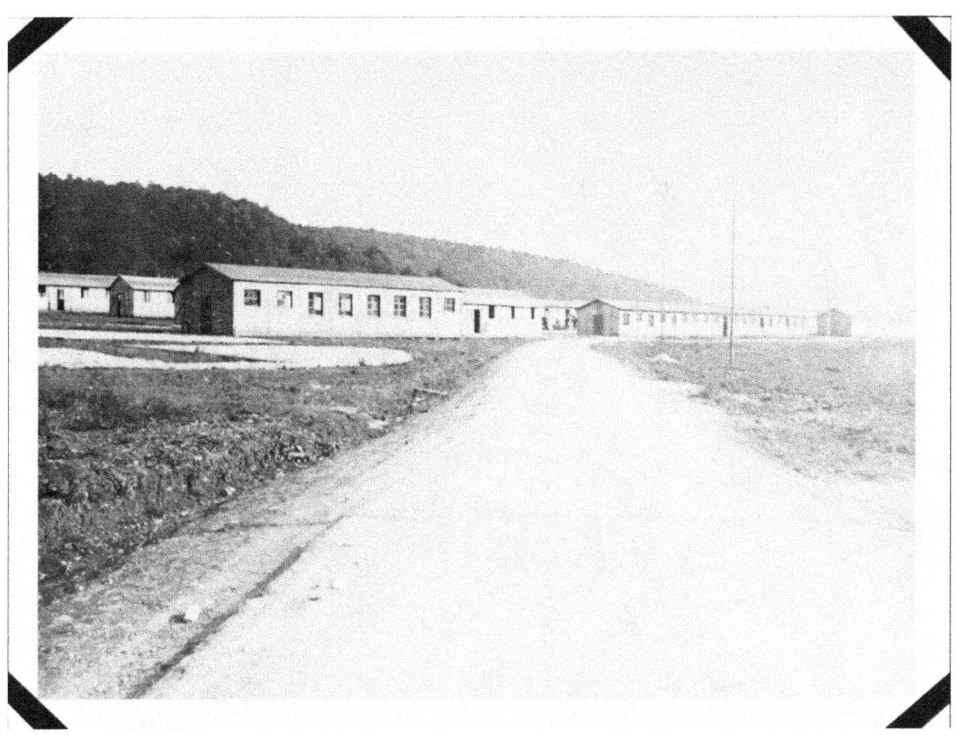

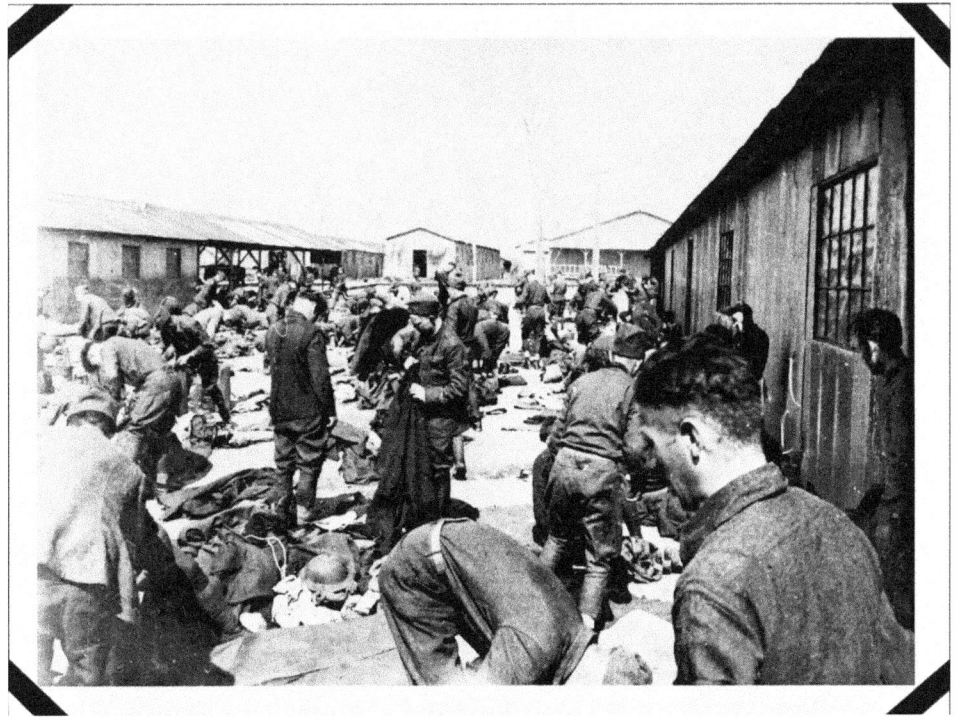

Two photographs from the album of Major Theodore J. Abbott. The caption for the top photograph reads "Entrance to 116." The caption for the bottom photograph reads "June 1918, arrival of first large convoy" (author's collection).

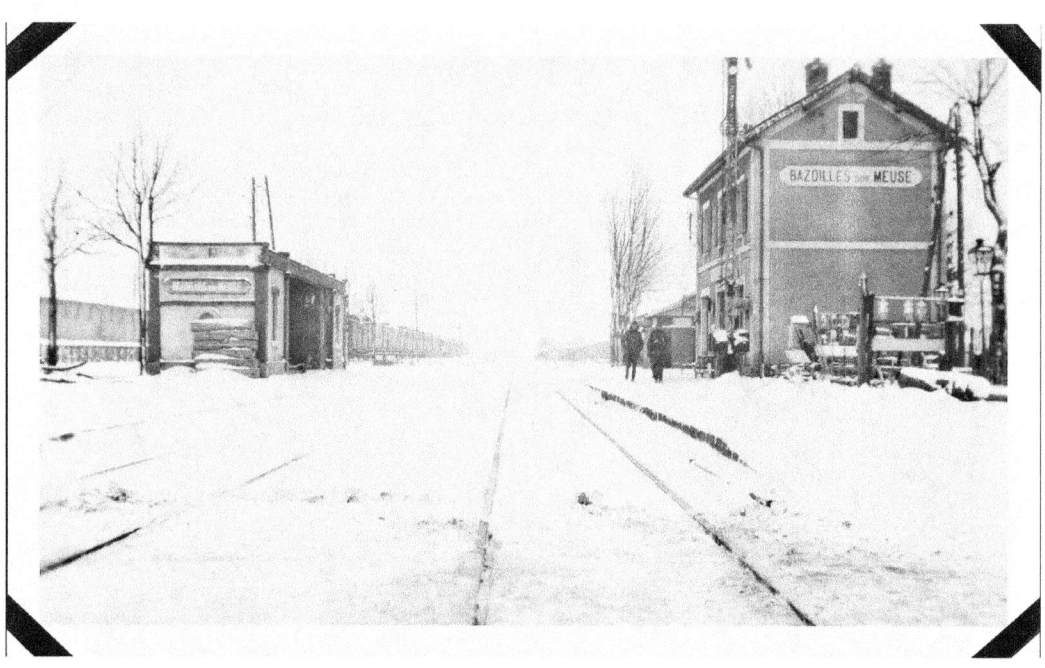

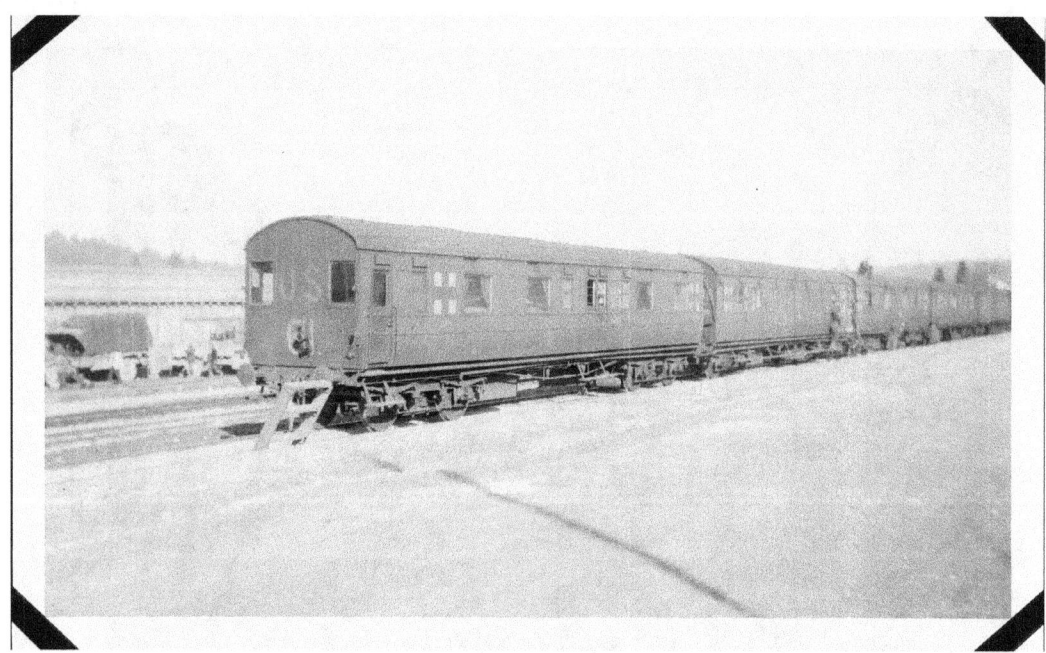

Two photographs from the album of Major Theodore J. Abbott. The caption for the top photograph reads "Railroad Station." The caption for the bottom photograph reads "American hospital train No. 61" (author's collection).

Eight. A Medical Officer's Photo Album

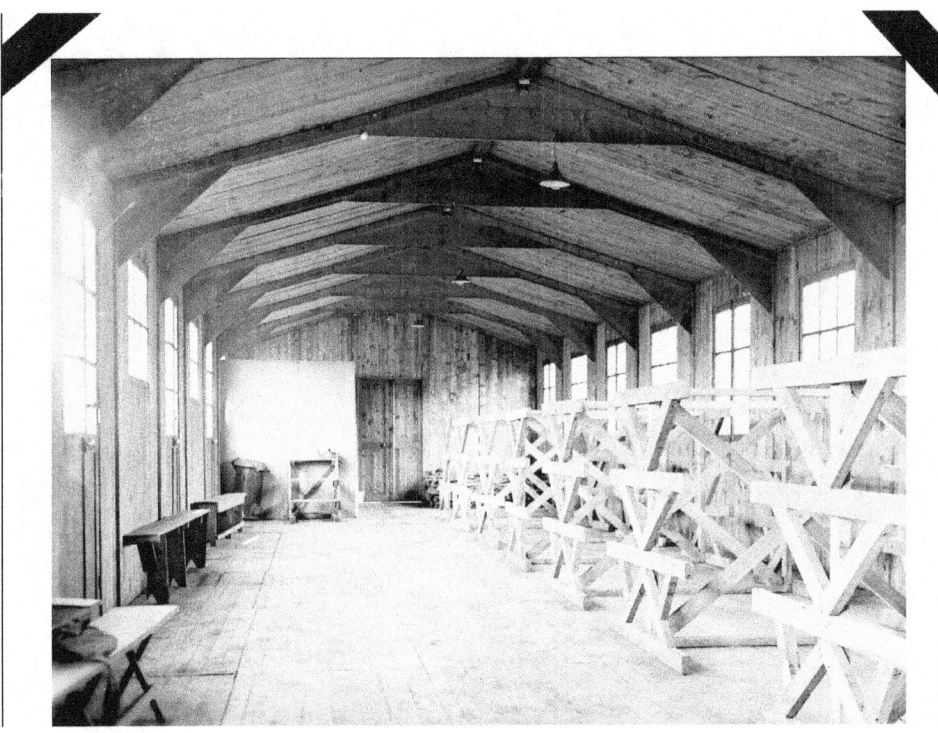

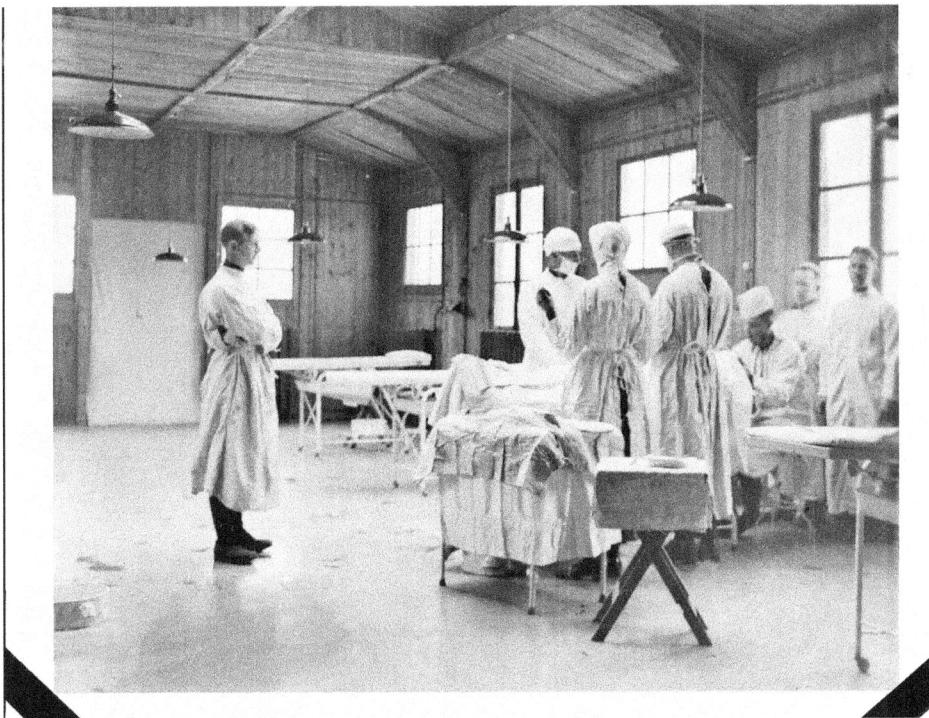

Two photographs from the album of Major Theodore J. Abbott. The caption for the top photograph reads "Receiving Ward." The caption for the bottom photograph reads "Operating Room" (author's collection).

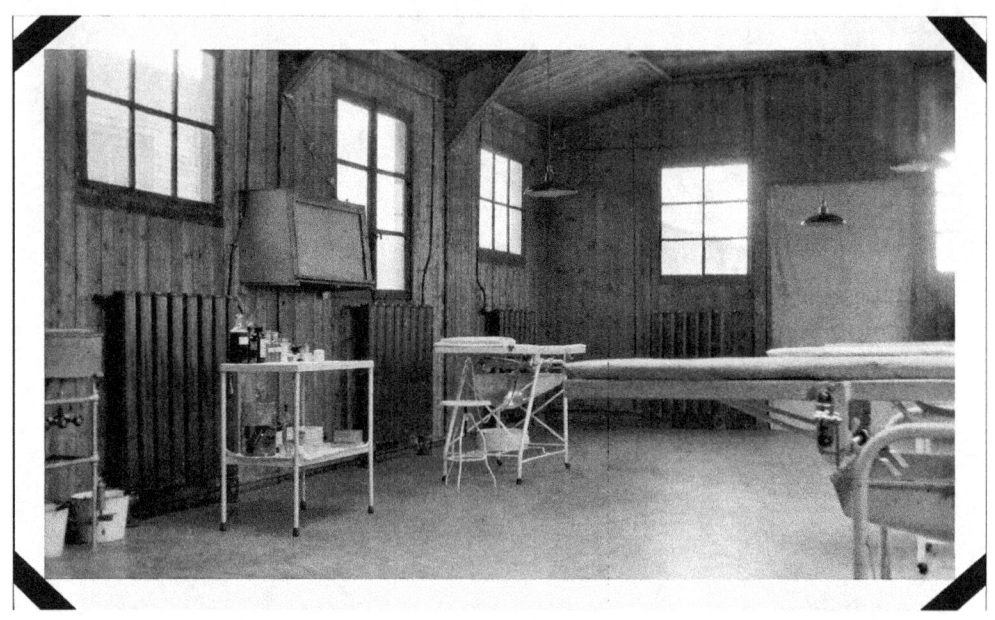

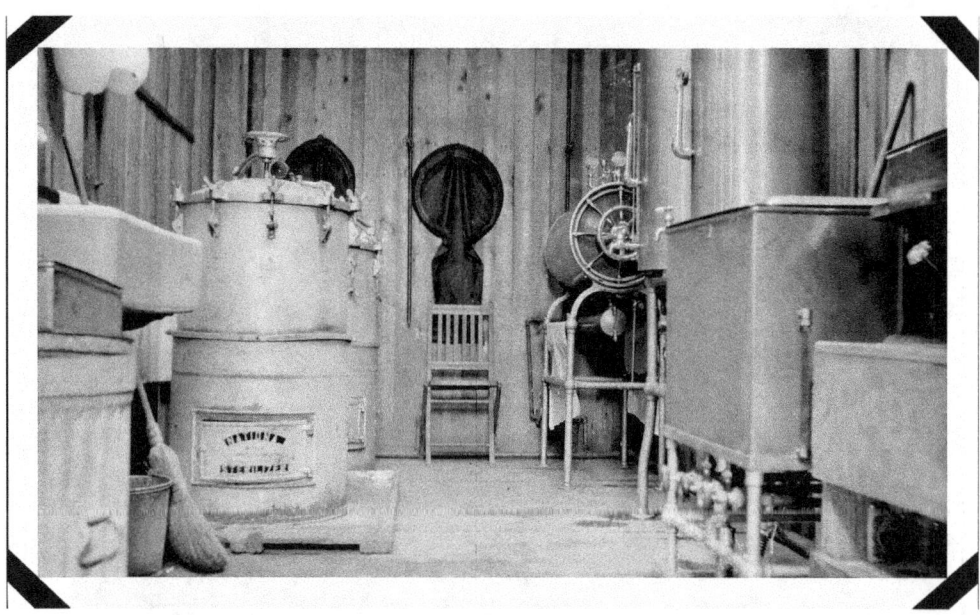

Two photographs from the album of Major Theodore J. Abbott. The caption for the top photograph reads "Operating Room." The caption for the bottom photograph reads "Sterilizing Room" (author's collection).

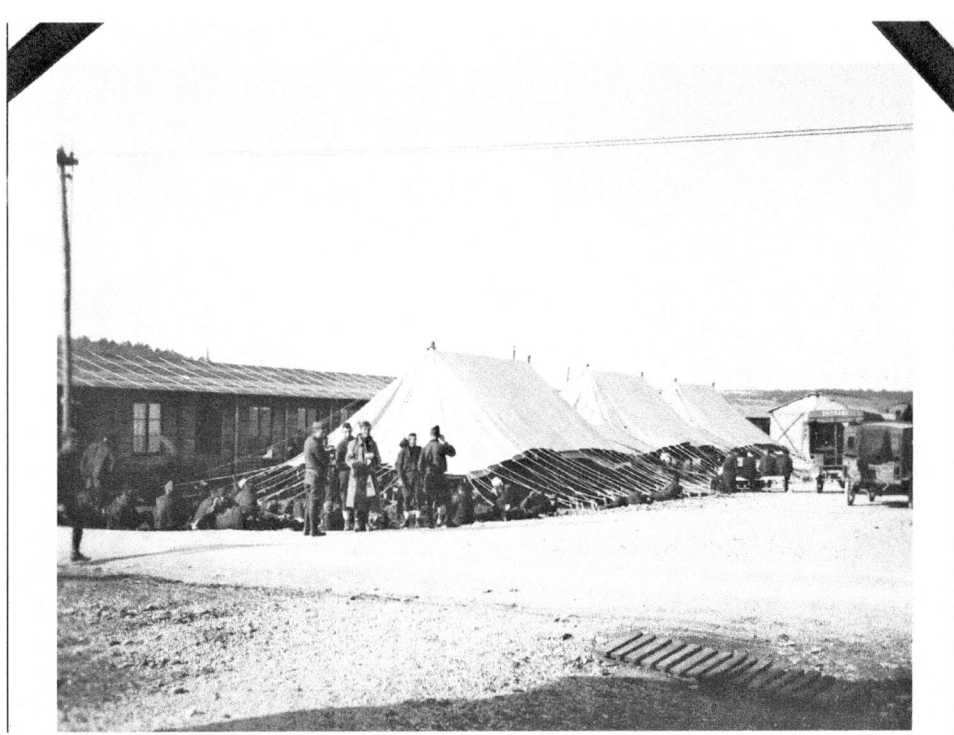

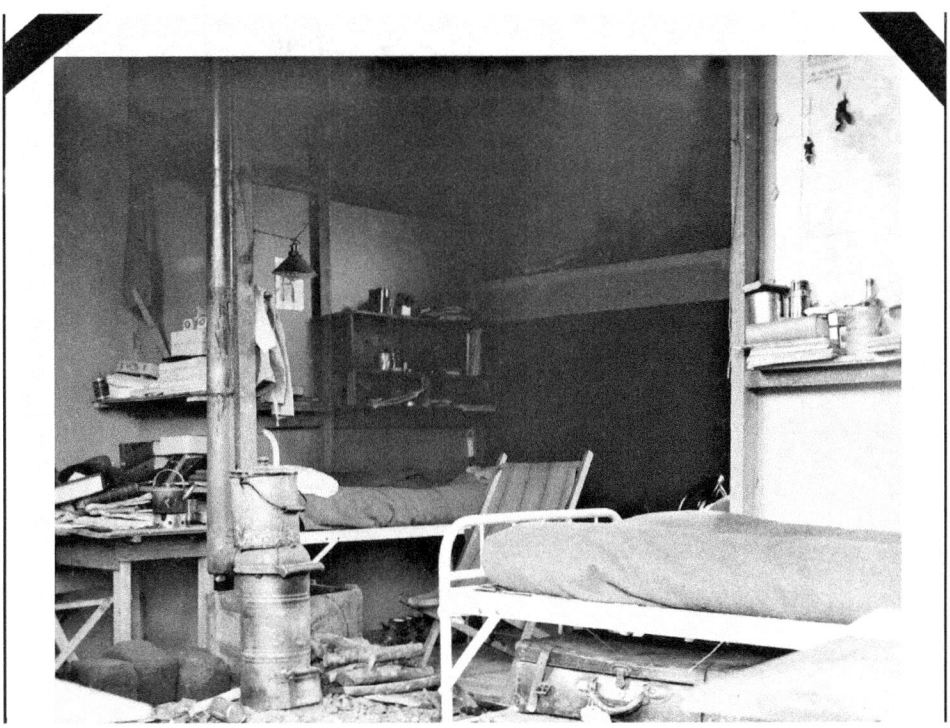

Two photographs from the album of Major Theodore J. Abbott. The caption for the top photograph reads "Convoy from Chateau-Thierry." The caption for the bottom photograph reads "Officers' Room. (Osgood, Lavelle and Youland)" (author's collection).

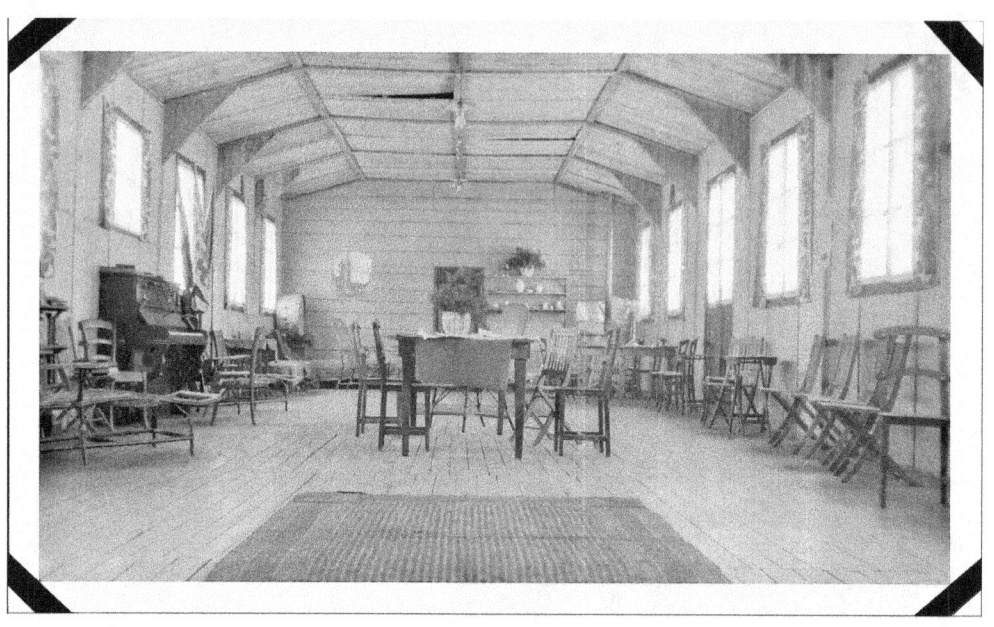

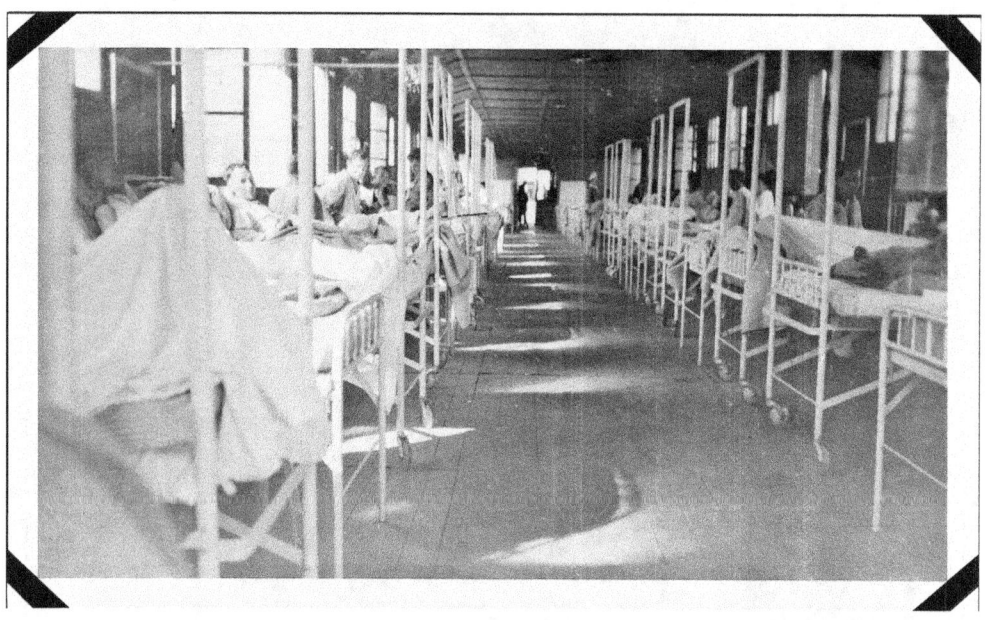

Two photographs from the album of Major Theodore J. Abbott. The caption for the top photograph reads "Nurses' Hut." The caption for the bottom photograph reads "Ward 8" (author's collection).

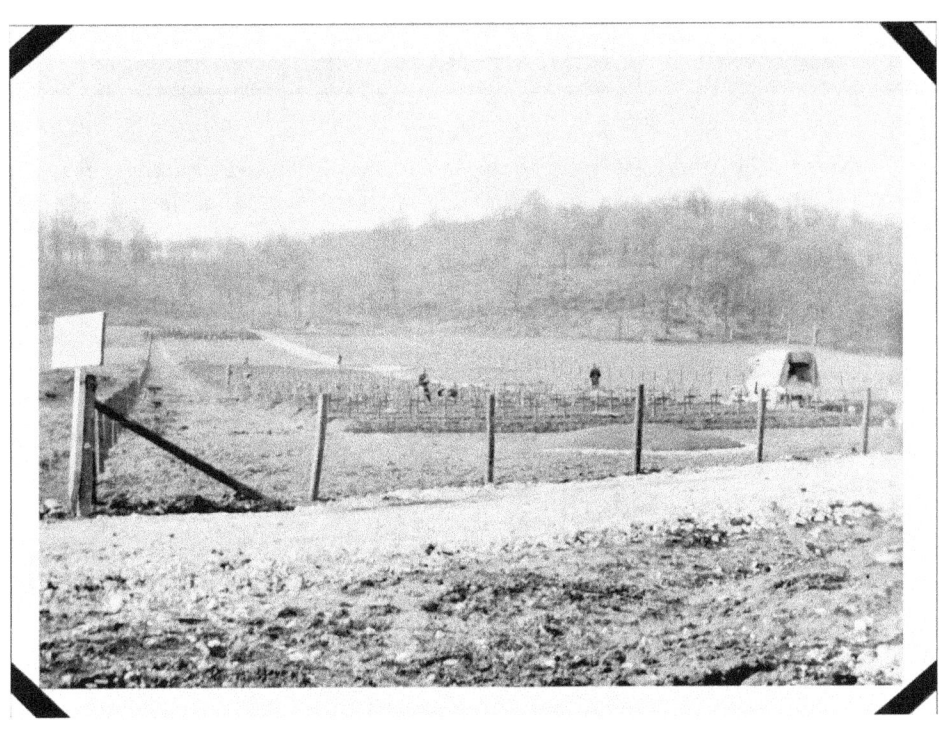

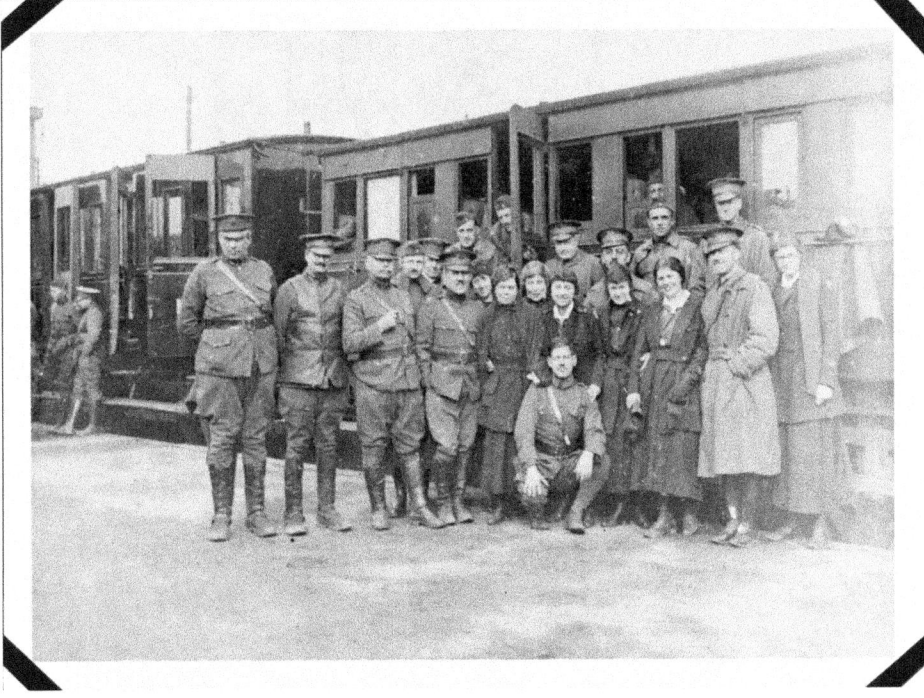

Two photographs from the album of Major Theodore J. Abbott. The caption for the top photograph reads "Bazoilles Cemetery." The caption for the bottom photograph reads "March 1919, en route to coast. Headed home?" (author's collection).

Christmas Overseas

The overseas Christmas celebration brought about many sentiments among the medical personnel of Bazoilles Hospital Center. Longing for home was set aside to bring joy to patients and fellow hospital workers regardless of a rainy Christmas Day. Printed below are the memories of Christmas 1918 of Nurse Sarah Sand and the diary entries of First Lieutenant Howard Osgood for December 25, 1918.

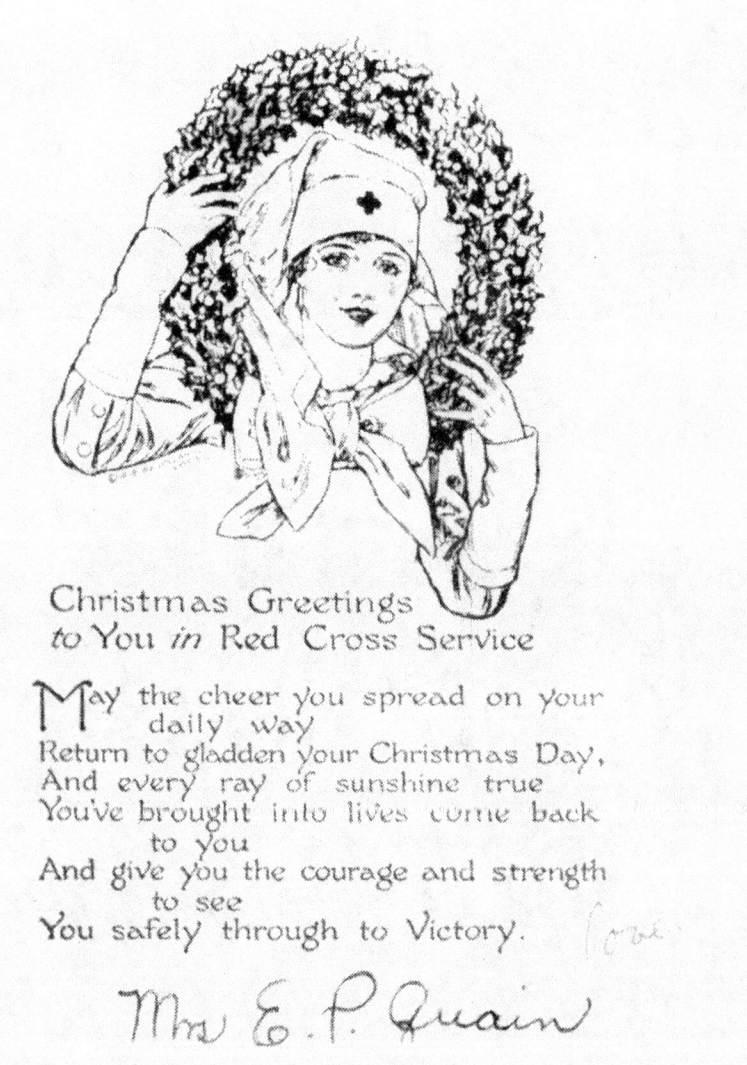

A Christmas greeting presumably presented in 1918 to Nurse Sarah Sand by Mrs. Quain, the wife of Lieutenant Colonel Eric P. Quain, Chief of Surgical Service at Base Hospital No. 60 (Sand, Stevenson S. *Lamp for a Soldier: The Caring Story of a Nurse in World War I*. North Dakota: North Dakota State Nurses' Association, 1976: 54).

Eight. A Medical Officer's Photo Album

In the book *Lamp for a Soldier: The Caring Story of a Nurse in World War I*, Nurse Sarah Sand described the Christmas celebration of 1918 in the pneumonia ward of Base Hospital No. 60.

Never shall I forget our Christmas celebration of 1918 in the pneumonia ward of Base Hospital 60, Bazoilles sur Meuse. We nurses planned it in great detail, even to our own personal adornment. When things quieted down in the night, I went to put on my white uniform and new shoes in preparation for our Christmas morning surprise. Everything seemed favorable until I made close inspection of my issued shoes and lo, they were both for one foot! This may be listed as one of my greatest disappointments as I was forced to wear my old muddy shoes with my nice white uniform and Red Cross cape, ordinarily we wore limp grey issued uniforms.

For days we had busied ourselves every spare moment off duty making baskets of English ivy and decorating the wards with green sprays and wreaths.

When morning came we surprised the boys with individual baskets containing cigarettes, cigars, apples, oranges and homemade candies. We also had a few sprays of flowers and champagne and orangeade for each patient that we felt would never see Christmas on earth again. Oh! The sad, sweet smile of gratitude as we tried to encourage them! The chaplains came early to administer Holy Communion to those desiring it. The chaplains were tireless workers who came whenever called, day or night. They realized the men's spiritual needs as they had themselves seen service at the Front for months and our patients were very fond of them.

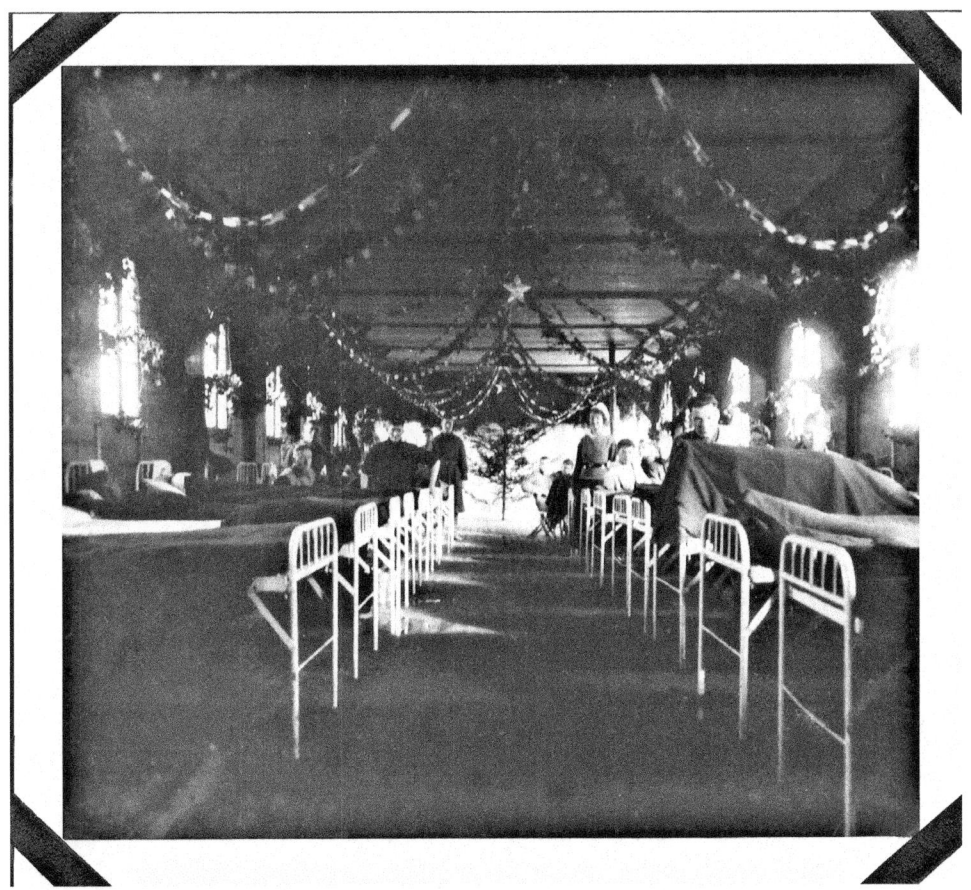

A patient ward of Base Hospital No. 116 at Bazoilles Hospital Center during Christmas 1918 (author's collection).

The Christmas program that we started in the early morning continued. The day nurses helped prepare a good dinner with many extras that the kitchen department knew nothing of and there were rumors afloat that the ward surgeon had ordered a wine glass full of something not required by the War Department. He had paid for it out of his own pocket and had sent it with his Christmas greetings; he suspected the boys would enjoy it and they surely did. Many silly little gifts were exchanged. The Red Cross and the Y.M.C.A. brought in a Christmas tree, nicely decorated, and presented a good Christmas program. This program was repeated in each of the wards as far as I know.

It seemed that the sick men actually were happy in the rain and mud of Bazoilles during this Christmas because they had done their duty for their country and were proud of it in their hearts. The nurses tried to forget their own heartaches and longings for home by trying to make others happy. The majority of them spent about all the money they had during this time buying little Christmas cheers.[1]

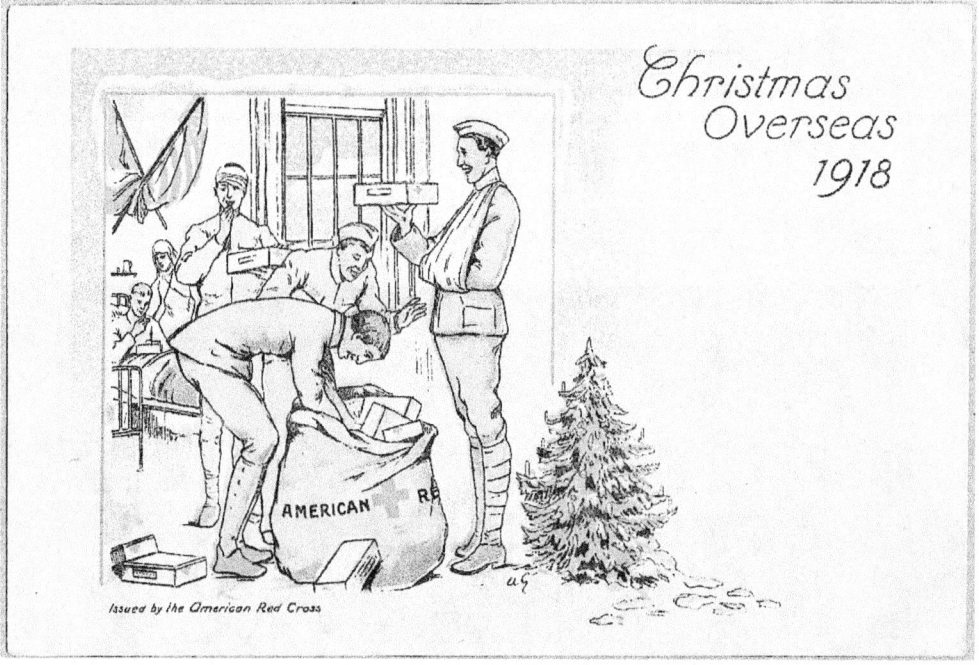

A postcard issued in 1918 by the American Red Cross depicts patients at an overseas U.S. Army hospital receiving boxes with Christmas gifts (author's collection).

In his diary entry for December 25, 1918, First Lieutenant Howard Osgood from Base Hospital No. 116 describes his Christmas Day sentiments and the gifts he received from a fellow officer and from home.

Wednesday Dec 25

Cold & rainy

Wakened by Father Compal [the Reverend Frederick P. Coupal, Chaplain, American Red Cross] & some enlisted men & nurses singing carols between barracks. Made me a bit home sick for a moment.

Capt. Newhall, A.R.C. [American Red Cross] came in & laid a pair of socks on each of our four beds. One contained a pound of nuts, cornucopia of candy & two postals cards showing U.S. troops in Paris on July 4. The other contained a tin of jam, a tin of buillon [bouillon] cubes a tooth brush & several packages of chewing gum & two boxes of cigarettes. Opened photo of [nephew] Emory! Opened box from home—socks from mother, manicure set, bridge set, shaving stick & cream, [the book] "Dere Mabel," & a sprig of holly & a little Santa Claus—a most satisfactory sort of Xmas prize. Loafed all day. Several letters from home. Excellent dinner c [with] nurses—Xmas telegrams & cards from Pershing & B.H. [Base Hospital] 53 read. Show in evening—One act play "Getting the Bird" from Punch—Minstrels c quartette—local songs & jokes. We had a lot of fun & audience seemed to also. Dance afterwards.[2]

Nine

Patients of Bazoilles Hospital Center
Three Soldiers Admitted Because of Physical and Mental Disease

During its period of operation, 37,165 patients were treated for disease at Bazoilles Hospital Center, outnumbering patients treated for injuries by a ratio of 1.4 to one. The center was also selected as the site of the main psychiatric collecting station. Its neuropsychiatric department began to function on July 20, 1918, as part of Base Hospital No. 116. Up to April 30, 1919, 1,654 neuropsychiatric patients were admitted. This chapter describes three soldiers admitted for physical or mental disease whose identification tags were recovered in 2016 at the former site of Bazoilles Hospital Center.

Private Frederick Loeffel, Army Service Number 2705744, Approximate Date of Admission September 30, 1918

Frederick Loeffel was born on November 9, 1892, in Pittsburgh, Pennsylvania, as a son of Swiss immigrants. His father passed away in 1915.[1] At the time of his registration for the World War I draft, on June 5, 1917, he lived in Carrick, Pennsylvania, and worked as a truck driver for the Jones and Laughlin Steel Company in Pittsburg.[2]

On April 27, 1918, Frederick Loeffel was inducted as a private in the U.S. Army.[3] In the evening of May 2, 1918, he left from Pittsburgh to train at Fort Thomas, Newport, Kentucky, in a contingent of 353 selectives.[4] Training was received in the 11th Company, 3rd Training Battalion, 155th Depot Brigade until May 12, 1918, after which he was transferred to Battery D, 315th Field Artillery, 80th Division. His overseas service started on May 26, 1918.[5]

Frederick Loeffel was hospitalized from September 30, 1918, onwards.[6] At that time, the 80th Division was engaged in the first phase of the Meuse-Argonne Offensive.[7] He returned from overseas at the port of Newport News, Virginia, on November 9, 1918, two days before the signing of the Armistice.[8] This indicates he spent about a month in overseas hospitals before being transported back to the United States.

Frederick Loeffel was honorably discharged from the U.S. Army on August 15, 1919, and at that time reported 100 percent disabled because of Service Connected Disability (SCD).[9] He was diagnosed with dementia praecox [a psychiatric condition classified as a psychosis and currently known as schizophrenia][10] and had been under treatment at

Service card of Private Frederick Loeffel who had been assigned to Battery D, 315th Field Artillery, 80th Division and was hospitalized from September 30, 1918, onwards (Ancestry. Pennsylvania, World War I Veterans Service and Compensation Files, 1917–1919, 1934–1948 for Frederick Loeffel. https://www.ancestry.com; accessed October 16, 2016).

U.S. Army General Hospital No. 28 at Fort Sheridan, Illinois, until his army discharge.[11] Cases of dementia praecox were often observed in army psychiatric units during World War I, but it was stated that war did not create this type of psychosis.[12] A list of the hospitals to which mental and nervous soldiers were transferred from the ports of Hoboken and Newport News between April 1918 and June 30, 1919, mentioned that 65 mental cases were admitted to General Hospital No. 28 from Newport News among a total of 7108 mental and nervous cases received from the American Expeditionary Forces.[13] Frederick Loeffel is assumed to have been among these 65 mental cases. It was November 17, 1918, that the first patients from overseas began to arrive at General Hospital No. 28.[14]

On the day of his army discharge, August 15, 1919, Frederick Loeffel was transferred to Dixmont Hospital for the Insane at Kilbuck Township, just outside of Pittsburgh. The transfer was by request of the U.S. Bureau of War Risk Insurance which was charged a rate of ten dollars per week for his stay at Dixmont. On June 7, 1921, he was transferred to Allentown State Hospital in Allentown, Pennsylvania, by request of the U.S. Public Health Service. At that time, his condition was reported as improved.[15] On August 29, 1925, he was transferred to U.S. Veterans' Hospital No. 42 at Perry Point, Maryland, at that time a U.S. Veterans' Bureau institution focusing on neuropsychiatric care. Frederick Loeffel received register number 4287 and remained at Perry Point for the rest of his life. In 1930, he resided in Ward 2.[16] After 42 years of institutionalization, he died, aged 68, on August 18, 1961, from severe pulmonary edema and congestion due to arteriosclerotic

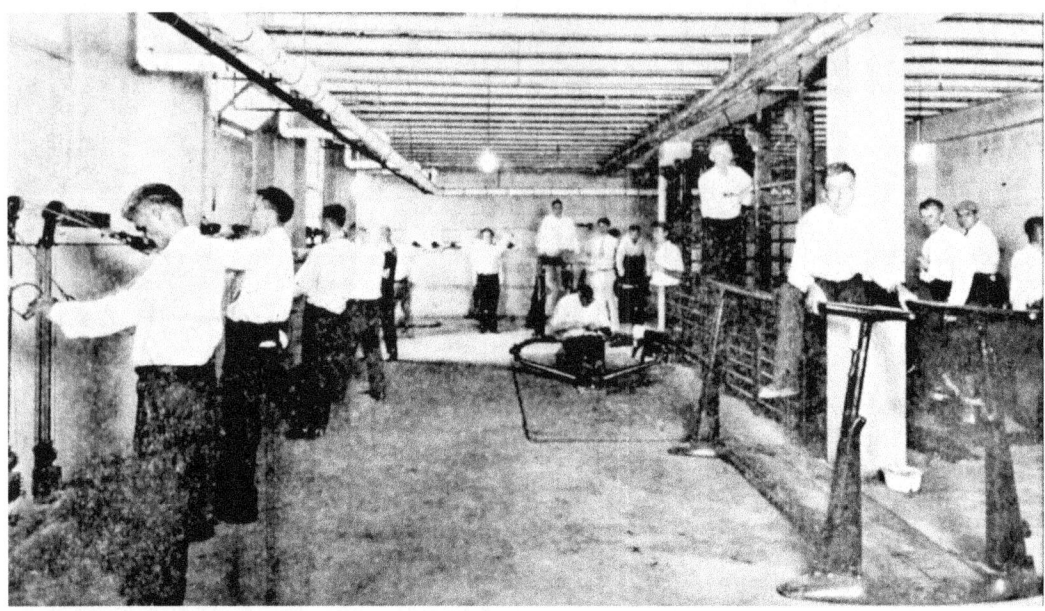

In 1930, Frederick Loeffel resided in Ward 2 of U.S. Veterans' Hospital No. 42 at Perry Point. This image from the August/September 1930 issue of *The Perry Point Bulletin* shows patients of Ward 2 working out in the gymnasium (Stinnett, S. *Pictorial History of Perry Point*. n.p.; n.d.: 281).

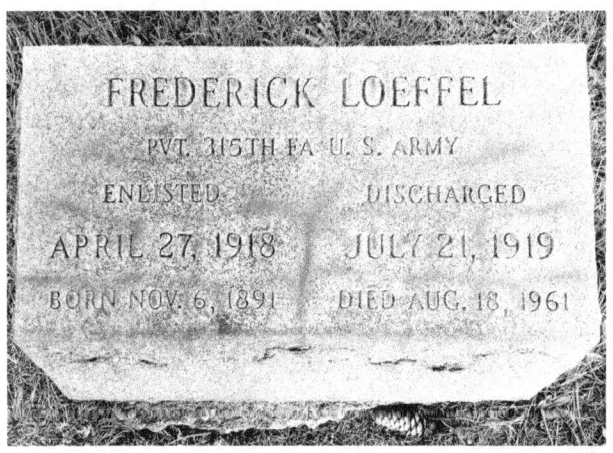

Frederick Loeffel is buried at Birmingham Cemetery in Pittsburgh, Pennsylvania. The headstone of his grave honors him as a veteran of World War I who served with the 315th Field Artillery and lists the dates of his enlistment and discharge in the U.S. Army (Find a Grave. Frederick Loeffel. https://www.findagrave.com/memorial/44539274; accessed November 8, 2017 (courtesy Jas).

heart disease.[17] He is buried at Birmingham Cemetery in Pittsburgh, formerly known as Zimmerman Cemetery.[18]

In September 2016, an identification tag was recovered at the former site of Bazoilles Hospital Center inscribed on one side with "FREDERICH. LOEFFEL" and on the other side with Army Service Number "2705744." The combination of name and Army Service Number provides certainty that this identification tag had belonged to Private Frederick Loeffel described above. The first name on the identification tag was either misspelled or written as a variant of the German name Friedrich.

It was planned by the U.S. Army Medical Department that, in general, soldiers who had been hospitalized with psychoses or other mental diseases would not return to duty but to transport them back to the United States for further treatment. In carrying this plan into effect, a psychiatric col-

Nine. Patients of Bazoilles Hospital Center   111

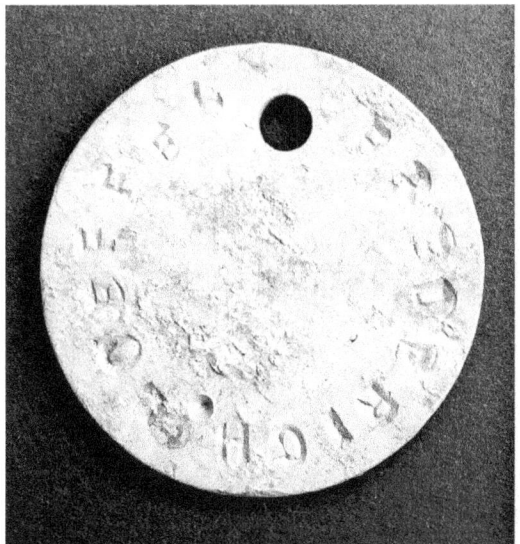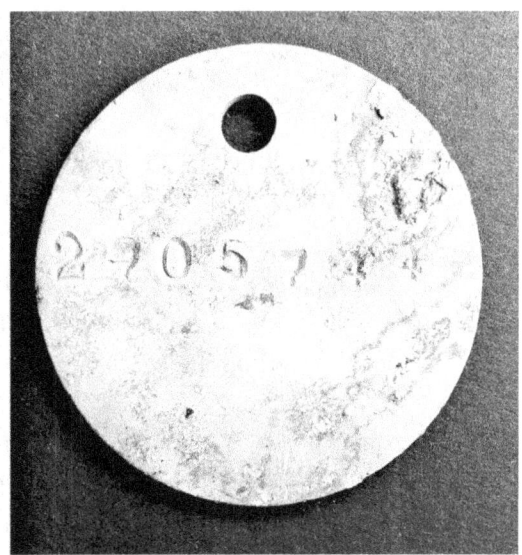

The identification tag of Frederick Loeffel recovered at the former site of Bazoilles Hospital Center in September 2016. It is inscribed on one side with "FREDERICH . LOEFFEL" and on the other side with Army Service Number "2705744" (author's collection).

lecting station had to be established for the forward area.[19] Bazoilles Hospital Center was selected as the site of the main psychiatric collecting station because of its proximity to the prospective site of the special hospital for war neuroses at La Fauche (Base Hospital No. 117), the headquarters of the professional services at Neufchâteau and its nearness to the front.[20] The neuropsychiatric department began to function on July 20, 1918, as part of Base Hospital No. 116. The department consisted of six wooden barracks located to the rear of the grounds occupied by Base Hospital No. 81. Four of the barracks were used for patients with a total normal bed capacity of 80. When the patient capacity of the department was inadequate, an additional neuropsychiatric ward was put into use at Base Hospital No. 116. From three to five medical officers were on duty during the greater part of the existence of

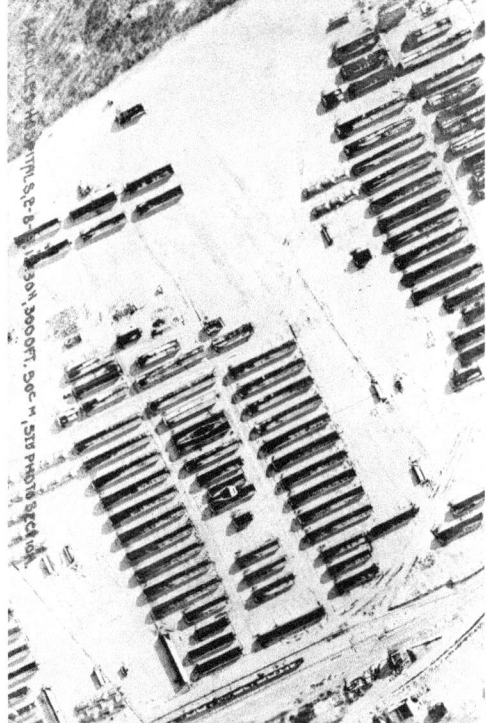

Aerial view obtained on February 8, 1919, of a snowed-under Bazoilles Hospital Center with Base Hospital No. 116 to the right and Base Hospital No. 81 to the left. The six barracks located to the rear of the grounds occupied by Base Hospital No. 81 made up the neuropsychiatric department. Presumably, Frederick Loeffel was admitted to one of the wards of this department (author's collection).

the neuropsychiatric department. The enlisted detachment consisted of four non-commissioned officers, two cooks and fourteen privates first class and privates. Ten nurses were required for the efficient service of the department. During the period from July 20, 1918, to April 30, 1919, 1,654 patients were admitted. The most common diagnoses among those admitted were psychosis (675 cases among which 395 cases of dementia praecox), defective mental development (morons and imbeciles; 263 cases), psychoneurosis (including war neurosis or "shell shock"; 204 cases), constitutional psychopathic state (198 cases) and idiopathic epilepsy (156 cases).[21] The majority of these cases, presumably including Frederick Loeffel, were evacuated to the United States through Savenay Hospital Center near the port of St. Nazaire.[22]

Private Harry H. McQuigg, Army Service Number 1967589, Approximate Date of Admission October 21, 1918

Harry Horace McQuigg was born on March 17, 1890, in Wooster, Ohio.[23] At the time of his registration for the World War I draft, on June 5, 1917, he lived in Wooster and was listed as a self-employed farmer. Notably, as ground for potential exemption from the draft it was listed that he was "just out of hospital."[24] He entered the U.S. Army on April 1, 1918, and was assigned as a private to Company M, 329th Infantry Regiment, 83rd Division.[25] His military training was received at Camp Sherman near Chillicothe, Ohio.[26] He qualified as an expert rifleman.[27]

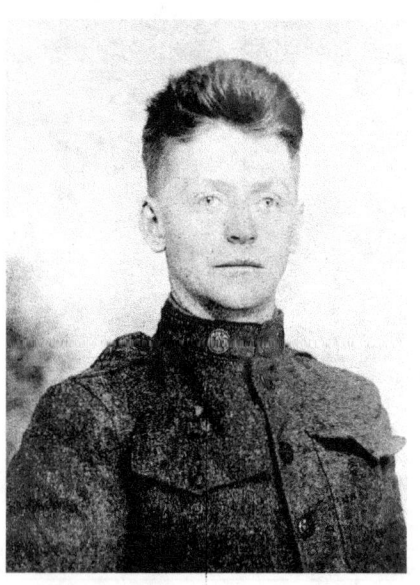

Harry H. McQuigg in uniform prior to shipping out for Europe in 1918. His uniform has a United States National Army collar disk attached to the left collar (courtesy Dave McQuigg, Delaware, Ohio).

Private McQuigg's unit sailed for Europe on board the *RMS Carmania* of the Cunard Line leaving New York, New York, on June 12.[28] The 83rd Division was designated a depot division supplying replacements to combat divisions in France.[29] On July 25, Private McQuigg was transferred to Company H, 101st Infantry Regiment, 26th Division. He served as runner and rifleman and was engaged in the Battle of St. Mihiel on September 12 and 13.[30] A runner was a military courier responsible for carrying messages and, therefore, important to military communications. As runners had to leave the relative safety of their shelters to carry messages to other positions, their job was among the most dangerous.[31]

Harry McQuigg was "dropped fr rolls per GO.111" on October 21.[32] General Order No. 111 states that officers and soldiers were dropped from the rolls of their organization (a) upon death; (b) when missing after an absence of ten days; (c) when discharged from the service; (d) when transferred to another unit; (e) when admitted to hospital.[33] It is assumed that Harry McQuigg dropped from rolls because of hospitalization. Although he had distinct mustard gas

Nine. Patients of Bazoilles Hospital Center

REPORT OF CHANGES OF ENLISTED MEN

France — 101st U.S. Infantry

For the twenty-four hours ending at midnight on Oct. 21, 1918.

Name	Army Serial Number	Grade	Company and Regiment, or Arm or Corps of Department	Remarks
Spillane, Paul	62304	Sgt	M, 101st	Apptd. 1st Sgt. per C.O. #1
Theault, Joseph	62321	Cpl	M, 101st	Fr duty to sk InHosp. InLD not result of misconduct Hosp. unknown.
Murphy, Frank E	62500	pvt	M, 101st	Fr A.W.O.L. to duty
Dickson, Walter	1678476	pvt	L, 101st	Fr duty to sk In hosp In LD not result of misconduct Hosp. unknown.
Halverson, Harold R	62204	pvt	L, 101st	Ass as repl per memo G-1 hqs. 26th Div.
Reddy, Edward R	61867	Mess Sgt	K, 101st	" " " " "
Foley, Thomas J.	63055	pvt	I, 101st	Fr duty to D.B. at 26th Div. Disciplinary Bct. per RSO 157
Wilbur, John	61815	pvt	I, 101st	" " " " "
Egan, John	61743	pvt	I, 101st	" " " " "
Bearzie, Joseph	1942460	pvt	I, 101st	" " " " "
Sardina, Anthony	61379	Cpl	H.Co. 101st	" " " " "
McQuigg, Harry	1967589	Wa-pvt	I, 101st	Dropped fr rolls per G.O. 111
Lipsic, Leo J.	61530	pvt	H, 101st	" " " " "
Lavers, William	2107245	pvt	H, 101st	" " " " "
O'Neil, Dewey F.	1596860	pvt	H, 101st	" " " " "
Riley, Thomas F.	61559	pvt	H, 101st	" " " " "
Goodwin, Eugene	61510	pvt	H, 101st	" " " " "
Spellman, Joseph	80074	pvt	H, 101st	" " " " "
Bilsky, Walter	1967482	pvt	H, 101st	" " " " "
Pitts, George W	61366	Cpl	A, 101st	" " " " "
Keene, Willis E	61379	pvt	A, 101st	Ass as repl per memo G-1 hqn. 26th Div.
Griffin, James L.	61513	pvt	E, 101st	" " " " "
Shaughnessy, Jas		Cpl	E, 101st	" " " " "
Kumberg, Bismark	260646	pvt	H, 101st	Trans. to Supply Co., 101st Inf. per S.O. 156
Haley, Thomas C	67061	Wagoner	Sup, 101st	Ass to duty
John J.	2850	Wagoner	Sup, 101st	" " " " "

The Report of Changes of October 21, 1918, for the 101st Infantry Regiment, 26th Division, lists that Harry H. McQuigg dropped from rolls per General Order No. 111 presumably indicating that he was admitted to hospital (National Personnel Records Center [Military], National Archives at St. Louis, St. Louis, Missouri [provided by Golden Arrow Military Research, St. Louis, Missouri]).

burns on both his arms,[34] his honorable discharge report mentions that he did not receive wounds while in service.[35] Correspondingly, his name has not been found on any casualty list. However, it is known that he suffered from acute gastrointestinal issues.[36] Moreover, half way through October, the Spanish flu swept through the ranks of the 26th Division leading to the loss of officers and men in every battalion and company.[37] Thus, there are several possible reasons for hospitalization of Harry McQuigg.

On December 9, Harry McQuigg was transferred from a replacement organization to his original company in the 26th Division. He was sent to the AEF University at Beaune in the east of France on March 11, 1919.[38] He left Beaune, however, before the end of the first term. On April 10, he sailed from Brest on the USS *New Jersey* with Casual Company No. 764 arriving in Boston, Massachusetts, on April 23.[39] Subsequently, he proceeded to Camp Sherman where he was honorably discharged on May 23 while with Detachment No. 303.[40]

After the war, Harry McQuigg was placed into work as a rural mail carrier.[41] He worked for 39 years on Wooster RD 5.[42] He did not openly discuss his World War I service and would admonish his children if he caught them playing or looking at the duffel bag that contained his uniform and other service items. When specifically asked about the war, he would only state "that he hated having wet feet." Throughout his life, he kept suffering from severe gastrointestinal issues, which might have been the result of unrecognized ulcerative colitis or Crohn's disease, and required several operations. His wife attributed all of his illnesses to his exposure to germs and rotted materials in the trenches of World War I. In the last year of his life, Harry McQuigg was diagnosed with amyotrophic lateral sclerosis (ALS) complicated by pneumonia in the last month.[43] On July 11, 1966, at the age of 76 years, Harry McQuigg died at a long-term care facility.[44] He is buried at Wooster Cemetery in Wooster. Next to his grave is a marker honoring him as a U.S. Army soldier during World War I.[45]

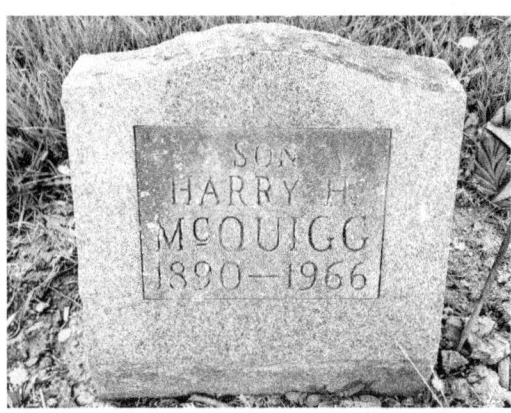

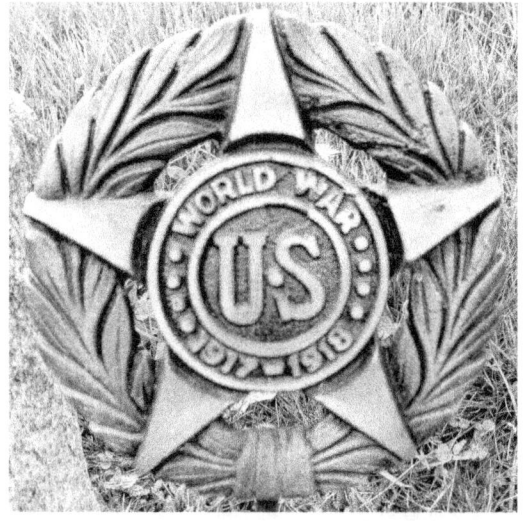

Left: Headstone of the grave of Harry H. McQuigg at Wooster Cemetery in Wooster, Ohio. *Right:* Next to the grave where Harry H. McQuigg is buried, stands a marker honoring him as a U.S. Army soldier during World War I (both photographs courtesy John E. Bastin, Wooster, Ohio).

In December 2016, a damaged identification tag was recovered at the former site of Bazoilles Hospital Center inscribed on one side with "…Y H. M^CQUIGG" "U. S. A." and on the other side with Army Service Number "…(?)67(?)89." The combination of name and Army Service Number provides certainty that this identification tag had belonged to Private Harry H. McQuigg described above.

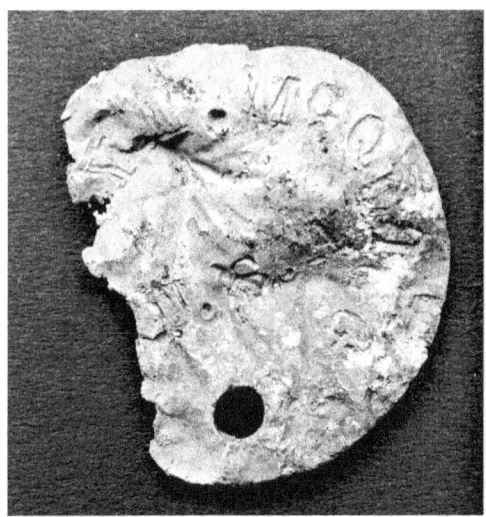 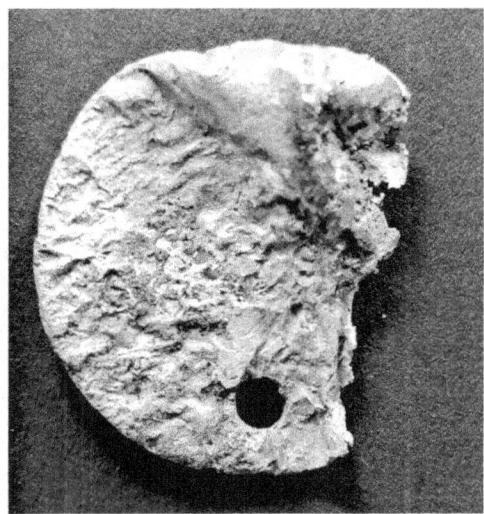

The identification tag of Harry H. McQuigg recovered at the former site of Bazoilles Hospital Center in December 2016. It is inscribed on one side with "…Y H. MCQUIGG" "U. S. A." and on the other side with Army Service Number "…(?)67(?)89" (author's collection; identification tag donated by author to McQuigg family).

In January 2017, the author set out to contact the next of kin of Harry McQuigg. A contact was established with his grandson Dave McQuigg, a detective at the Delaware City Police Department in Delaware, Ohio. Dave McQuigg provided input and an image for the history of Harry McQuigg. The author mailed him the identification tag of his grandfather in July 2017. Upon receipt, Dave McQuigg wrote that he was "speechless and overwhelmed" and that "the probability alone of Harry's grandson touching/holding his dog tag from WW1 is beyond belief." Dave McQuigg presented the identification tag in September 2017 to his cousin Staff Sergeant Paul McQuigg, United States Marine Corps, who resides in Oceanville, California. Staff Sergeant McQuigg nearly died in Iraq in 2006 from injuries inflicted by an improvised explosive device (EID) and continues to struggle with chronic pain.[46]

Private Morgan J. Magness, Army Service Number 2686980, Date of Admission April 19, 1919

Morgan James Magness was born on November 25, 1888, in Georgetown, Texas. At the time of his registration for the World War I draft, on June 4, 1917, he listed Casper, Wyoming, as home address, where he worked as a train conductor on the Burlington

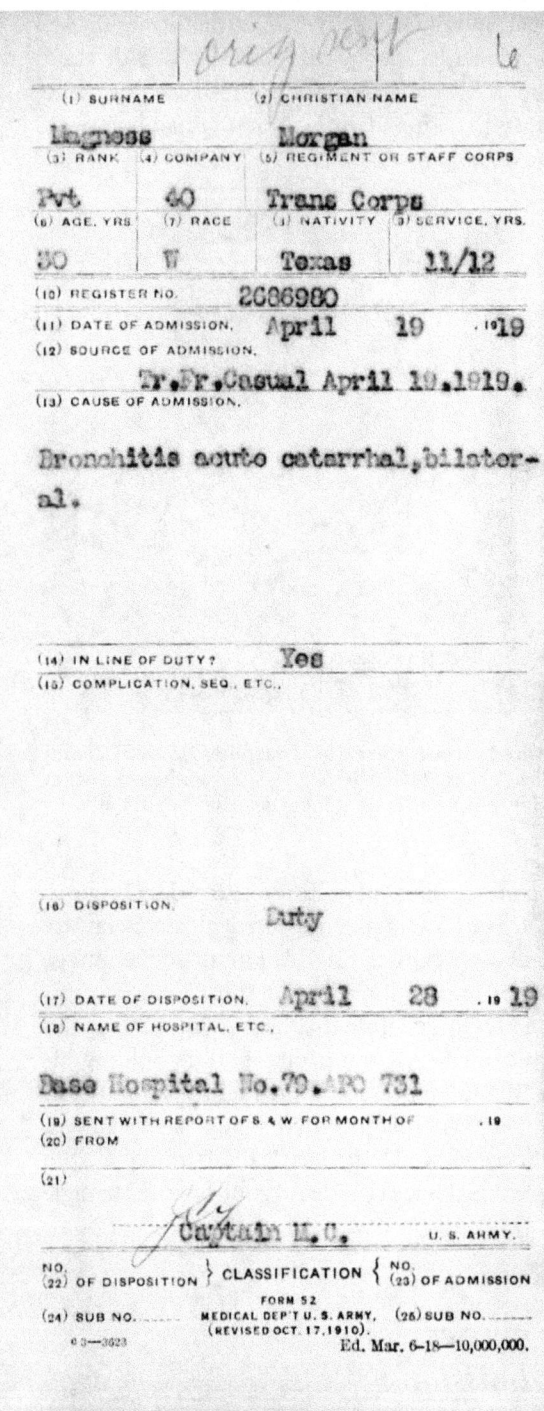

Route.[47] He entered the U.S. Army on May 17, 1918, and reported for military duty at Fort Benjamin Harrison, Lawrence Township, Indiana, on May 19, where he was assigned to Company B of the 62nd Engineer Regiment.[48] The personnel of the 62nd Engineers was filled by the enlistment and induction of railway operating men from practically every state. On July 14, the regiment set sail for Europe on the *Zealandia* of the Huddart Parker shipping company, landing in Liverpool on July 26. The trip to Cherbourg, France, was made on the channel boat *Antrim* on the night of July 28 to 29. From Cherbourg, the regiment entrained for the *Camp de Grasse* in Saint-Pierre-des-Corps which was reached on July 31.[49] There, the 62nd Engineers were used in railroad operation and car repair shops. On September 18, the designation of the 62nd Engineer Regiment was changed to the 62nd Regiment Transportation Corps.[50]

On November 11, a detachment of about 200 men, including Morgan Magness, and six officers of the 62nd Regiment Transportation Corps proceeded to Connantre in the *département* Marne for railroad duties. The 62nd Regiment Transportation Corps was abolished on November 12 and its Companies A, B and C became, respectively, the 86th, 87th and 88th Companies Transportation Corps. From December 12 to March 11, 1919, Morgan Magness was on detached service with the 67th Company Transportation Corps, while from March 11 onwards, he was on detached service with the 40th Company Transportation Corps.[51]

The Sick and Wounded Report Card (Form 52) for Private Morgan J. Magness lists details of his hospitalization from April 19 to April 28, 1919, at Base Hospital No. 79, Bazoilles Hospital Center, because of bilateral acute catarrhal bronchitis (National Personnel Records Center [Military], National Archives at St. Louis, St. Louis, Missouri [provided by Golden Arrow Military Research, St. Louis, Missouri]).

Morgan Magness was admitted to Base Hospital No. 79 of Bazoilles Hospital Center on April 19, 1919. He suffered from bilateral acute catarrhal bronchitis (double-sided acute lower respiratory tract inflammation with mucus production usually caused by viruses or bacteria). His disease might have been the result of the third wave of Spanish flu, which occurred during the initial months of 1919.[52] He was discharged and returned to duty on April 28.[53] Base Hospital No. 79 ceased to function on May 1 when its patients were evacuated to Angers and Nantes. On that date, Bazoilles Hospital Center ceased operation indicating that Morgan Magness was among the last patients treated at the center.[54]

After discharge from Base Hospital No. 79, Morgan Magness returned for detached service to the 40th Company Transportation Corps at Liffol-le-Grand, close to Bazoilles-sur-Meuse. While there, on May 13, he was involved in a railroad accident. While repairing an apron on a German coach, a French box-car was switched upon the same track. His forearm got caught and twisted between the aprons. He was admitted to Base Hospital No. 59, Rimaucourt Hospital Center at Rimaucourt, where he was initially diagnosed with a fracture of his left forearm. On May 15, the diagnosis was revised to a sprain wrist. After his discharge on May 28, he returned to the 40th Company Transportation Corps for detached service until May 31, following which he returned to his old unit which had been renamed the 87th Company Transportation Corps.[55]

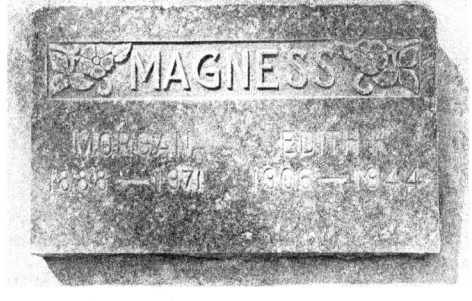

Left: Report of changes for Private Morgan J. Magness dated May 13, 1919, stating that he has been admitted to Base Hospital No. 59, Rimaucourt Hospital Center, because of an accidental fracture of his left forearm at Liffol-le-Grand (National Personnel Records Center [Military], National Archives at St. Louis, St. Louis, Missouri [provided by Golden Arrow Military Research, St. Louis, Missouri]). *Above:* Headstone of the grave of Morgan J. Magness and his second wife Edith M. King Magness at Lehi City Cemetery in Lehi, Utah (courtesy Lori Nielsen, Lehi, Utah).

Morgan Magness departed France on June 16 on the SS *Aeolus* arriving with the 87th Company Transportation Corps at Hoboken, New Jersey, on June 28. From there, he was subsequently forwarded to Camp Merrit, Creskill, New Jersey, and Fort Russel, Cheyenne, Wyoming, where he was honorably discharged on demobilization on July 11, 1919.[56]

After the war, Morgan Magness returned to railroad work with the Burlington Railroad and the Union Pacific Railroad, from which he retired in 1957. On October 24, 1971, at the age of 82 years, Morgan Magness died of natural causes in a hospital in Salt Lake City, Utah. He is buried at Lehi City Cemetery in Lehi, Utah.⁵⁷

In October 2016, an identification tag was recovered at the former site of Bazoilles Hospital Center inscribed on one side with "MORGAN J. MAGNESS" "U. S. A." and on the other side with Army Service Number "2686980." The combination of name and Army Service Number provides certainty that this identification tag had belonged to Private Morgan J. Magness described above.

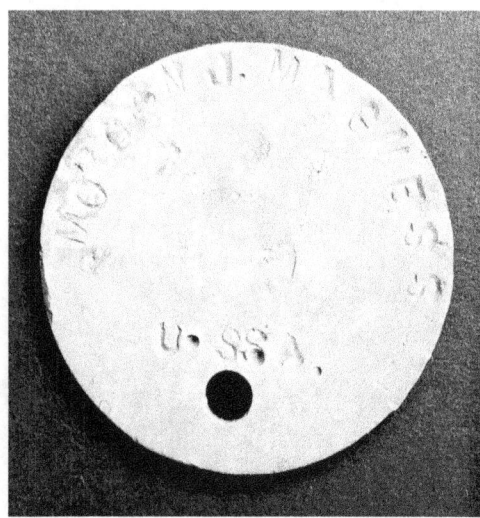 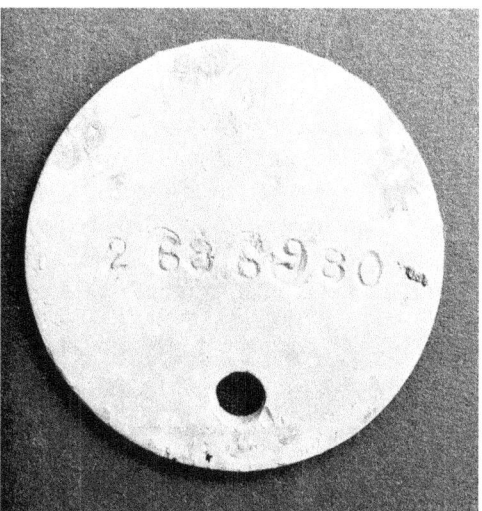

The identification tag of Morgan J. Magness recovered at the former site of Bazoilles Hospital Center in October 2016. It is inscribed on one side with "MORGAN J. MAGNESS" "U S A" and on the other side with Army Service Number "2686980" (author's collection).

Review of the Personnel by General Pershing

In April 1919, General John J. Pershing, Commander-in-Chief of the American Expeditionary Forces, was making an inspection tour reviewing American units that were still in France. On April 11, General Pershing inspected units from Bazoilles Hospital Center at Neufchâteau, while on April 13, he reviewed the men of Base Hospital No. 116 who were staying near Nantes awaiting orders for embarkation. Printed below are the memories of Nurse Sarah Sand and the diary entries of First Lieutenant Howard Osgood describing these occasions.

In the book *Lamp for a Soldier: The Caring Story of a Nurse in World War I*, Nurse Sarah Sand of Base Hospital No. 60 described the inspection by General Pershing of, among others, the nurses of Bazoilles Hospital Center on April 11, 1919.

> Notification of General Pershing's inspection was received in camp. The bugle called us at 5:00 a.m.; we had our breakfast at 5:45 a.m. and were in marching line by 7:00 a.m. We were taken to Neufchateau in ambulances and on to the French aviation camp. Here we found thousands of enlisted

Nine. Patients of Bazoilles Hospital Center

men in line with their officers. The nurses from Bazoilles sur Meuse formed two lines in front of the corpsmen of Base Hospital No. 60 and behind them, as far as the eye could see, were American soldiers. Here we waited from 8:00 a.m. until 11.00 a.m. in a steady drizzling rain. A large truck with a ladder decorated the center of the aviation field. Alongside this truck was a beautiful American flag belonging to the Second Cavalry.

We thought General Pershing was coming at 10:00 a.m. Three cavalrymen on their beautiful prancing horses watched for him. The bugler sounded the call; the messenger called his orders; the acting lieutenant colonel called attention and aboutface for all first lines. Well, we thought General Pershing was coming but it was merely a practice. He came at 11:00 a.m. in a beautiful gray automobile decorated with gold stars.

General Pershing's immediate attendants were a major, a lieutenant colonel, and a colonel. As soon as he arrived, the three horses were led up to his car but he must have refused them; he handed his overcoat to the major, who passed it on to the orderly. Then the General shook hands with the receiving officer, Colonel Dale. He immediately came over to us, inspecting the nurses' lines first. General Pershing smiled; his face dimpled in a very pleasing manner and he said, "Good morning, girls. I would like to meet each one individually but that is impossible." He turned to the officer with him and asked where our rubber[boot]s and raincoats were. The answer was not audible, but, as a matter of fact, they had been taken from us at Bazoilles and we had stood in the rain from 8:00 a.m. to 11.00 a.m.

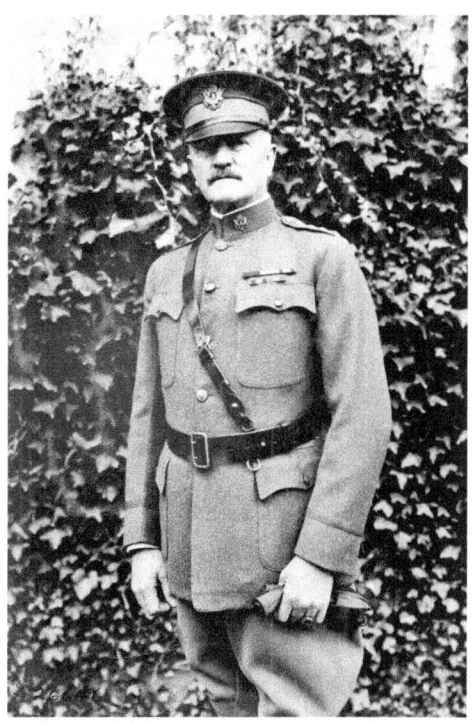

General John J. "Blackjack" Pershing, Commander-in-Chief of the American Expeditionary Forces in October 1918 (Wikipedia. Pershing at General Headquarters in Chaumont, France, October 1918, accessed March 19, 2017).

General Pershing seemed to me to be the nicest, cleanest man I had met in France. He fairly captured my heart with his careworn face and husky, much abused voice; he looked that day like a man who had almost reached the limit of his strength, although in passing down the line after line of men he walked so fast that the rest of the officers could scarcely keep up with him. He spoke to each man who wore a Distinguished Service Medal. We were told to gather close to the truck as General Pershing was returning to give us a speech. He came back in a short time and, as he was about to step onto the ladder of the truck, his attendant officer said, "Be careful, General, or you will lose your dignity!" This seemed to be a point of humor with them, as each smiled. Then one of the nurses caught his hand and they shook hands as he stepped onto the truck. Looking around, he spied an army photographer on top of a large airplane hangar nearby. He called to him to come down. The sergeant saluted and quickly folded his camera but in the meantime he had taken a number of pictures of the General. General Pershing looked at his two colonels stationed behind him as much as to say, "I knew he would make it."

It continued to rain. General Pershing had a bad cold and was very hoarse; he coughed frequently and talking seemed an effort. He said in part, "Go home to every hamlet and village and city of America and be proud you have had a part in this great struggle. Yes, let it be a modest pride, the kind that raises your head and squares your shoulders for America has played a part in turning the tide of failure to one of success and victory." Then he told the nurses he would always appreciate their efforts in caring for the wounded.

In the audience were French officers and several French Red Cross nurses who came out in the rain to hear what the great American General had to say. After his speech we dispersed and returned to

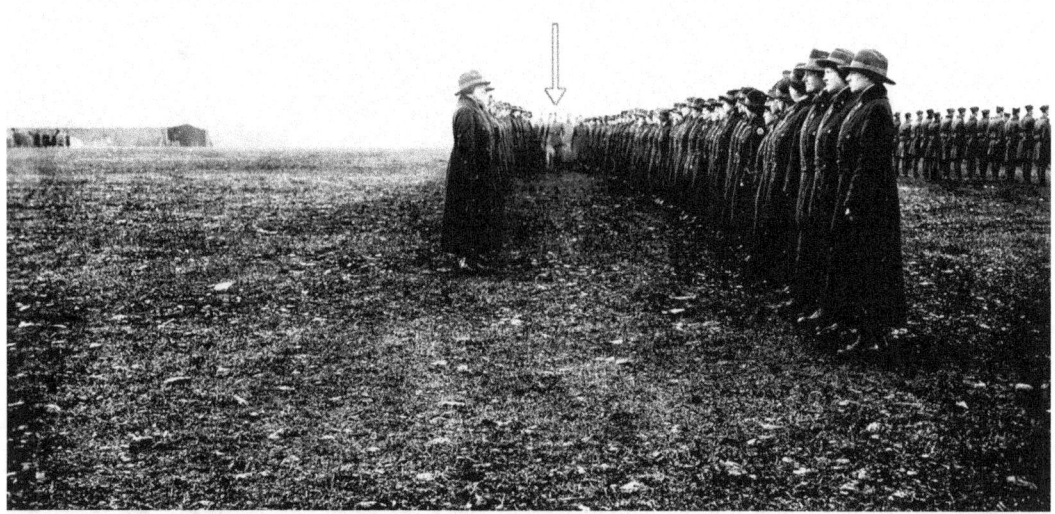

Nurses from Bazoilles Hospital Center stand in two lines during the inspection by General Pershing at the French aviation camp of Neufchâteau on April 11, 1919. The general and his party can be seen at the rear in-between the two lines (courtesy Oregon Health & Science University, Portland, Oregon [Historical Collections & Archives, Grace Phelps Papers, Accession No. 20100-05, box 1 folder 1]).

camp, wet and tired but satisfied that our group had been properly inspected before going back to the United States.[1]

The men of Base Hospital No. 116 were inspected by General Pershing on April 13, 1919, while staying near the city of Nantes where they were awaiting orders for embarkation. First Lieutenant Howard Osgood wrote to his mother about the inspection in a letter dated April 16, 1919.

My dear Mother,

We are still in the reserve area waiting for orders to go to the port, probably St. Nazaire. Base Hosp. 46 which came down from Bazoilles with us left for St. Nazaire nearly a week ago and according to the papers has already sailed for home. We thought we were S.O.L. [shit out of luck], as the expression is, meaning out of luck. But Saturday night we learned why we were detained; we received orders to be ready at 8:30 A.M. Sunday [April 13, 1919] to go in trucks to a certain rendez-vous and there be inspected by Gen'l Pershing. That evening there was much polishing of leather & brushing up of uniforms.

We had breakfast at 7:30 and then stood for inspection by our C.O. [Commanding Officer] before getting into the trucks. There were several other Units to be inspected at the rendez-vous. We got all lined up to wait for the General when a headquarters colonel came up in his car and said the inspection was postponed until 12:30. As there was a long wait the trucks took us back to our billets for lunch.

All the Units were lined up again at the rendezvous on time. Presently five or six cars came over the long bridge nearby and then things began to happen. We were called sharply to attention & the men faced around so that we officers were standing behind them. Personally I was scared still for Pershing has a reputation of being very severe. Well, he started up the left end of the line with our C.O. at his shoulder and a line of staff officers following behind. When he came opposite us, he pushed through the line & inspected the officers. [Lieutenant] Vic Seidler had permission to stand out of the

Nine. Patients of Bazoilles Hospital Center

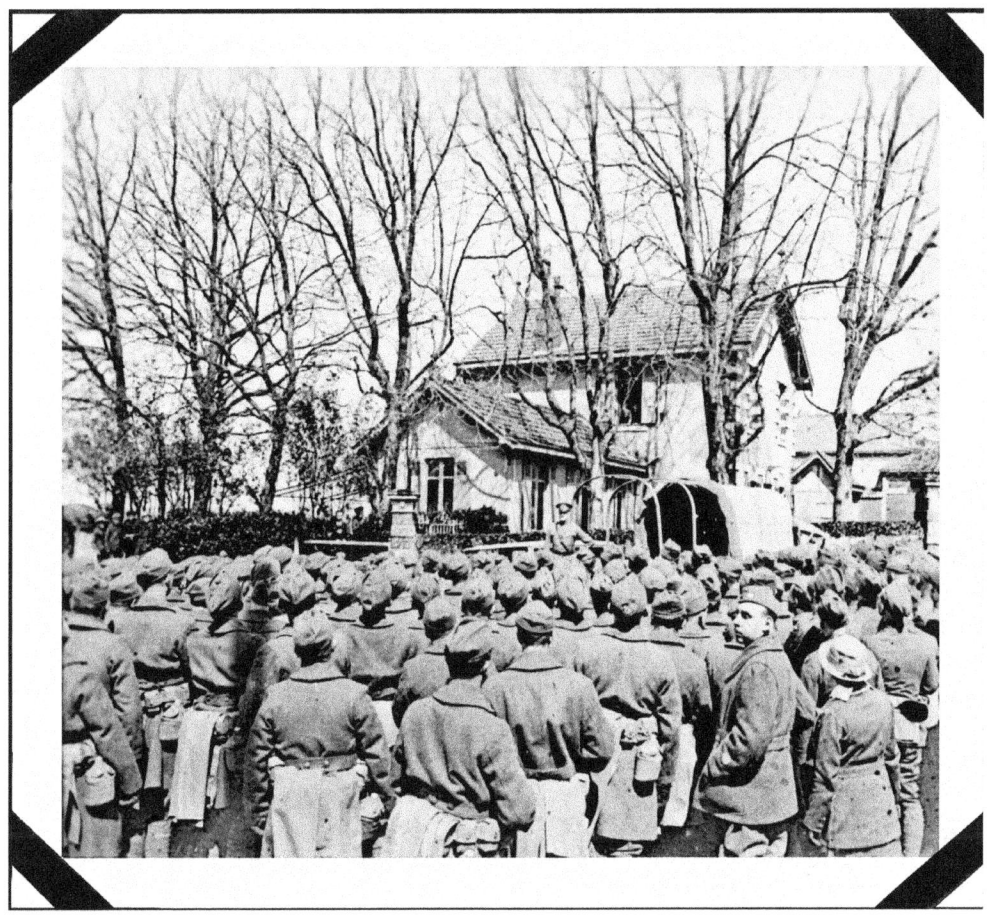

General Pershing addresses the men of Base Hospital No. 116 from a truck on April 13, 1919, at Saint-Sébastien-sur-Loire near the city of Nantes (author's collection).

inspection and take some photos of us. He said our line was very funny, everyone standing up so straight & rigid. Pershing stopped in front and said "Good morning, gentlemen" whereat in their excitement and entirely against regulations two of the officers replied "Good morning." Afterwards one of them denied having said it & the other was sore because the rest of us did not reply too. However Gen'l Pershing told our C.O. that the Unit looked very well, & that he was pleased with it. When he had finished reviewing all the Units present he made a little speech in which he thanked us for what we had done individually, hoped we would keep on with the high ideals after returning to civil life, and wished us a good trip home. The whole thing was soon over, but it is something to have been inspected by the C. in C. [Commander-in-Chief] Now all we want is to get home.[2]

Ten

Capital Punishment at Bazoilles-sur-Meuse
The Execution of Two American Soldiers

Officially, 11 American soldiers were sentenced to death by court-martial and executed in France during World War I. Two of these soldiers were executed by hanging at Bazoilles Hospital Center. Following charges from Senator Watson of Georgia in 1921 that American soldiers in France were executed without court-martial, several witnesses came forward with stories related to the hangings at Bazoilles-sur-Meuse. These accounts have been gathered in this chapter. They provide a picture of an entertainment-like atmosphere to which soldiers were invited to attend and thousands showed up. In addition, insight is provided in burial procedures following such executions. In 1923, the Senatorial committee appointed to investigate the charges of Senator Watson unanimously reported that it found the allegations unfounded.

The Hanging of an American Soldier at Bazoilles-sur-Meuse

On July 13, 1918, an American soldier was executed by hanging at Bazoilles-sur-Meuse after being sentenced to death by court-martial for the rape of an 68-year-old French peasant woman. The soldier had been identified by an identification tag, which the woman had snatched from his wrist. While waiting for the sentence to be approved, the soldier was confined in a military prison at Neufchâteau, some four miles north of Bazoilles-sur-Meuse.[1] A first-hand detailed account of the hanging was provided by U.S. Army chauffeur William B. West in his 1919 book *The Fight for the Argonne*:

> On July 12 it was rumored that a soldier had been sentenced to be hung the next day at ten o'clock for an unspeakable crime. The gallows was already built on the edge of the camp at Bazoilles. I saw it on my afternoon trip and knew that the report was true. Being interested in the psychology of such a scene on the men present, I put aside my inward rebellion at so gruesome a sight and arranged my trip so as to be present. I reached the camp at nine forty-five and was the last man admitted. The gallows was built in the center of the semicircle facing two hills which came abruptly together, leaving a large grass plot at their base. This formed a natural amphitheater. About two thousand soldiers, both white and colored, were seated on the grass inside a rope inclosure. A company of soldiers from another camp had been marched in to act as guards, and they formed a complete circle standing just outside the ropes and extending down to the gallows on either side.
>
> Many French civilians and visiting soldiers lined the edges or looked down from points of vantage

Ten. Capital Punishment at Bazoilles-sur-Meuse

on the hillside. I stood on one side about one hundred feet from the "trap." At nine fifty a Red Cross ambulance drove up, and the prisoner, his hands bound behind him, alighted, and accompanied by a guard and the officials, walked up a dozen wooden steps to the platform. He was escorted to the front of the platform, and in a clear, strong voice spoke to the almost breathless crowd. He acknowledged with sorrow his crime, and urged upon all the necessity of being true to God and their country. He stepped back on the "trap," the black cap was drawn over his head, the noose placed about his neck, the "trap" sprung, and with a sickening thud he dropped to his doom. For twenty minutes, from nine fifty to ten ten, his body hung there before he was pronounced by the attending surgeon officially dead.

I never witnessed a twenty minutes of such deathly silence. Two guards fainted, and the effect on the crowd was indescribable. I overheard a colored fellow say, "I never want to do anything bad again as long as I live."

The body was immediately cut down, placed in a coffin, and taken in the ambulance to its burial. It was a silent, thoughtful company that went out from the tragic scene.[2]

The execution is also described in the diary of First Lieutenant Howard Osgood from Base Hospital No. 116:

> The hanging is in everyone's mind this morning. The gallows was built in a little ravine back of one of the unoccupied Units; three nooses & traps. At the proper time all the men in a certain command to which the prisoner belonged were paraded about the gallows; there were others present, and an armed guard thrown around the whole group. The prisoner made a short speech saying he was sorry for what he had done; then the noose was adjusted & the three traps sprung by three different men, so neither knew which string was the one that dropped the man.[3]

This account describes the site where the gallows was built as "back of one of the unoccupied Units."[4] On the date of the execution, July 13, 1918, the hospital units that had not yet arrived at Bazoilles Hospital Center were Base Hospitals Nos. 42, 60, 79 and 81, which were all to be situated on the east bank of the Meuse River.[5] In addition this account describes the site as located "in a little ravine [a small narrow steep-sided valley]," where the other account describes the location of the gallows as "in the center of the semicircle facing two hills which came abruptly together, leaving a large grass plot at their base" thus forming "a natural amphitheater" situated "on the edge of the camp at Bazoilles."[6] These descriptions indicate that the site of the gallows was situated on the east bank of the Meuse River on a narrow grass strip between two forested hills next to the field to be occupied by Base Hospital No. 42. This strip of land is still discernable today.

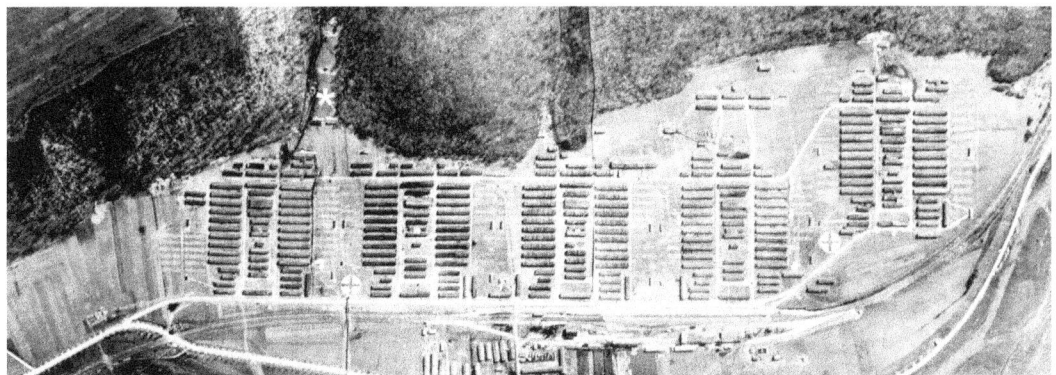

Aerial view of the five base hospitals of Bazoilles Hospital Center on the east bank of the Meuse River. The presumed location of the gallows where a black American soldier was executed by hanging on July 13, 1918, is marked (upper left) with an asterisk (author's collection).

Another detailed account of the hanging was provided in 1922 by former personnel of Base Hospital No. 46:

> Men who served with the unit recall distinctly how, soon after its arrival, word was given out that the unit was to be ordered to parade to a hanging at the hospital center at Bazoilles-sur-Meuse. The report, first considered an idle rumor, was given credence when at the edge of the camp a high scaffold was erected, on the east side of the river Meuse. ...
>
> The condemned man, it soon became known, was a private in a negro labor battalion attached to the hospital center, which at that time included three hospitals, and lay on both sides of the river. It was reported that this soldier had attacked an aged French woman, causing her death.
>
> The hanging was set for July 13, the day before Bastille day. At about 9 o'clock that morning all units in the camp formed on their own parade grounds preparatory to marching to the scene of the hanging. The scaffold had been erected at the edge of the woods skirting the hospital center. A company of infantry, bayonets fixed, formed a hollow square, into which the labor battalion, of which the condemned man was attached, and other units filled. ...
>
> Up from the American military prison in Neufchateau sped an army truck, its sides and ends covered with tarpaulin, an odd sight at that area in July, where every breeze is welcome. The truck was driven close to the scaffold. Its covering at the rear was thrown up and a half dozen American military police sprang out, the last two guiding between the prisoner, his hands bound.
>
> Up the steps of the scaffold the prisoner was led. At the wide trap opening he halted. A chaplain conferred with the doomed man and the latter turned to the silent assembly. In a halting voice that in the deathly stillness sufficed to carry to the rear rank of infantry, he expressed regret for his misdeed. ...
>
> A note of unconscious irony crept into his short talk when he said: "I've learned a lesson from this, boys." But no one smiled.
>
> The attending guards stepped forward to adjust the black cap and noose. Watchers, shifting their eyes from the scaffold, saw the low wooded hills about the scene dotted with the blue and white uniforms of nurses of the center, who had made their way to points of vantage to witness the hanging.
>
> Cap and noose adjusted, the guards sprang aside. From behind his black cap the prisoner spoke again.
>
> "Don't do what I did, boys," he said. "I hope you all get back home."
>
> The guards sprang back. The condemned man uttered a muffled shriek. The trap fell with a resounding clang, and the body in olive drab twitched and swung.
>
> A Portland physician, Dr. R. F. Benson, an officer of base hospital 46, took his stand beside the body to determine when death had claimed the dangling figure. Occasionally he touched the pulse. The fall had evidently not broken the man's neck. Eleven minutes had elapsed before the word was given, the body cut down and the burden again loaded into the truck and driven off.
>
> No ceremonies accompanied the burial of the soldier in the American cemetery on the west side of the river–the same cemetery in which Corporal Ernest Stout and two nurses of base hospital 46 were buried.
>
> The identification tag on the cross bore the simple, ironic legend, "George E. Chambers, died, July 13, 1918 [incorrect first name]."[7]

Presumably, the hanged soldier was interred in the small French military cemetery next to the *Château de Bazoilles-sur-Meuse*, which was occupied by Base Hospital No. 18. This cemetery was closed on July 15, 1918, two days following the execution, after which the new cemetery for Bazoilles Hospital Center was opened that was officially known as U.S. Military Cemetery No. 6.[8]

Rumors of Lynchings of American Soldiers

The execution on July 13, 1918, at Bazoilles-sur-Meuse is officially one of the 11 cases in which American soldiers were sentenced to death by court-martial and executed in

France during World War I. Eight of these soldiers were black. All the cases involved charges of rape while three incidents also included charges of murder.⁹

There were, however, persistent rumors, both during and after World War I, of lynchings—executions without trial—of American soldiers.¹⁰ National headlines were made by the infamous charges from Democratic Senator Thomas E. Watson of Georgia in 1921, that American soldiers in France were hanged without court-martial or other form of trial. Senator Watson asked the Senate:

> How many Senators know ... that a private soldier was frequently shot by his officers because of some complaint against officers' insolence; and that they had gallows upon which men were hanged day after day, without court martial or any other form of trial? I had and have the photograph of one of those gallows, upon which twenty-one white boys had already been executed at sunrise when the photograph was taken; and there were others waiting in the camp jails to be hanged morning after morning.

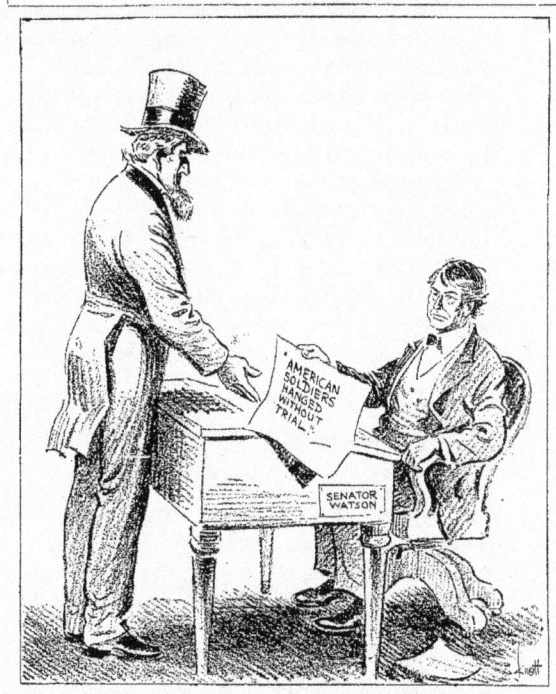

A cartoon from the front page of *The Galveston Daily News* of November 5, 1921, illustrating the request to Senator Watson to provide proof of his charges that American soldiers in France were hanged without trial ("The Proof, Senator?" *The Galveston Daily News*. November 5, 1921: 1).

The Senate characterized Watson's charges as "monstrous." On November 1, 1921, by unanimous vote, a committee of five Senators was ordered to investigate the facts, specifically the charge that men were executed without trial.¹¹

Pictures Obtained in Defiance of Army Regulations

Senator Watson received aid to substantiate his charges among others from J. Danby Conwell. Serving as a private first class with Evacuation Hospital No. 6, Conwell had been stationed at Bazoilles Hospital Center until the hospital's departure on July 18, 1918.¹² Conwell forwarded to Senator Watson two pictures and the story of the hanging of an American soldier in uniform before thousands of his comrades. The *New York Times* published his story on November 4, 1921"

> "We were with Evacuation Hospital Detachment No. 6, ... when news of the proposed hanging was made public, some time in June or July, 1918. We, with the members of another hospital detachment and a large number of infantrymen, were invited to attend the execution.

"Thousands of us turned out to witness it. A hastily built scaffold was erected at Bazoilles-sur-Meuse, where my outfit was stationed at the time. Although the hanging had all the aspects of the execution of an official court-martial, we were never told officially why the man had to die. Many rumors were current among the doughboys, and the one given the most weight was that the man had committed a murder following an attack on a girl.

"Many officers, including an army chaplain, were present at the execution, but what surprised me most was the fact that the man was hung in his uniform. It had always been my belief that hanging was a disgrace and, therefore, the man should be shorn of his insignia before going to the gallows."

The photographs sent to Senator Watson showed the soldier swinging from the gallows and preparations for the execution.

In explaining how the pictures were obtained in defiance of the army regulations, Conwell said:

"We hid our cameras under our coats and selected positions where the crowd was densest. Then when all eyes were riveted on the hanging, Private Cohn and myself reached our cameras over the shoulders of the men in front of us and made the snapshots. Cohn's films turned out all right, but mine were blurred. He has the film in his possession now."[13]

Asger G. Cohn, who was also attached as private first class with Evacuation Hospital No. 6 and had taken the photos sent to Senator Watson, also told his story to the *New York Times*.

Asgar [Asger] Cohn ... showed a Times reporter last night photographs of the hanging of a negro soldier, which Cohn said he and 700 other soldiers witnessed at Bezoilles [Bazoilles] in the Vosges Mountains on July 13, 1918. Cohn, who was attached to Evacuation Hospital 6, said that he had taken the photographs himself. He did not remember whether the negro had a court-martial, but said that all soldiers in the vicinity were informed that the negro was to be hung.

Cohn referred to his diary and said that the negro's name was Jeffries [incorrect name] and that he had attacked and killed a French woman 65 years old. Just before the trap was sprung, according to Cohn's diary, the soldier asked permission to say something to the onlookers. When permission was given, he said:

"Brothers, all I can say is that I am very sorry for what I have done. I hope none of you ever commit the same things. I only hope that America will win the war and that you all will return safely to America."

Cohn said that he had heard stories of other hangings, but had never seen but one.[14]

According to a picture submitted to the Senatorial committee by Senator Watson, "a huge gallows" was erected at Bazoilles-sur-Meuse.[15] It is assumed that this refers to one of the pictures taken by Asger Cohn.

The Hanging of a Second American Soldier at Bazoilles-sur-Meuse

The next day, November 5, 1921, various newspapers printed statements from Irving D. Porter, former Captain in the U.S. Army Corps of Engineers,[16] who had been in charge of the first of two executions at Bazoilles-sur-Meuse.

I personally hanged one negro on my station. Two negroes were hanged on the station, but I was away at the time of the second execution.... The first negro was hanged on July 24, 1918 [incorrect date].... The prisoner was tried and convicted by due process of court-martial. His sentence was approved by the commander in chief [U.S. Commander-in-Chief General John J. Pershing].[17]

According to Porter, the hanging of a second soldier at Bazoilles-sur-Meuse, after conviction by court-martial for assault on a white woman, was conducted by First Lieutenant Carl M. Hoskinson.[18]

That same day, controversy was further stirred by Senator Watson, who announced that he would present an affidavit to the Senatorial committee charging that the bodies of four black soldiers were found with ropes tied around their necks when they were dug up in the cemetery at Bazoilles-sur-Meuse.

> In the case of these four men, my evidence tends to show that [they] were hanged without trial and that an effort was made to "cover up."
>
> I have evidence that is categorical and unequivocable in disclosing instances, officers and places connected with outrages against American soldiers.
>
> The most startling [evidence] is that concerning the four bodies. The man who gave it returned from France two weeks ago and is now in Washington. In France he was engaged in the preparation of the bodies of Yanks for shipment home.
>
> The bodies were dug up in a cemetery at Bazoilles and there is still a scaffold on the hill nearby large enough to hang three soldiers at a time, my witness tells me.
>
> Although the bodies of all soldiers, even in cases where they have been executed, were identified by records placed in a bottle within the coffins, there was no identification in these four cases, and the evidence indicated irregular and hasty burial.[19]

Indeed, at least at Bazoilles-sur-Meuse, it was custom that graves were marked with a bottle containing a report of death.[20]

Assistant Embalmer Rufus P. Hubbard Testifies

On January 4, 1922, the witness supposedly referred to by Senator Watson was heard by the Senatorial committee. Rufus P. Hubbard was employed by the American Graves Registration Service. Working as an assistant embalmer, his task had been to prepare bodies of American soldiers for shipment from France.[21]

Hubbard testified that in January 1921 the bodies of three (instead of four as stated by Senator Watson) American soldiers had been disinterred at Bazoilles-sur-Meuse with black caps over their heads and ropes around their necks.[22] The bodies were exhumed in different parts of the cemetery on the same day. There was nothing within the coffins by which the bodies could be identified, but it had been possible to identify them by markings on the crosses. Also, there were no tags on the bodies. He stated that he thought "two of the bodies were of black men and one of a white man but was not certain." Hubbard had been ordered to remove the ropes, which were about three feet long, but was not ordered to take off the black caps. Thus, the bodies were shipped to the U.S. for burial with the black caps still over the heads [at least one body was transported to the Meuse-Argonne American Cemetery at Romagne-sous-Montfaucon]. He told the committee that he had protested against allowing the bodies of the three soldiers to lie on

On January 4, 1922, *The Wichita Beacon* headlined on the front page with the statement of assistant embalmer Rufus P. Hubbard that soldiers had been disinterred at the cemetery of Bazoilles Hospital Center with ropes around their necks (Soldiers Necks Bore Nooses. *The Wichita Beacon*. January 4, 1922: 1).

the ground overnight in the rain. He also thought it was a disgrace to the army that the bodies went to the parents without the black caps being removed.[23]

Don L. Jacobson was called to testify next. He was questioned about illegal hangings at the town of Gièvres, but had no knowledge thereof. He did tell the Senatorial committee about the execution by hanging of a court-martialed black soldier:

> Jacobson then told how he had put the noose around the neck of a negro soldier hanked [hanged] after courtmartial conviction [for rape]. After the hanging the body was cut down and a short stretch of rope left around the neck, he said.
> "It was customary to bury a man hanged with the rope and a black cap in place," he declared.
> He testified that the soldier at whose execution he assisted was buried in the cemetery at Bazoille [Bazoilles] where Hubbard previously had testified that three bodies were dug up.[24]

This anecdote seemingly explains why, according to Porter, two executions had taken place at Bazoilles-sur-Meuse, but, according to Hubbard, three bodies with black caps and ropes were disinterred from the cemetery. Yet, in contradiction to Jacobson's testimony, it has also been stated that only one execution took place in Gièvres. This concerned the hanging of a white soldier convicted for murder on June 20, 1919, which occurred in secrecy to avoid causing a disturbance in a nearby camp.[25] In addition, in contradiction to the testimony of Hubbard, Major Samuel J. Heidner of the Graves Registration Service stated during a later hearing "that a rope and black cap were found on two bodies dug up at Bazoilles. "The body of only one of the men hanged was shipped to the United States and in both instances the cap and rope were removed, ..."[26]

Colonel Edwin E. Lamb Testifies

Captain Porter's statement regarding a second hanging was confirmed on January 17, 1922, during a hearing by the Senatorial committee of Colonel Edwin E. Lamb, who had been the commander of the Military Police in the northern section of France.[27]

> Col. Edwin E. Lamb…, who directed the hangings of two negroes at Bazoilles, described these hangings.
> "The first was July 13, 1918, and the second on January 24, 1919. The first man's name was Chambers and the second Jones."
> "Were any drugs given these men to compose their nerves?" asked Senator Brandegee.
> "It was suggested to me at the second hanging, and I said, 'Yes, go ahead,'" replied Lamb.
> Lamb said that he knew in the case of the first hanging that the black cap and rope were left on the boy, but he was not certain about what was done in the second case.[28]

Senator Watson asked Colonel Lamb if the executed men were buried together with other soldiers.

> "And you mean to say that these men hanged for an almost unmentionable crime were buried with the honorable dead?" Senator Watson asked.
> "Yes. They were our men who had fallen and paid the extreme penalty."
> Some of the doctors later suggested, he added, that in future executions the bodies be buried in separate lots, but there were no other executions at that post.[29]

Senatorial Committee Finds Allegations Unfounded

The hearings by the Senatorial committee into the incidents at Bazoilles-sur-Meuse were part of a much larger investigation that came to be known as "the Watson inquiry."[30]

During this inquiry, Senator Watson himself suddenly died of cerebral bleeding on September 26, 1922, at the age of 66 years.[31]

On March 2, 1923, the five-member Senatorial committee appointed to investigate the charges of Senator Watson reported that it had unanimously found the allegations unfounded. The committee's findings were embodied in one of the briefest reports ever submitted as it was scarcely a dozen lines in length. It stated merely that, in pursuance of the order of the Senate, the committee had held hearings and inquired into the allegations of Senator Watson and had determined that they were "not sustained by the testimony."

The hearings were referred to by a newspaper as a "sensational chapter of senate history" featuring "many sensational incidents ... at which some of the highest officers of the army and of the war department were called to testify."[32]

The information upon which Senator Watson based his charges has been regarded as largely a fabrication of army rumors.

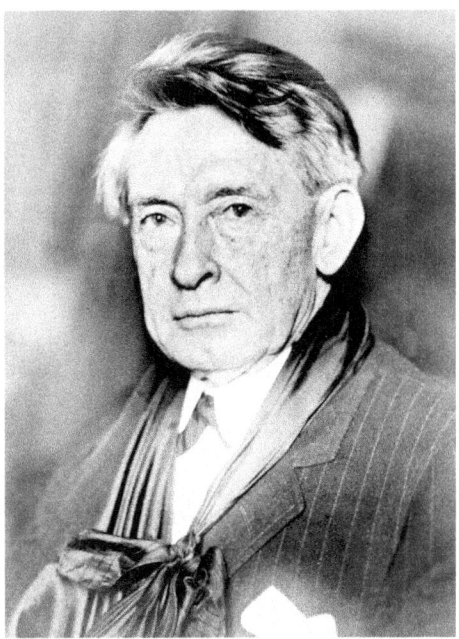

Democratic Senator Thomas E. Watson, who suddenly died of cerebral bleeding on September 26, 1922, during the Senatorial investigation into his charges that American soldiers were executed in France without trial. This investigation came to be known as "the Watson inquiry" (Library of Congress).

Men who were in the service well know how these rumors started on the merest conjecture of some one in the confidence of some one in the authority, and spread with almost incredible rapidity, gathering bulk and detail as they went. The rumors took root in and sustenance from the fact that military necessity demanded a certain degree of secrecy as to the official news of the army. ...

It is easy to see how eleven official hangings in the American forces overseas grew into a rumor of many hangings, and it is equally clear that the indiscretion or even the mental collapse of a few officers in the heat and anxiety of battle might result in numerous reports of summary executions by gunfire in the interest of discipline. No apology for this sort of thing is needed. It is merely one of the horrors of the most horrible of mankind's inventions. The inexplicable feature of the whole affair is how a man of enough intelligence and force to gain a seat in the United States senate, and separated by three years and 3,000 miles from the war, was duped as it appears the Georgia senator has been duped.[33]

Synopsis

Despite the sometimes sensational and contradictory statements, the consulted historical sources indicate that two black soldiers, convicted by court-martial, were executed by hanging at Bazoilles-sur-Meuse and buried with the black caps over their heads and the ropes still around their necks. Records of death customary contained within a bottle were not added to the coffins, while no tags were attached to the bodies. There is, however, no evidence of illegal hangings of American soldiers during or after World War I at Bazoilles-sur-Meuse.

```
                Chambers,         Charles  E.           233,054              X White  * Colored.
                (Surname)         (Christian name)      (Army serial number)

Residence:      1327 Pott St.     PHILADELPHIA,                              PENNSYLVANIA
                (Street and house number)  (Town or city)  (County)          (State)

* Enlisted R A N G E R C  *Inducted at  Columbus Bks. Ohio      on  Nov 1  , 1917
Place of birth: Philadelphia, Pa.           Age or date of birth:   19 10/12 yrs
Organizations served in, with dates of assignments and transfers:  Co E 304 Stevedore
     Regt. Nov 6/17 to Dec. 10/17;  Co G 305 Stev. Regt. to Dec 10/17
     to -- 12 Co 301 Stev. Regt to July 13/18
Grades, with date of appointment:                 Private.


Engagements: _____


Wounds or other injuries received in action: * None.
Served overseas from † Dec 26/17  to †  July 13/18 from † _____ to †_____
Died X  result of execution                              July 13       , 1918
                         (Cause and date of death)
Person notified of death:  Miss Jones,              Friend,
                           (Name)
        1327 Potts Street,       Philadelphia,                        Pa
        (No. and street or rural route)  (City, town, or post office) (State or country)
Remarks: _____
Form No. 724-8, A. G. O.    * Strike out words not applicable.  † Dates of departure from and arrival in the U. S.
       Nov. 22, 1919.
                                         3—7369
```

Service card of Private Charles E. Chambers who had been assigned to several regiments of black laborers. He died at the age of 20 years as the "result of execution" on July 13, 1918, while serving with 12th Company, 301st Stevedore Regiment. He was the first of the two black soldiers executed by hanging at Bazoilles-sur-Meuse (Ancestry. Pennsylvania, World War I Veterans Service and Compensation Files, 1917–1919, 1934–1948 for Charles E Chambers. https://www.ancestry.com; accessed September 28, 2016).

The cited first-hand accounts of the first hanging at Bazoilles-sur-Meuse provide a picture of an entertainment-like atmosphere to which men were invited to attend and thousands of soldiers and nurses showed up. Likewise, the Watson inquiry revealed a similar atmosphere at Is-sur-Tille, where soldiers were reportedly also ordered out to see the hangings and French locals, seemingly happy over it, were clapping and yelling.[34] Similarly, in the United States, at least 17 executions were performed outdoors, within the confines of a military camp before several, if not all, of the soldiers stationed thereby.[35]

A search in an online military records database revealed the service card of Private Charles E. Chambers, Army Service Number 233054, from Philadelphia, Pennsylvania. He was inducted in the U.S. Army on November 1, 1917, and served overseas with several regiments of black laborers from December 26, 1917, to July 13, 1918. On the latter date, while serving with 12th Company, 301st Stevedore Regiment, he died as the "result of execution," at the age of 20 years.[36] His family name, race, cause and date of death match with the first soldier executed by hanging at Bazoilles-sur-Meuse. Private Chambers is buried in Plot E, Row 26, Grave 9 at the Meuse-Argonne American Cemetery in Romagne-sous-Montfaucon.[37]

A search in an online card register of burials of deceased American soldiers revealed the Grave Registration Form of Private John Wesley Jones, Army Service Number 196774, from Plumerville, Arkansas. He served overseas with Company D, 508th Engineers,

Ten. Capital Punishment at Bazoilles-sur-Meuse

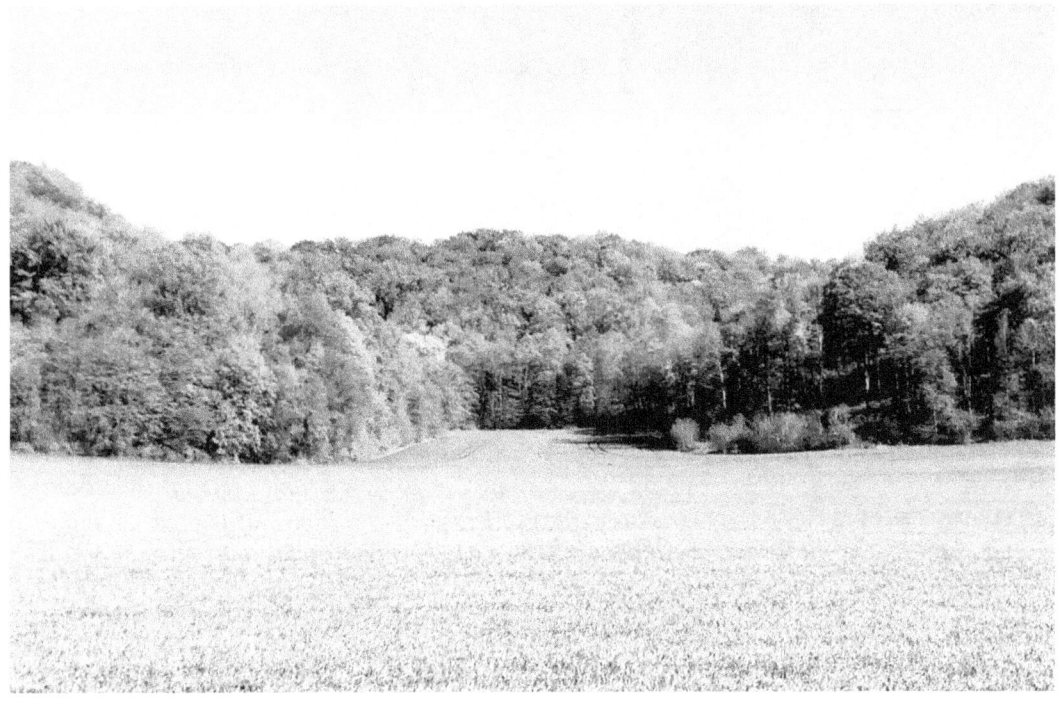

Present-day view showing the presumed location of the gallows where Private Charles E. Chambers was executed by hanging on July 13, 1918. This site was described as "a little ravine ... facing two hills which came abruptly together, leaving a large grass plot at their base" thus forming "a natural amphitheater" (photograph by author).

which was a black service battalion, until January 24, 1919. On that date, he was "executed by hanging" at "Bozoilles-sur-Meuse."[38] His family name, race, cause and date of death match with the second soldier executed by hanging at Bazoilles-sur-Meuse. In 1921, the body of Private Jones was repatriated to Plumerville. It is not known where he is currently buried.

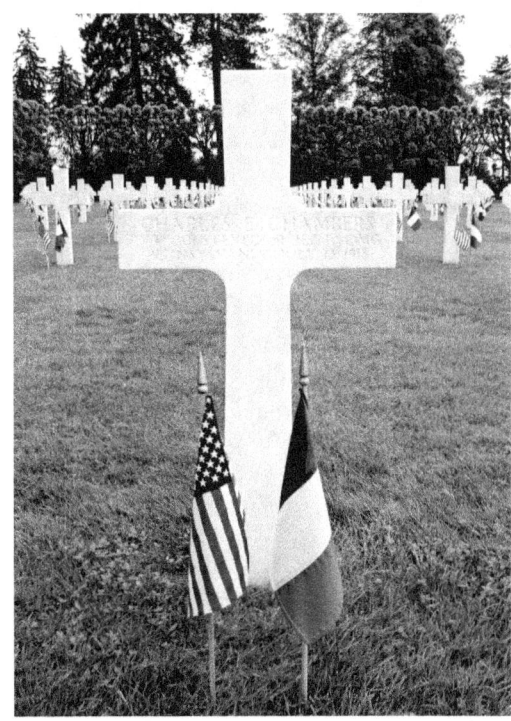

Headstone of the grave of Private Charles E. Chambers at the Meuse-Argonne American Cemetery in Romagne-sous-Montfaucon. This picture was taken on May 22, 2016, when all headstones were decorated with miniature U.S. and French flags on the occasion of the annual Memorial Day Ceremony (courtesy American Battle Monuments Commission [Overseas Operations Office, Paris, France; photograph by Maarten Otte, Nantillois, France]).

Eleven

Traces of Medical Care at Bazoilles Hospital Center
Items from Institutional and Personal Collections

Bazoilles Hospital Center ceased operation on April 30, 1919. Since then, items reminiscent of its existence have found their way into institutional and personal collections. Among these are objects recovered from the former site of the center. Such tangible reminders provide a confrontation with daily life at a U.S. Army hospital center during World War I.

Johns Hopkins Base Hospital Flag

The Alan Mason Chesney Medical Archives of The Johns Hopkins Medical Institutions in Baltimore, Maryland, holds this cloth flag (8 feet/2.4 m long by 5 feet/1.5 m wide) which flew over Base Hospital No. 18 at Bazoilles-sur-Meuse during World War I.[1] Base Hospital No. 18 was organized at Johns Hopkins Hospital, Baltimore, and, therefore, also referred to as the Johns Hopkins Unit. After mobilization on May 24, 1917, it sailed from New York for St. Nazaire, France, on June 14, where it arrived June 28. Toward the end of July, it proceeded to Bazoilles-sur-Meuse, where it arrived on July 26, being the farthest advanced hospital in the American Expeditionary Forces at that time. The unit began operation on July 31, 1917, functioning independently until July 1, 1918, when it became part of Bazoilles Hospital Center. On January 9, 1919, it ceased operation.[2]

There are no known photos depicting this flag at Bazoilles-sur-Meuse, but it can be seen on pictures of the nursing staff presumably taken in New York in the beginning of June 1917, shortly before leaving for Europe.[3] The flag is considered representative not only of the medical accomplishments of the Johns Hopkins Unit, but also of the broader successes the medical community achieved against the challenging environment of World War I.[4]

Glass Syringe

This 10 cc glass syringe with a scale in one-fifths was recovered at the former site of Bazoilles Hospital Center. The tip of the syringe has broken off. An identical syringe is listed in the *Illustrated Catalogue of Standard Surgical Instruments and Allied Lines*

Eleven. Traces of Medical Care at Bazoilles Hospital Center 133

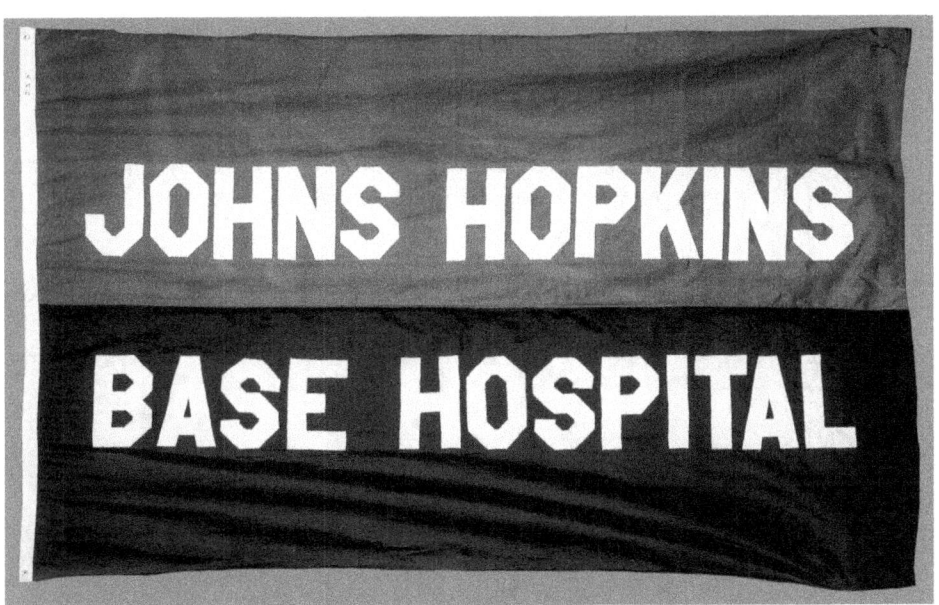

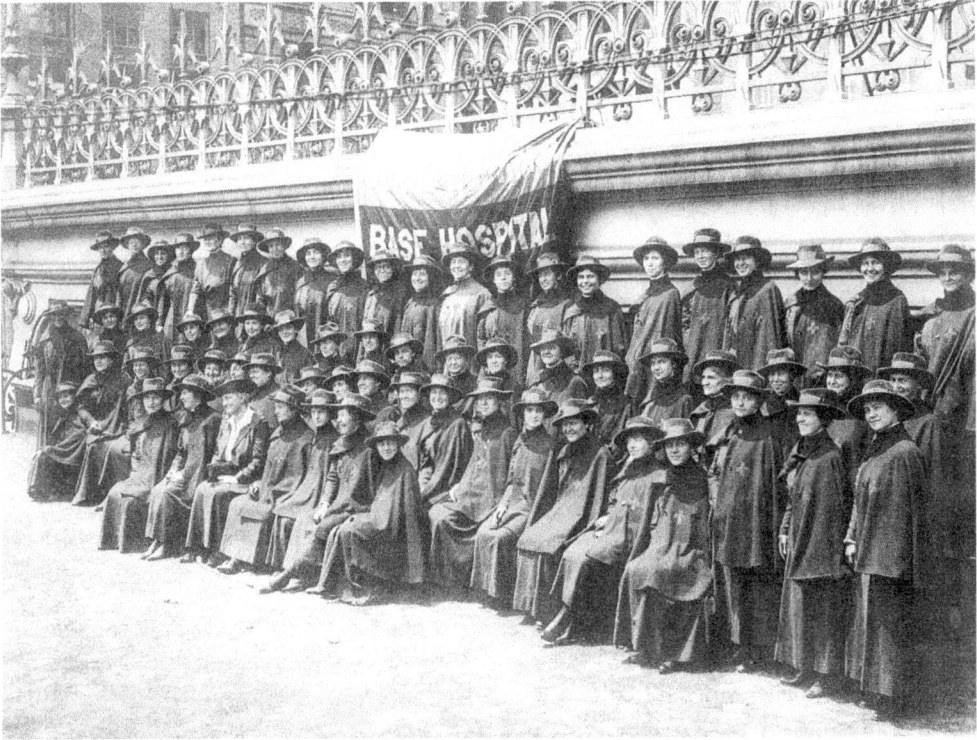

Top: Cloth flag which flew over Base Hospital No. 18 at Bazoilles-sur-Meuse. Currently, the flag is held by the Alan Mason Chesney Medical Archives of the Johns Hopkins Medical Institutions, Baltimore, Maryland (courtesy The Alan Mason Chesney Medical Archives of the Johns Hopkins Medical Institutions). *Bottom:* A photograph depicting the nursing staff of Base Hospital No. 18 presumably taken in New York in the beginning of June 1917, shortly before leaving for Europe. The Johns Hopkins Base Hospital flag is attached to the railing in the background (Library of Congress; courtesy Bridget Chandonnet DeSimone, Washington, D.C.).

from Hudson Surgical Co., Inc. located in Union Hill, New Jersey.[5] On April 2, 1918, the Chief Surgeon of the American Expeditionary Forces recommended a list of medical supplies for the initial equipment of an overseas 1,000-bed base hospital (revised on May 18, 1918, by the Surgeon General's Office). Among the listed laboratory supplies are "syringes: ... 10 c.c. in one-fifths," which description fits the recovered syringe. The initial allowance for 10 cc syringes was 12 dozen for a 1,000 bed base hospital. Other listed syringe sizes were 1 cc, 2 cc and 20 cc.[6]

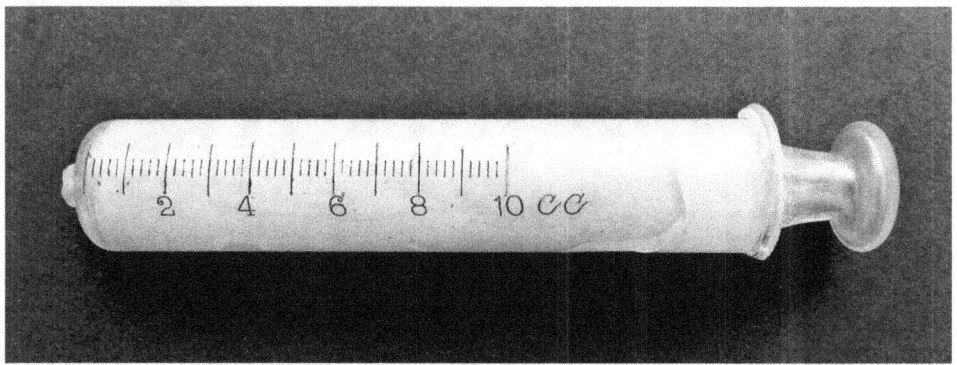

A 10 cc glass syringe with a scale in one-fifths recovered at the former site of Bazoilles Hospital Center. Such syringes were listed among the medical supplies for the initial equipment of an overseas 1,000-bed base hospital (author's collection).

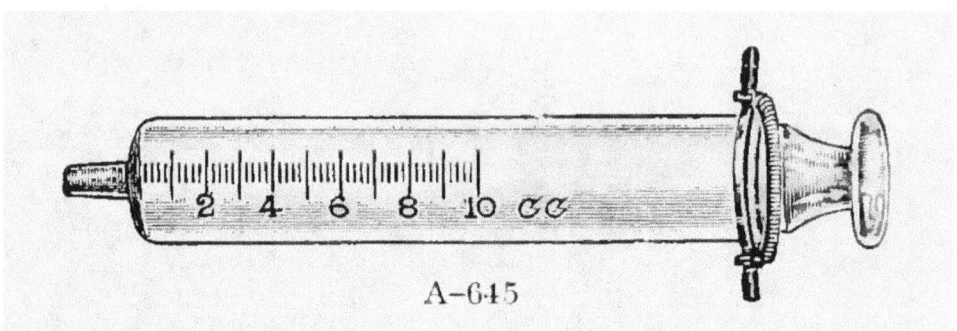

A 10 cc glass syringe with a scale in one-fifths listed in the *Illustrated Catalogue of Standard Surgical Instruments and Allied Lines* from Hudson Surgical Co. (*Illustrated Catalogue of Standard Surgical Instruments and Allied Lines*. Union Hill, NJ: Hudson Surgical Co., n.d.: 17).

The complete equipment of an overseas 1,000-bed base hospital was bulky and heavy. It occupied approximately 30,000 ft^3 (850 m^3) of space and weighed "120 short tons" (108,862 kg). Considerable difficulty was experienced in assembling it. Part of the equipment required packing, especially surgical instruments and other small articles. The quantities of many articles on the standard list were less than commercial case lots. The assembly was carried out at the New York medical supply depot. More bulky articles could not be carried in stock for lack of space and had to be ordered in from manufacturers as needed.[7]

Base Hospital No. 46 Baseball Team

This undated photo depicts members of the baseball team of Base Hospital No. 46. Notably, the man crouching outermost left wears a shirt with the designation MTC indicating he served with the Motor Transport Corps. This corps was formed on August 15, 1918,[8] indicating that this photo was taken after the arrival of Base Hospital No. 46 at Bazoilles Hospital Center on July 2, 1918.[9] The baseball team of Base Hospital No. 46 consisted of 11 players besides their manager Private Garret "Garry" Stelsel of the registrar's office and director of athletics First Lieutenant Dorwin L. Palmer, who was in charge of the X-ray service at the Surgical Department. The latter two might be the men pictured in uniform since the soldier holding the dog is wearing a lieutenant's bar on his shoulder straps and overseas cap and an officer's Sam Browne belt over his tunic.

Baseball was about the only game for which the personnel of Base Hospital No. 46 found much time. Already on July 4, 1918, two days after arrival at Bazoilles Hospital Center, Base Hospital No. 46 played against and defeated Base Hospital No. 116. The team had the advantage of a real pitcher in the person of Private Harry K. "Slim" Kackley. Several more games were played throughout the season of which the great majority was won, making Base Hospital No. 46 champion among the several hospitals at Bazoilles Hospital Center.[10]

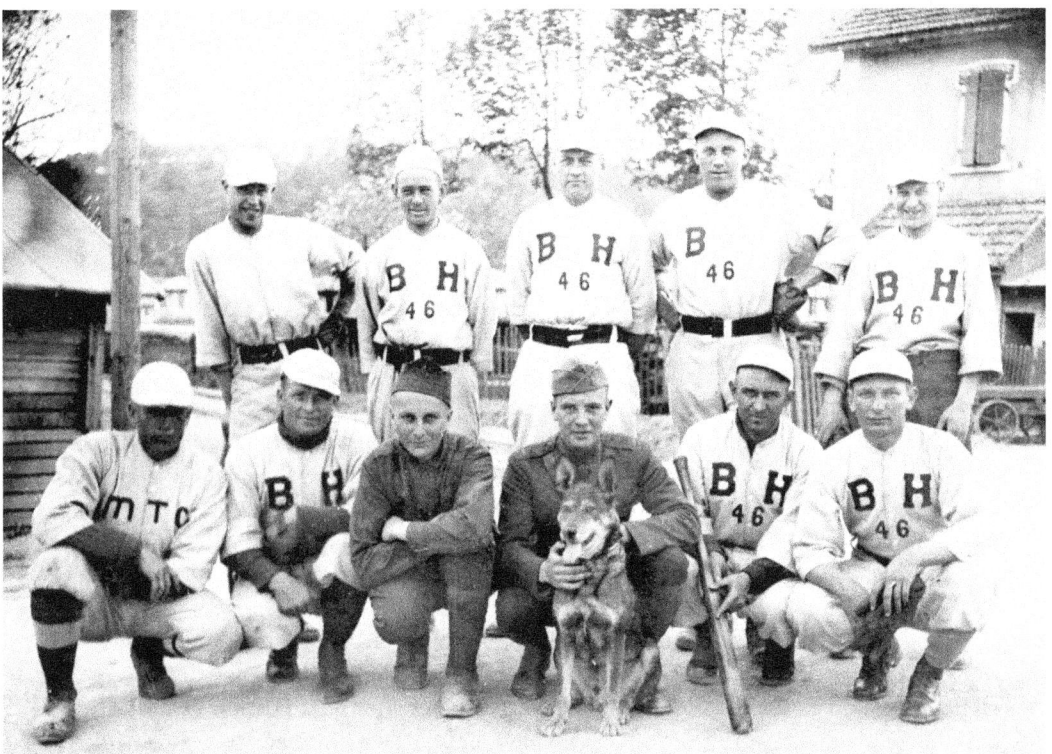

A photograph depicting members of the baseball team of Base Hospital No. 46 at Bazoilles Hospital Center. Presumably, the uniformed soldier holding the dog is the team's director of athletics First Lieutenant Dorwin L. Palmer with manager Private Garret Stelsel to his right (author's collection).

Officer Garrison Hat

This officer garrison hat was made by Charles Coopey, a tailor from Portland, Oregon. It has the name A.S. Rosenfeld written on the inside leather band. Its original owner was First Lieutenant Arthur S. Rosenfeld, Medical Corps, who served with the Medical Department of Base Hospital No. 46.

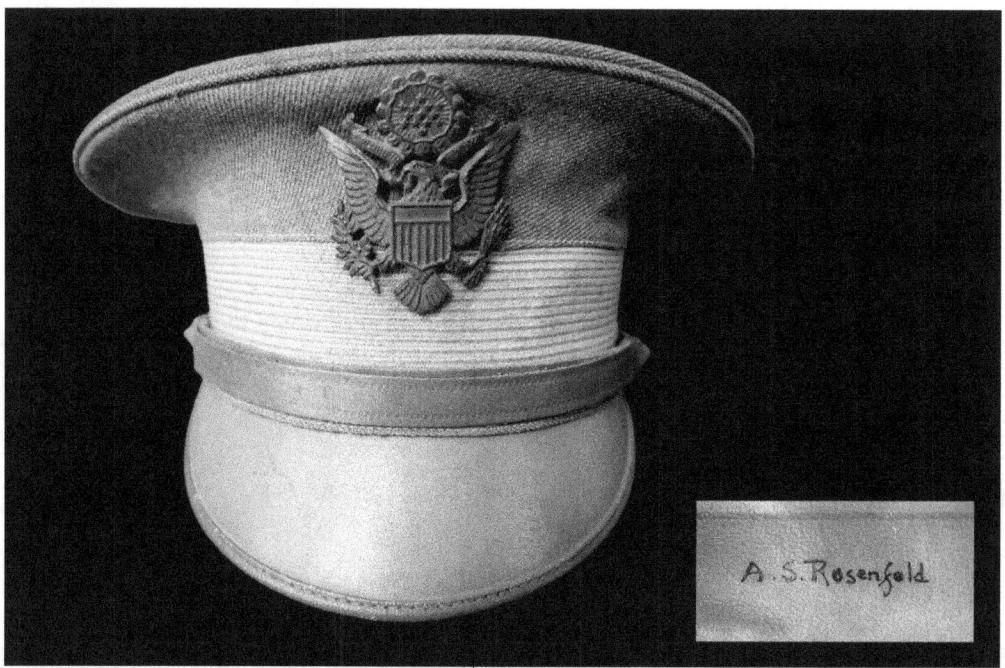

Officer garrison hat of First Lieutenant Arthur S. Rosenfeld who served as receiving officer at Base Hospital No. 46. The inset depicts the name A.S. Rosenfeld written on the inside leather band of the hat (author's collection).

Arthur Samuel Rosenfeld was born on January 28, 1886, in Portland. He graduated from Stanford University, A.B., in 1907 and from Johns Hopkins Medical School in 1911. Subsequently, he became a staff member at the University of Oregon in Portland. On June 20, 1917, Dr. Rosenfeld was among the first staff members named by the Faculty of the Medical School as officers for a base hospital furnished by the University of Oregon. He was commissioned First Lieutenant on September 17, 1917. At Bazoilles Hospital Center, he served as receiving officer in charge of the Receiving and Evacuating Department of Base Hospital No. 46. This department was responsible for the admission, evacuation and transfer of patients, and, therefore, in complete control of the movement of patients.

In general, cases reached Bazoilles Hospital Center in three ways, namely by hospital trains (capacity of 400 to 600 patients), by motor ambulance convoy (capacity of 50 to 60 patients) and as "casuals." The distribution and apportioning of patients to the different base hospitals constituting Bazoilles Hospital Center was directed from a central evacuation office.

In the Receiving and Evacuating Department of Base Hospital No. 46, a permanent staff consisting of five examining officers and five enlisted men was present. Depending

Eleven. Traces of Medical Care at Bazoilles Hospital Center

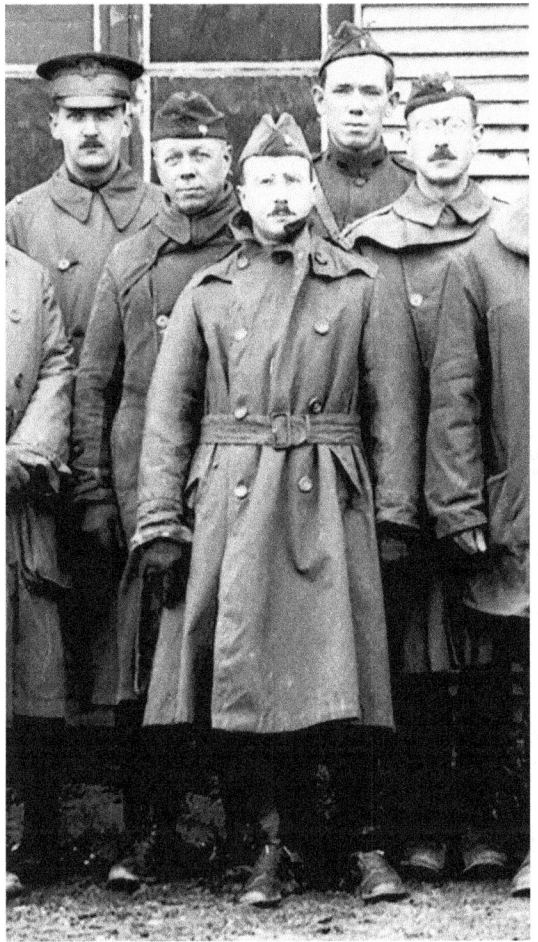

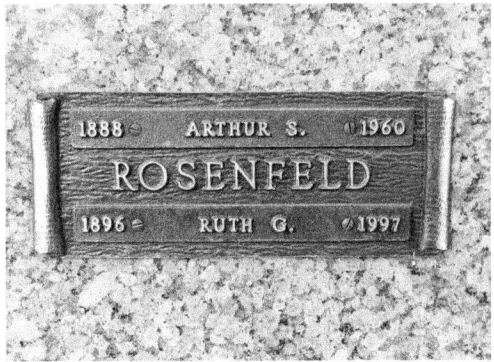

Left: This photograph shows First Lieutenant Arthur S. Rosenfeld in front of other officers of Base Hospital No. 46 at Bazoilles Hospital Center (courtesy Oregon Health & Science University, Portland, Oregon [Historical Collections & Archives, Otis B. Wight Base Hospital 46: Glass Plate Negative Collection, Accession No. 20060-12, box 1]). *Above:* Arthur S. Rosenfeld is interred at Beth Israel Cemetery, Portland, Oregon. The cover plate lists an erroneous year of birth of 1888 (photograph by author).

on the size of an incoming convoy of patients and the number of litter cases, a detail of 20 to 60 men was supplied to support the receiving ward. Patients were registered and given a serial number, undressed, examined, differentiated as to their underlying condition and as to the presence or absence of "cooties" (lice), deloused if necessary, assigned to a ward, bathed and clothed in fresh hospital garments. Their clothes were put in sacks, labeled, sent to the "Cootie Kitchen" for sterilization and, later, put in separate bins in the clothing and effects building. Most of this work was done in the bath house which was joined to the receiving ward by a covered runway. A steady procession of patients entered at one end of the building and left at the other, from where they were conducted to their assigned wards.[11]

Signet Bottles

These oval apothecary bottles were recovered at the former site of Bazoilles Hospital Center. All bottles have a so-called "I inside a diamond" mark on the base indicating that they were produced by the Illinois Glass Company from Alton, Illinois. In order from the smallest to the largest size, the apothecary measures "℥ii," "℥iii" and "℥vi" are embossed at the base of the neck of the bottles. As the ℥ symbol represents fluid ounce (fl. oz.),[12] these marks indicate that the bottles have a volume of two, three and six fl. oz., respectively. These machine-made bottles came in 15 different sizes ranging from ½ to 32 fl. oz. and were sold under the name "Signet." Intact examples and fragments from five different sizes of Signet bottles have been recovered at the former site of Bazoilles Hospital Center.

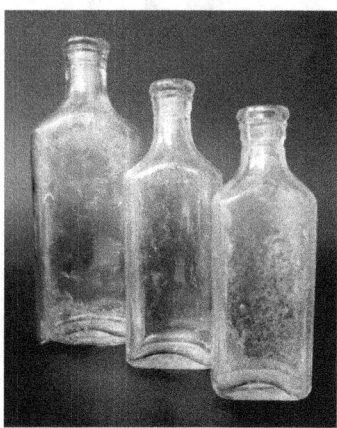
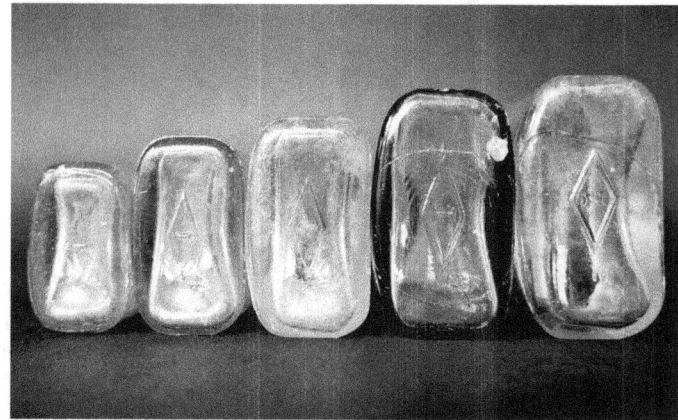

Left: Three oval apothecary bottles recovered at the former site of Bazoilles Hospital Center. These bottles were produced by the Illinois Glass Company and sold under the factory name "Signet" (author's collection). *Right:* The bases of five different sizes of Signet bottles recovered at the former site of Bazoilles Hospital Center. The "I inside a diamond" mark indicates that the bottles were produced by the Illinois Glass Company. The embossed numbers may be mold identification marks for quality control (author's collection). *Below:* Two partially filled Signet bottles are visible on a shelf in the meningitis laboratory of Base Hospital No. 66. Situated at nearby Neufchâteau, this hospital was part of Bazoilles Hospital Center from August 11, 1918, to November 10, 1918 (U.S. National Library of Medicine. Digital Collections. http://resource.nlm.nih.gov/101397756; accessed May 25, 2017).

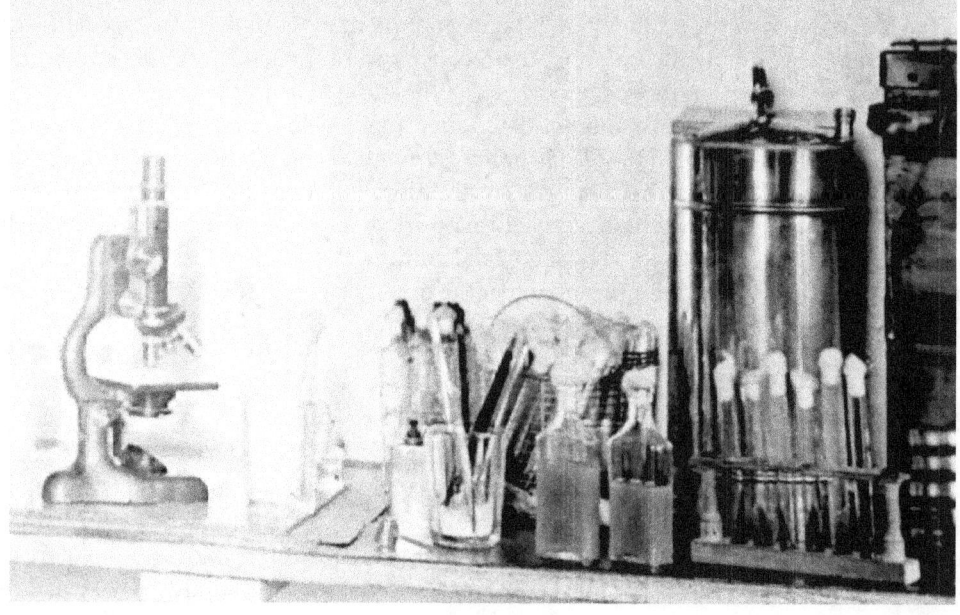

Eleven. Traces of Medical Care at Bazoilles Hospital Center

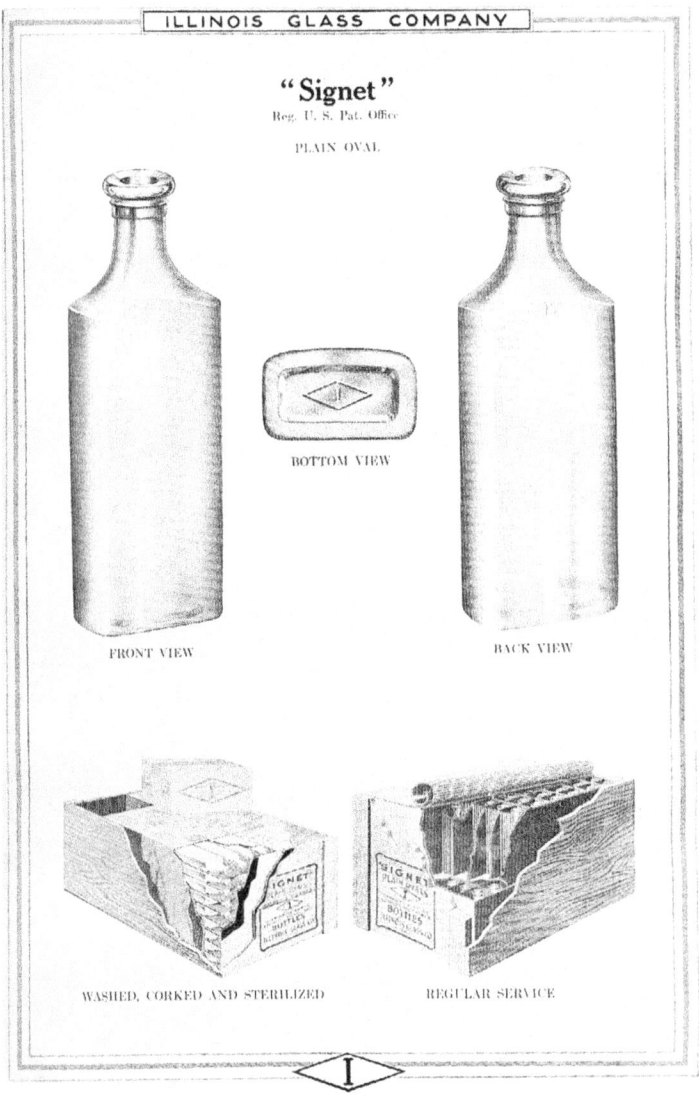

A page from the *1920 Illinois Glass Company Bottle Catalog* depicting the Signet bottle and the method of its packing in cardboard cartons and a wooden shipping case (*Illinois Glass Co. Bottles of Every Description: Diamond Products, General Cataloque "A."* n.p.; n.d.: 17).

The Signet bottle was listed in the *1920 Illinois Glass Company Bottle Catalog*. It was supplied in either "Regular Service" or in "Washed, Corked and Sterilized Service." Although designed principally for prescription purposes, the fact that the bottles could be easily labeled made them also adaptable to other uses. Two fl. oz. Signet bottles were sold in a quantity of 720 (five gross) per wooden shipping case with a list price of U.S. $ 7.75 per gross, three fl. oz. bottles at a quantity of 432 (three gross) per case with a list price of U.S. $ 9.50 per gross and six fl. oz. bottles at a quantity of 288 (2 gross) per case with a list price of U.S. $ 12.25 per gross. The Illinois Glass Company produced hundreds of different bottles used for a multitude of products like medicines, foods, sauces, extracts, flavorings, chemicals, bleach, vinegar and cosmetics.[13]

Report of Death

The National Archives at Kansas City in Kansas City, Missouri, holds 23 reports of death of German prisoners of war who died at Bazoilles Hospital Center from September 30 to November 18, 1918. Many of these men died of wound infections.[14] Deceased German prisoners of war were buried at U.S. Military Cemetery No. 6, the cemetery of Bazoilles Hospital Center, which held 27 German graves on December 17, 1918.[15]

> Base Hospital #42, A.P.O. #731.
> October 14, 1918.
>
> From: Commanding Officer.
>
> To: Commanding Officer, Hospital Center APO #731.
>
> Subject: Report of death.
>
> 1. Private Sebastian Binning, 125th.Infantry, German Prisoner of War, died at Base Hospital #42, at 1.15 A.M., October 14, 1918.
>
> 2. I.Cause of death: GSW,S,right buttock,IA, 9/29/18. Complications: Septicaemia (fulminating gas bacillus)
>
> 3. The remains of the deceased are at the morgue of this hospital awaiting burial. It is requested that the Group Quartermaster, Hospital Center APO #731, be notified so the proper disposition can be made of the remains.
>
> 4. Additional information relative to the deceased is furnished herewith: Age- 36yrs. Race-White. Service- 3/12. Nativity-Germany. Religion: Catholic.
>
> 5. The Quartermaster, Base Hospital #42, has been notified to this effect.
>
> A.C.Harrison,
> Lt.Col.,M.C.,U.S.A.
> Commanding.

Report of death of *Leutnant* Sebastian Binnig who served with *Württembergische Landwehr-Infanterie-Regiment Nr. 120*. Binnig died on October 14, 1918, as a German prisoner of war at Base Hospital No. 42 of septicemia (blood poisoning) and gas gangrene infection complicating a gunshot wound (GSW) sustained in action (IA) on October 1, 1918. The family name, rank, unit and date of injury on this report of death are inconsistent with other sources and presumably inaccurate (National Archives at Kansas City, Kansas City, Missouri [Record Group 120: Records of the American Expeditionary Forces (World War I), 1848–1942, Correspondence of the Hospital Center at Bazoilles, 1918–1919, National Archives Identifier 6636481, box 2 folder 383.6 Enemy Prisoners of War]).

Among the German prisoners of war who died at Bazoilles-sur-Meuse was *Leutnant* (Lieutenant) Sebastian Binnig from Ellwangen an der Jagst, Germany. Sebastian Binnig served with the *Württembergische Landwehr-Infanterie-Regiment Nr. 120*. He received a gunshot wound in the right buttock on October 1, 1918, during an American tank attack near Apremont amid the first phase of the Meuse-Argonne Offensive. After being captured by the U.S. Army, he was transported to Bazoilles Hospital Center and admitted to Base Hospital No. 42. Sebastian Binnig died, aged 36, on October 14, 1918, of septicemia (blood poisoning) and gas gangrene infection of his wound. On October 16, he was buried in grave No. 13 of the German section of the hospital's cemetery. He left a four-month-old son without a father.[16]

After the war, the remains of Sebastian Binnig were exhumed and re-buried at the nearby *Cimetière Militaire de Neufchâteau* (Military Cemetery of Neufchâteau), where a total of 120 German soldiers are resting.

A Nurse's Personal Items

The National World War I Museum and Memorial in Kansas City, Missouri, holds personal items of Nurse Ruth Regina Shields. In September 1917, Nurse Shields graduated from St. Vincent's Hospital Training School in Portland, Oregon. She then joined the American Red Cross, which at that time was a reserve for the Army Nurse Corps. Nurse Shields volunteered for overseas duty and was assigned to Base Hospital No. 46. She arrived at Bazoilles Hospital Center on July 16, 1918.

In her letters home, she wrote "Everything is going so smoothly for a

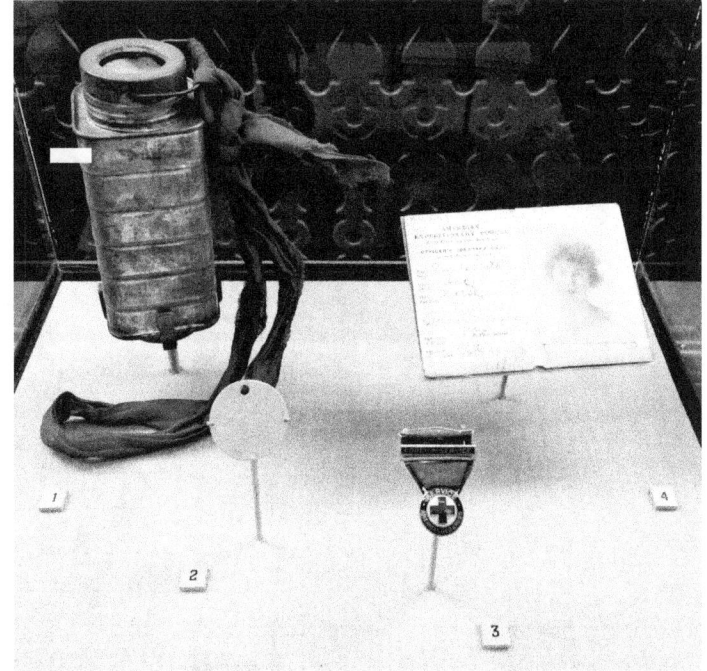

Top: Headstone of the current grave of *Leutnant* Sebastian Binnig at the *Cimetière Militaire de Neufchâteau* (Military Cemetery of Neufchâteau). German war graves are maintained by the *Volksbund Deutsche Kriegsgräberfürsorge e.V.*, Kassel, Germany (photograph by author). *Bottom:* In November 2016, various personal items of Nurse Ruth R. Shields, who had been assigned to Base Hospital No. 46, were on display in the Memory Hall of the National World War I Museum and Memorial: her identification tag, identity card, condiment can (to transport coffee, sugar and salt) and Red Cross badge for overseas service (courtesy the National World War I Museum and Memorial, Kansas City, Missouri [photograph by author]).

new place. We opened under some difficulties ... but now we can accommodate 1900 patients. Each ward is in a long frame building with 50 beds. Another nurse and I am in the officer's ward and we have 30 of these young heroes just now. My admiration for them grows deeper each day when I see such grit and pluck shown."[17]

In November 2016, various of Nurse Shields' personal items were on display in the Memory Hall of the National World War I Museum and Memorial: her identification tag, identity card, condiment can (to transport coffee, sugar and salt) and Red Cross badge for overseas service.[18]

Victims of Disease

Within the Meuse-Argonne American Cemetery at Romagne-sous-Montfaucon rest the largest number of American military dead in Europe, a total of 14,246 men and women. Most of those buried lost their lives during the Meuse-Argonne Offensive.[19] The Meuse-Argonne American Cemetery is also the final resting place of two hospital staff members of Bazoilles Hospital Center who died during its period of operation.

Army Nurse Charlotte A. Cox from Baltimore, Maryland, served with Base Hospital

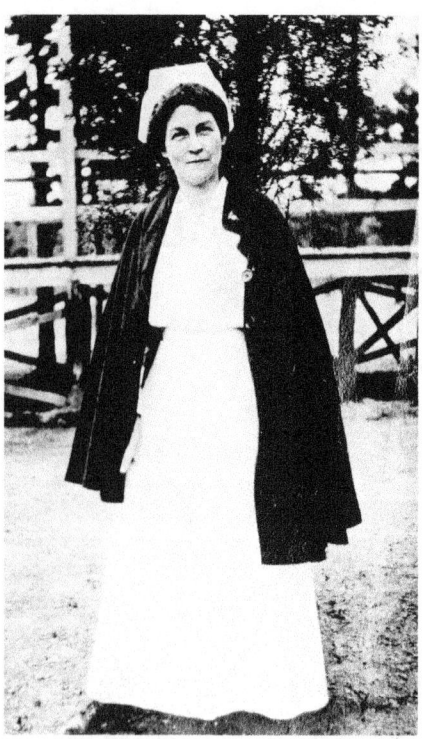
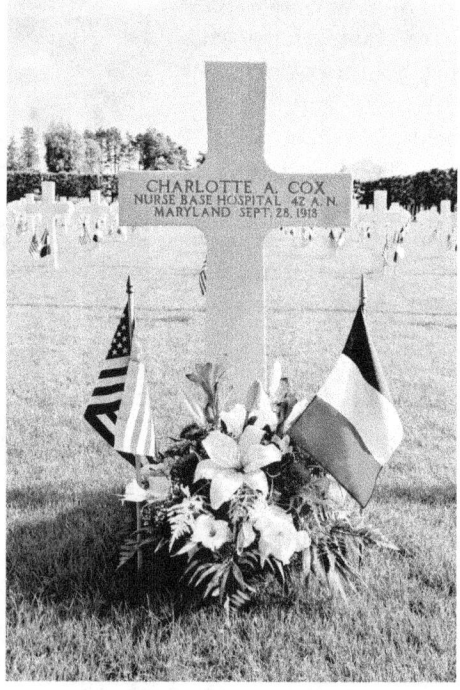

Left: Nurse Charlotte A. Cox from Baltimore, Maryland, served with Base Hospital No. 42. She died on September 28, 1918, of dysentery (Library of Congress). *Right:* Headstone of the grave of Nurse Charlotte A. Cox at the Meuse-Argonne American Cemetery in Romagne-sous-Montfaucon. This picture was taken on May 28, 2017, when all headstones were decorated with miniature U.S. and French flags on the occasion of the annual Memorial Day Ceremony (courtesy American Battle Monuments Commission [Overseas Operations Office, Paris, France; photograph by Maarten Otte, Nantillois, France]).

No. 42. The day before she was to be sent to an evacuation hospital at the front, she fell ill with dysentery. She did not recover and died, aged 37, on September 28, 1918. She was buried with military honors in U.S. Military Cemetery No. 6 at Bazoilles Hospital Center on September 30.[20] Nurse Cox was re-buried at the Meuse-Argonne American Cemetery in Plot F, Row 1, Grave 25.[21] Private First Class Guy Harley Criss from Little Birch, West Virginia, served with Base Hospital No. 60. He died of an unspecified disease, aged 22, on October 17, 1918, and is buried at the Meuse-Argonne American Cemetery in Plot C, Row 39, Grave 21.[22]

The American Battle Monuments Commission operates and maintains 25 American cemeteries and 26 memorials, monuments and markers in 16 countries.

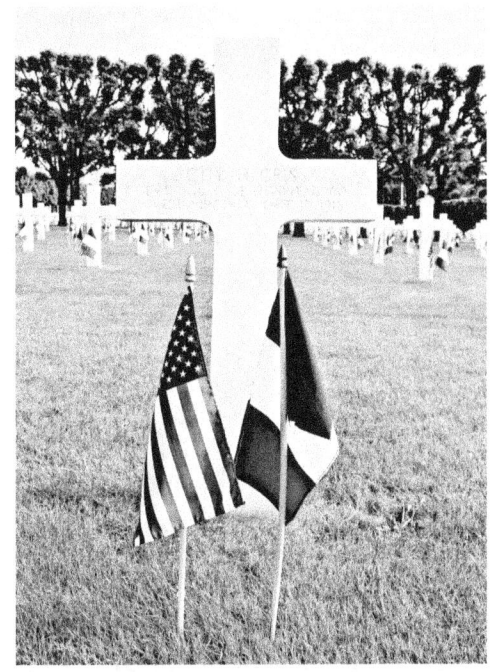

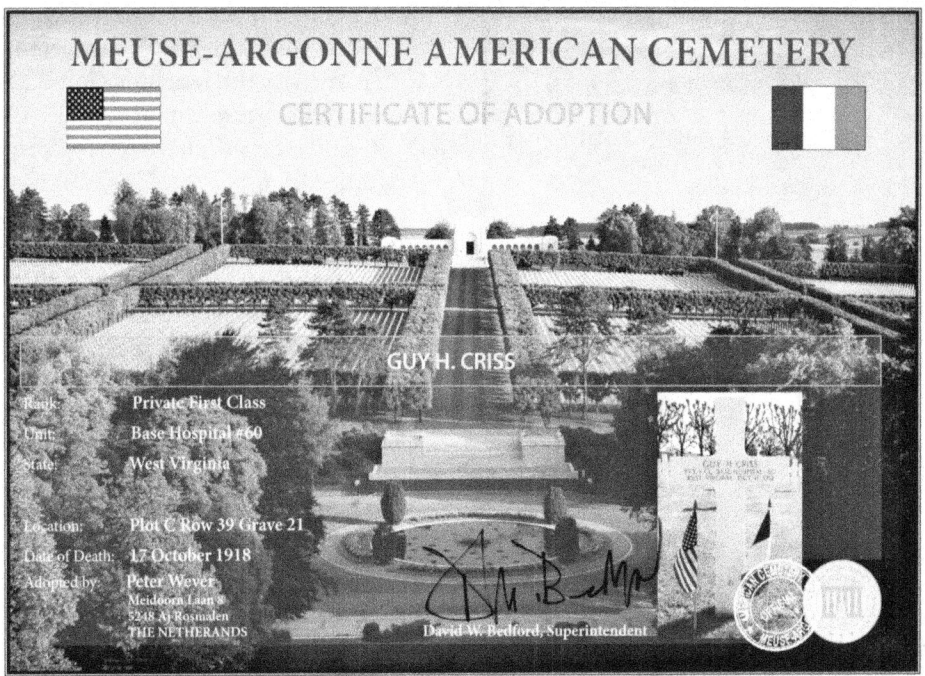

Top: Headstone of the grave of Private First Class Guy H. Criss at the Meuse-Argonne American Cemetery in Romagne-sous-Montfaucon. This picture was taken on May 28, 2017, on the occasion of the annual Memorial Day Ceremony (courtesy American Battle Monuments Commission [Overseas Operations Office, Paris, France; photograph by Maarten Otte, Nantillois, France]). *Bottom:* Certificate of Adoption of the grave of Private First Class Guy H. Criss issued by the Meuse-Argonne American Cemetery to the author on June 8, 2017 (author's collection).

The land on which the Meuse-Argonne American Cemetery rests has been granted free use by the French government as a permanent burial ground in perpetuity without charge or taxation.[23]

The Convalescent Entertainers

The Connecticut State Library in Hartford, Connecticut, holds a publicity poster for The Convalescent Entertainers issued by the American Young Men's Christian Association (Y.M.C.A.) in Paris, France.[24] The Convalescent Entertainers were promoted as "a group of eleven privates organized while all its members were patients in Base Hospital No. 46 at Bazoilles."[25] In reality, only seven of its members were convalescent, as the other four worked in Base Hospitals Nos. 18 (accordionist Valentino Gazzola, also known under the stage name Val Marconi, and Conrad L. "Jack" Wayman) and 46 (opera singer Victor M.W. Orr and singer and entertainer Charles W. Bauer).[26] Moreover, its members included a sergeant and a corporal.[27]

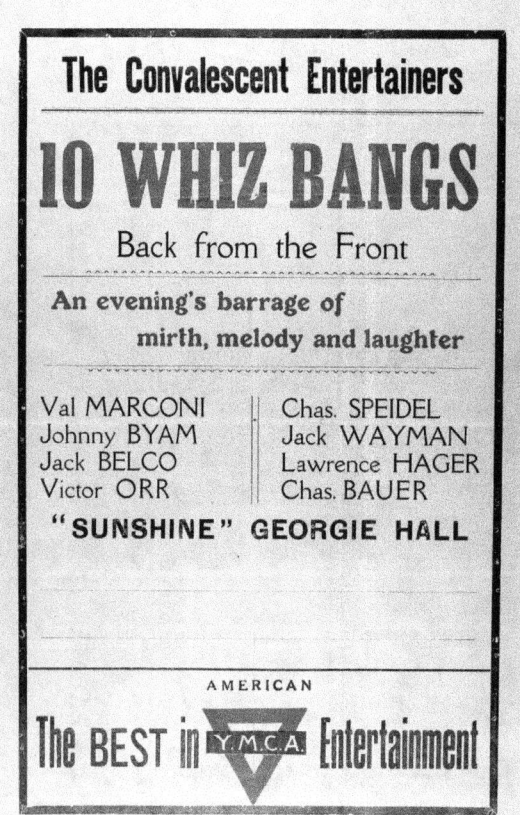

One of the wounded men in The Convalescent Entertainers was Private Lawrence Thomas Hager from Danbury, Connecticut, who worked as an actor and singer before the war. He was inducted into service on March 29, 1918, and went overseas while assigned to Company A, 320th Machine Gun Battalion, 82nd Division. On October 15, 1918, during the second phase of the Meuse-Argonne Offensive, he received shrapnel wounds during fighting near the village of Grandpré. Later, he stated: I "had my forehead and part of chin blown off." He made his way to a dressing station, received first aid and was placed on a Red Cross train to Bazoilles Hospital Center, where he was admitted to Base Hospital No. 46 on October 16.[28] His face was patched up with the eyebrow of a dead soldier, grafted above his right eye, and two silver plates supporting his forehead bone and replacing his chinbone.[29]

During his convalescence at Base Hospital No. 46, Lawrence Hager met accordionist Val Marconi, who spent his spare time playing for the sick and

Publicity poster for The Convalescent Entertainers issued by the American Young Men's Christian Association in Paris, France. The poster lists nine names of the original eleven members of the company (Ancestry. Connecticut, Military Questionnaires, 1919–1920 for Lawrence Thomas Hager. https://www.ancestry.com; accessed June 26, 2017).

Eleven. Traces of Medical Care at Bazoilles Hospital Center   145

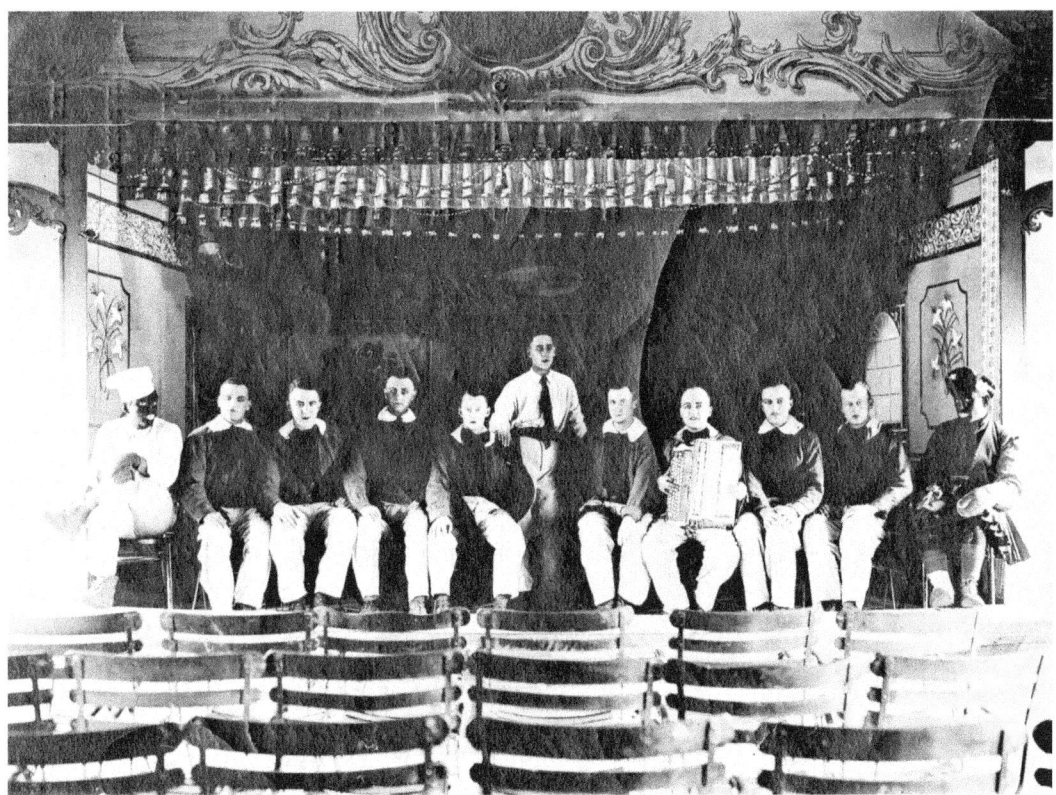

Group photograph portraying the eleven members of The Convalescent Entertainers at the Red Cross Recreation Hut of Base Hospital No. 46. From left to right: "Sunshine" George H. Hall, Lawrence T. Hager, Mayne W. McKee, Charles W. Bauer, Conrad L. "Jack" Wayman, Charles A. Speidel, Victor M.W. Orr, Valentino Gazzola (stage name Val Marconi), John W. Byam, John J. "Jack" Belco and Bert Bowman (courtesy Oregon Health & Science University, Portland, Oregon [Historical Collections & Archives, Grace Phelps Papers, Accession No. 20100-05, box 2 folder 3]).

wounded. The two men had known each other professionally in the United States. Soon, it was learned that other well-known professional entertainers were present at Bazoilles Hospital Center. It was then decided to give a vaudeville show (stage entertainment consisting of various acts) to entertain the patients of Base Hospital No. 46.[30]

After several weeks of rehearsing, the first shows were put on at the Personnel Club (Red Cross Recreation Hut) of Base Hospital No. 46 and at the Y.M.C.A.[31] The program consisted of sentimental and patriotic songs, dancing, blackface performances and general jazz added "to give zest."[32] The show was a tremendous hit. Additional performances under the auspices of the Y.M.C.A. were given in the area. The Y.M.C.A made a request to General Headquarters that the men should be detached so "all the boys in France might see their performance."[33] Their four-month tour brought them to hospitals, theaters, rest camps, embarkation camps and places like Aix-les-Bains, Chamonix and Grenoble. Their show was witnessed by members of royalty of Romania and Spain. In Monte Carlo, they played at the Casino for the Prince of Monaco.[34] After touring France, they played at the *Théâtre des Champs-Élysées* in Paris on 17, 18 and April 19, 1919, together with the Army Ambulance Service Jazz Band, as well as in other Paris centers and hospitals.[35]

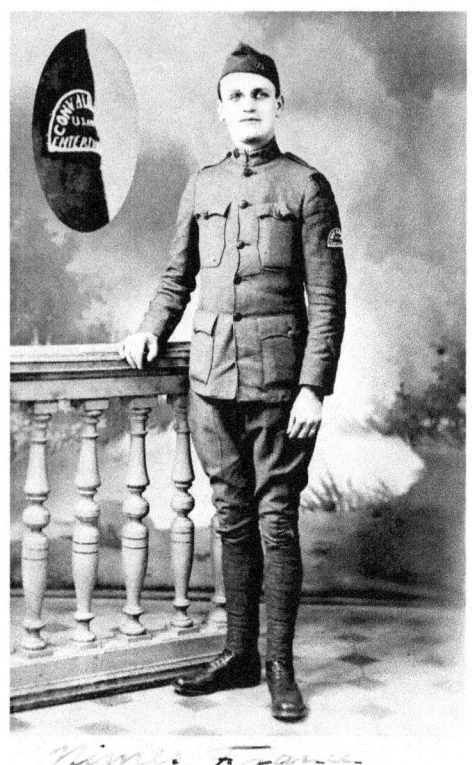

The Convalescent Entertainers were reportedly the hit of the Y.M.C.A.'s theatrical season overseas and the most popular of all the groups of hospital entertainers employed.[36] On May 11, 1919, the group set sail for the United States on board the USS *Artemis* bringing an end to its existence.[37]

Thanksgiving Dinner Menu

In 1918, Thanksgiving Day was celebrated on Thursday, November 28. This Thanksgiving Dinner menu belonged to Nurse Gertrude Hayden Bowling from Baltimore, Maryland,[38] who served with Base Hospital No. 18. On July 15, 1918, Nurse Bowling was temporarily detached to the front as part of a so-called "shock team." This team was composed of a medical officer, two nurses and two privates.[39] Its task was to improve the condition of the severely wounded to such an extent that operation would be possible.[40] To compensate for the loss of blood, salt solutions and blood transfusions were given. The team was sleeping so near to the front that it was at times necessary to take refuge in dugouts.[41] For her actions, Nurse Bowling was cited for bravery and coolness.[42]

Thanksgiving Day at Bazoilles Hospital Center was celebrated with sumptuous meals at the different base hospitals. At Base Hospital No. 46, preparation of the Thanksgiving Dinner started the day before with two shifts of cooks and it was served at 12.30 on Thanksgiving Day. It was stated that the memory of that dinner would always bring a smile to the lips of the hospital's personnel.[43] Nurse Bowling's Thanksgiving

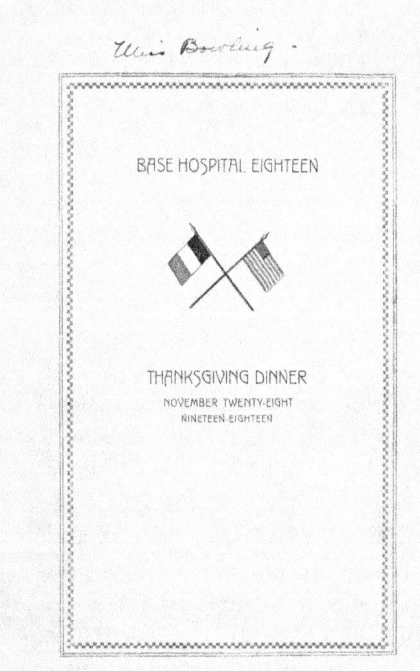

Top: A studio photograph of Private Lawrence T. Hager taken in southern France while he was touring with The Convalescent Entertainers. The handwritten caption reads: "Nimes, France March 15, 1919." The inset depicts the patch on the left sleeve of his uniform which reads "Convalescent Entertainers U.S. Army" (Ancestry. Connecticut, Military Questionnaires, 1919–1920 for Lawrence Thomas Hager. https://www.ancestry.com; accessed June 26, 2017). *Bottom:* Thanksgiving Dinner menu of Nurse Gertrude H. Bowling of Base Hospital No. 18. The menu is signed "Miss Bowling" (author's collection).

Dinner menu lists the abundance of food served at Base Hospital No. 18: sardines, celery, herring, bologna, olives, cold slaw, homemade pickles, minced tenderloin of beef, fresh mushrooms, Madeira sauce, mashed potatoes, Brussels sprouts, roasted spring turkey, dressing and gravy, way-down south sweet potatoes, cauliflower, hollandaise, lettuce salad, plum pudding, hard sauce, assorted fruits, nuts, demi-tasse [half the size of a full coffee cup], beer, cigars and cigarettes. Clearly, every effort was taken to celebrate cherished American traditions despite difficult conditions and being far from home.[44]

Songbook for Soldiers and Sailors

This songbook was issued by the Commissions on Training Camp Activities of the Army and Navy Departments.[45] It came from the estate of Nurse Eleanor Donaldson,[46] who was appointed temporary chief nurse of Base Hospital No. 46 on February 1, 1919. On that date, the former hospital's Chief Nurse Grace Phelps was transferred to head the nursing work at Base Hospital No. 81.[47] Base Hospital No. 46 had ceased operation already on January 19, while Base Hospital No. 81 remained functioning until March 31.[48]

Although the Base Hospital No. 46 unit sailed for the U.S. from St. Nazaire on April 20,[49] the hospital's nurses departed for New York from Brest already on April 9 under the command of Major William H. Skene,

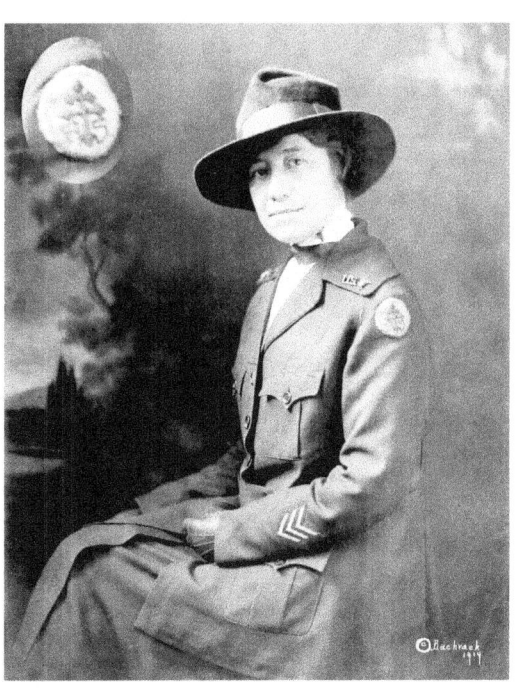

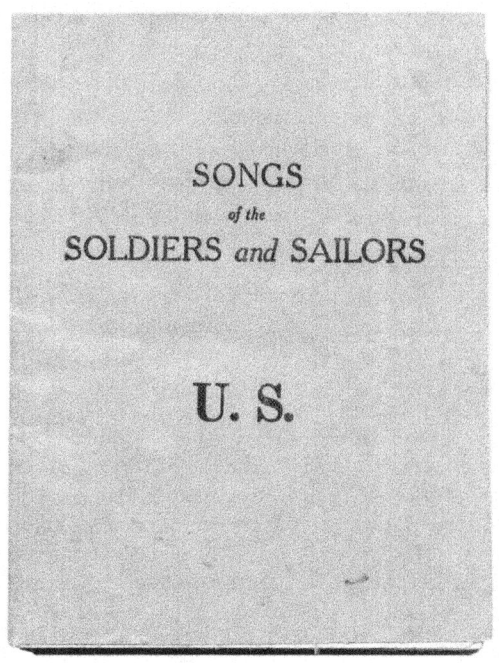

Top: A 1919-dated studio photograph of Nurse Gertrude H. Bowling who was temporarily detached from Base Hospital No. 18 to serve near the front as part of a shock team. The inset depicts her shoulder patch with Advance Section, Services of Supply insignia, which consisted of the French cross of Lorraine, flanked by the initials "A" and "S" in red on a white wool background surrounded by a blue ring (Ancestry. U.S., American Red Cross Nurse Files, 1916–1959 for Gertrude Hayden Bowling. https://www.ancestry.com; accessed March 15, 2018). *Bottom:* This songbook for soldiers and sailors belonged to Nurse Eleanor Donaldson, who was appointed temporary chief nurse of Base Hospital No. 46 at Bazoilles Hospital Center on February 1, 1919 (author's collection; generously donated by Greg Donaldson, Mountain View, California).

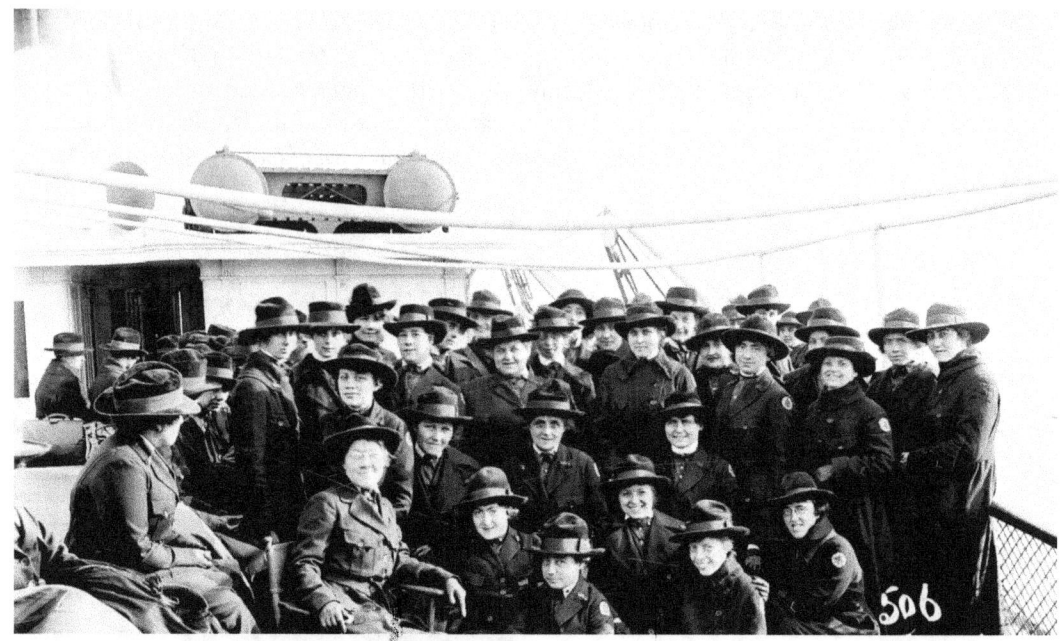

A picture of the nurses of Base Hospital No. 46 on their way home from Brest to New York on board of the ship *Kaiserin Auguste Victoria*. Chief Nurse Donaldson is seated centrally amidst the other nurses (courtesy Oregon Health & Science University, Portland, Oregon [Historical Collections & Archives, Eleanor Donaldson Papers, Accession No. 20080-20, Oversized Photographic Prints]).

Assistant Chief of the Surgical Department.[50] An undated photo shows Chief Nurse Donaldson on board ship seated centrally amidst the other nurses of Base Hospital No. 46. This picture was taken during the trip home to the U.S. because several nurses are wearing War Service Chevrons ("overseas stripes") on the sleeves of their coats, with each stripe denoting a six month period of service in the Zone of the Advance.[51] Furthermore, the nurses are wearing shoulder patches with the so-called Advance Section, Services of Supply insignia, which consisted of the French cross of Lorraine, flanked by the initials "A" and "S" in red on a white wool background surrounded by a blue ring.[52]

Chief Nurse Donaldson authored a two-page account titled *Our Trip Home* in which she voiced her frustration with the way the nurses were treated during the transatlantic journey.

> At five we were on board ship [the German ship *Kaiserin Auguste Victoria* which had been turned over to the British after the war][53] in the harbor at Brest. At first we thought a mistake had been made, so terribly dirty and unprepared were our quarters.... Our quarters were decks down and in the sick room[.They] were unswept [with] the waste water of the former occupant still in their recepticles. Fortunately the notices for venereal diseases ... were still posted in bath and toilet, [so] one of the chief nurses sent to Brest for lysol and took personal charge of the cleaning. Major W.H. Skene still in the belief that it was a mistake and not of Uncle Sams.... some of us protested to those in command and were promptly told that this was military law, nurses had no standing in the army and etc. It was some time before we accepted our fate, although we set to work at once to clean things up. These girls who had worked gladly and uncomplainingly and without adequate rest, when the work was required felt the injustice keenly, they still do.[54]

Distinguished Service Medal

This Distinguished Service Medal belonged to Colonel Elmer Anderson Dean, who was born in Centerville, Tennessee, on August 18, 1871. He graduated with a medical degree from the University of Pennsylvania on June 8, 1898.[55] That same year, he accepted a position as assistant surgeon in the U.S. Army.[56] In 1900, during the Philippine-American War (1899–1902), he was sent to the Philippine Islands.[57] His name is also on the roll for the Mexican Border Service Medal,[58] indicating he performed military service on the U.S.-Mexico border between January 1, 1916, and April 6, 1917, when the U.S. was on the verge of war with Mexico.[59] On May 15, 1917, shortly after the United States' declaration of war on Germany, Dean rose to the rank of colonel.[60] As its Commanding Officer from November 21, 1917, to June 15, 1918, he took Base Hospital No. 30 over to France, where it was stationed at the small town of Royat in the Auvergne Mountains. The hospital received its first patients on June 12.[61] Shortly thereafter, Colonel Dean was transferred to Bazoilles-sur-Meuse, where he arrived on June 30. There, he became Commanding Officer of Bazoilles Hospital Center, which started functioning on July 1.[62]

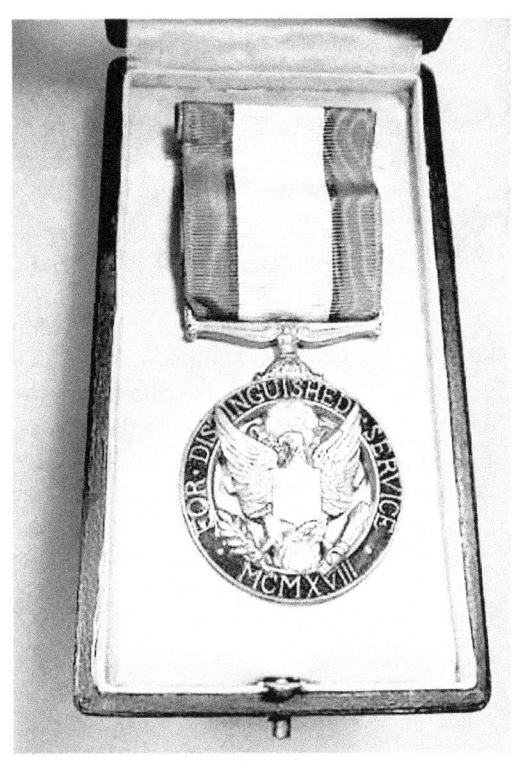

Boxed Distinguished Service Medal of Colonel Elmer A. Dean, who was Commanding Officer of Bazoilles Hospital Center (courtesy Dave Sleeper, Bangor, Maine [private collection]).

After the war, on September 19, 1919, Colonel Dean received the Distinguished Service Medal (edge number 1767), which is awarded for exceptionally meritorious and distinguished services, in a position of great responsibility.[63] His citation reads as follows.

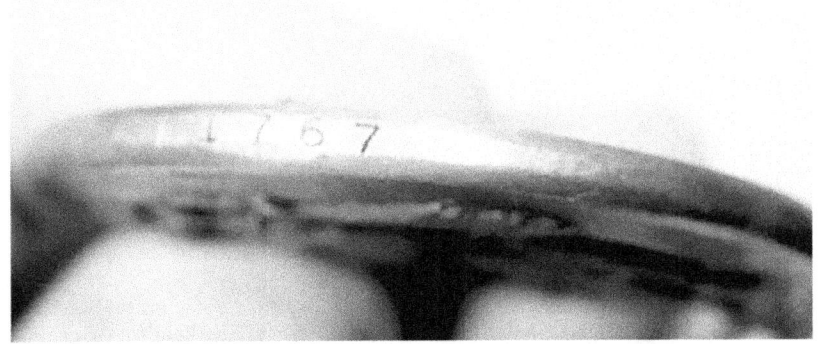

Colonel Elmer A. Dean's Distinguished Service Medal bears the edge number 1767 (courtesy Dave Sleeper, Bangor, Maine [private collection]).

He came to France with a base hospital unit, which he established. Later he organized and commanded the first large hospital center at Bazoilles. The success of this center in caring for a large number of sick and wounded was due in a large measure to his high professional attainments, zeal, and extraordinary executive ability.[64]

Colonel Dean died on December 21, 1965, and is buried in Arlington National Cemetery in Arlington, Virginia. Pictures of his Distinguished Service Medal and its box were posted in February 2013 on usmilitariaforum.com.[65]

United States Military Cemetery No. 6

The Historical Collections & Archives of the Oregon Health & Science University in Portland, Oregon, holds a photo of U.S. Military Cemetery No. 6 at Bazoilles Hospital Center. The cemetery was situated on the west bank of the Meuse River in a field located just north of Base Hospital No. 46. It was capable of containing 1932 graves.[66] In the written history of Base Hospital No. 46, Chief Nurse Eleanor Donaldson described the three roads on which soldiers went to and from Bazoilles Hospital Center, the first being the motorway and the second the railroad. "The third road ran just a few yards from our tent door, with the river beyond–the last road of all, for the boys we left in France. It was

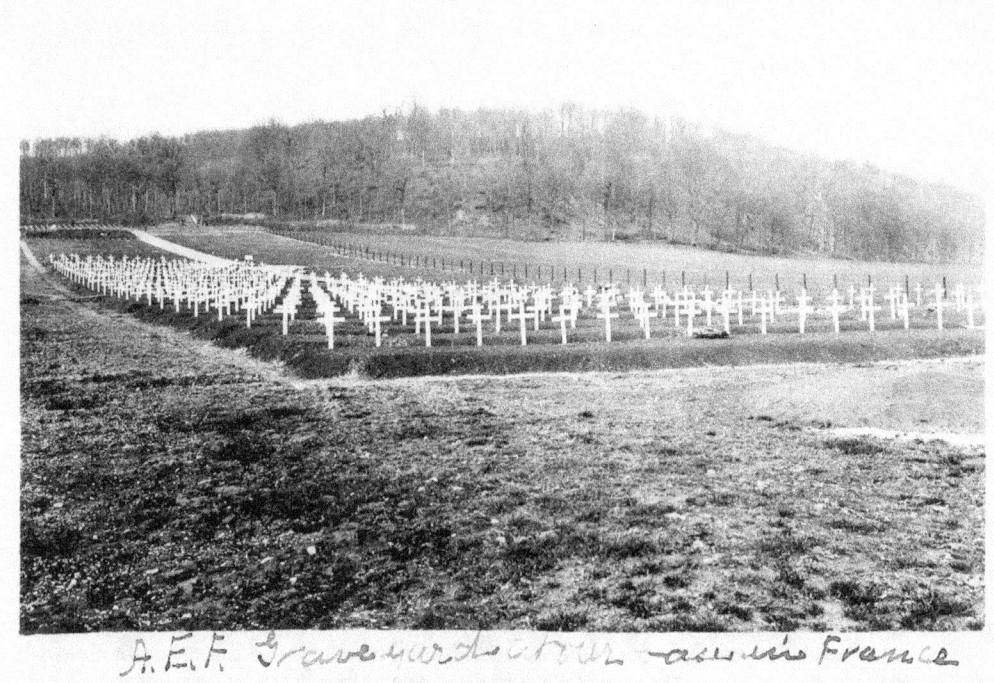

View toward U.S. Military Cemetery No. 6 at Bazoilles Hospital Center on the west bank of the Meuse River in a field located just north of Base Hospital No. 46. The handwritten caption reads: "A.E.F. Graveyard at our base in France" (courtesy Oregon Health & Science University, Portland, Oregon [Historical Collections & Archives, Eleanor Donaldson Papers, Accession No. 20080-20, box 1 folder 6 Photographic prints-Base Hospital 46]).

a short road, ending in a plot at the foot of the hill where the sun's last light touched the white crosses "row on row.""[67]

A little over five months after its opening, on December 17, 1918, nine officers, four nurses, 486 soldiers and 27 German prisoners of war were buried at U.S. Military Cemetery No. 6 (in total 526 burials).[68] Presumably, the cemetery provided a grave for most of the 850 deaths at Bazoilles Hospital Center, while additional graves might have been occupied by fatalities from accidents or executions. Indeed, Sergeant Basil L. Kiste, Unit No. 308, Motor Repair Department, died from drowning on February 15, 1919, and was buried in grave No. 856.[69]

Somewhat macabre, a memorandum issued January 2, 1919, requested all base hospital commanders to notify any proposed burials to Chaplain Thomas A. Dinan of Base Hospital No. 46, giving date and hour of each case. The flooded condition of the cemetery by water from the Meuse River made it necessary to have the grave detail pump the water from each grave before it could be used. But it was recognized that the water could not be permanently kept out, until something like a dike was made.[70] A different solution for the flooding problem was found, however. Photos of the cemetery indicate that at some point graves in higher ground at the opposite end of the field were used for burials. The Appendix shows that these graves, which had numbers in the 900s and 800s and were occupied in descending order, were used from January 1919 onwards.

Around January 1921,[71] the bodies buried at Bazoilles-sur-Meuse were exhumed for re-burial in the United States or at the Meuse-Argonne American Cemetery at Romagne-

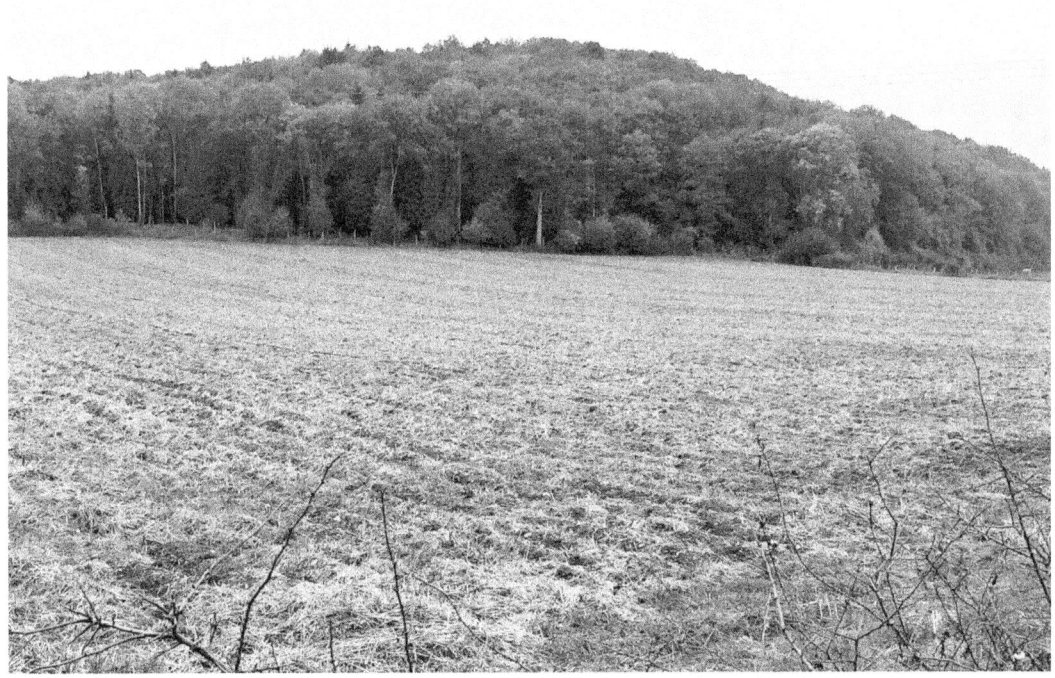

Present-day view of the field where U.S. Military Cemetery No. 6 was situated. Today, nothing bears witness to the one-time presence of the cemetery (photograph by author).

sous-Montfaucon. Today, nothing in the small village of Bazoilles-sur-Meuse bears witness to the presence of Bazoilles Hospital Center or U.S. Military Cemetery No. 6. A small monument next to the church with the names of nine local Frenchmen who gave their life is the sole remembrance of the Great War.

A Mother's Grief

Nettie Graves watched her only son leave for the war. Delbert Dee Graves served with Company H, 351st Infantry, 88th Division. The 88th Division did not participate as a whole in the major offensives and suffered only a small number of battle casualties.[72] Yet, Nettie Graves did not see her son again. Delbert Graves was admitted to Base Hospital No. 18 on December 5, 1918, with scarlet fever. He died, aged 27,[73] on December 12 and was buried in grave No. 422 of U.S. Military Cemetery No. 6 at Bazoilles Hospital Center. As reports kept surfacing that Delbert was seen after this time, the family was left with both anxiety and hope. Military investigations confirmed his death in April 1919. His body was exhumed and transported back to the United States in 1921. He was re-buried with full military honors in his hometown Carthage, South Dakota, with the Delbert Graves Post of the American Legion in charge of the funeral services.

The death of her son Delbert affected the remainder of Nettie Graves' life. In the 1990s, a family member coincidentally found a piece of paper in one of Delbert's childhood books, undisturbed until its discovery.[74] On the paper, the following poem was typed.

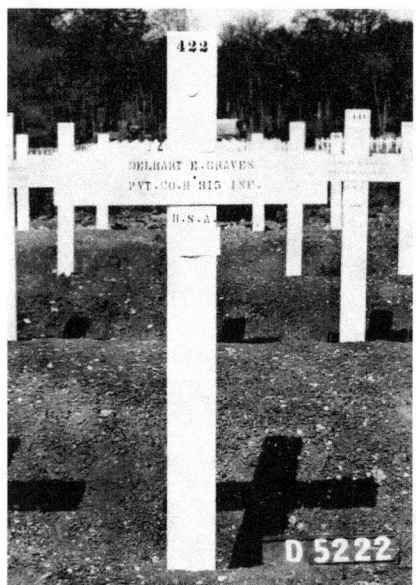

Left: The grave marker of Private Delbert D. Graves at U.S. Military Cemetery No. 6 at Bazoilles Hospital Center where he was buried in grave No 422 (courtesy Karen Seeman, Rochester, Minnesota [private collection]). *Right:* Nettie Graves kept this piece of paper in one of the childhood books of her son Delbert D. Graves who died from scarlet fever at Base Hospital No. 18. It remained undisturbed until the 1990s when it was coincidentally discovered by a family member (courtesy Don Knutz, Las Vegas, Nevada [private collection]).

Eleven. Traces of Medical Care at Bazoilles Hospital Center

IN LOVING MEMORY

In loving memory of our dear son and brother
and nephew, Delbert Dee Graves. who departed from
this life in the hospital in France, ten years ago
the fifth day of December 1918, In our hearts there
comes a longing,
If you only could come home, Friends may think
we have forgotten, when at times they see xx us smile,
But they little know the heart aches that our
smiles hide all the while, Sweet and peaceful be
thy rest, Forget you, we can never; God called
thee, he knows best, His will be done forever.
His loving Father, Mother, Sisters,
Nephews, and Neice,
Mother

Appendix

Unofficial List (Incomplete) of American Servicemen and Women Who Died at Bazoilles Hospital Center and/or Were Buried at U.S. Military Cemetery No. 6 from July 1, 1918, to April 30, 1919

156　　　　　　　　　　Appendix: Servicemen and Women Who Died

Date of Death	Name	Residence	Rank	Unit	Cause of Death	Hospital Unit	Grave Number at U.S. Military Cemetery No. 6	Grave Location at Meuse-Argonne American Cemetery
7/13/18	Charles E. Chambers	Philadelphia, PA	PVT	12th Co, 301st Stevedore Regt	execution			Plot E, Row 26, Grave 9
7/23/18	Frederick P. Taggart	Whittier, CA	SGT	5th Reg USMC, 2nd Div	wounds (gsw)		11	Plot D, Row 41, Grave 5
7/25/18	William F. Coale	Baltimore, MD	PVT	BH No. 42, Medical Dept	appendicitis			
7/29/18	Albert P. Kuttig	Lancaster, OH	SGT	Co L, 166th Inf, 42nd Div	wounds (shell)	BH No. 116		
8/6/18	Arthur F. Harris Jr.	Louisville, KY	1LT	341st Machine Gun Batt, 89th Div	accidental injuries	BH No. 18		
8/11/18	Harry V. Bossard	Papillion, NE	CPL	Co C, 314th Field Signal Batt, 89th Div	gassed	BH No. 116		Plot B, Row 38, Grave 36
8/13/18	Arthur W. Goecks	Windsor, WI	PVT	Co A, 355th Inf, 89th Div	gassed	BH No. 116		
8/13/18	Edgar W. Sykes	South Groveland, MA	CPL	Hdqrs Co, 101st Inf, 26th Div	wounds	BH No. 116		Plot C, Row 38, Grave 2
9/2/18	Henry B. Hall	Michigan	CPL	Co D, 125th Inf, 32nd Div	wounds	BH No. 18		Plot B, Row 41, Grave 15
9/10/18	Roy L. Heimbaugh	Akron, OH	PVT	101st Inf, 26th Div	pneumonia	BH No. 66		
9/13/18	John G. Van Dyke	Prairie View, KS	PVT	Co C, 314th, Engineers 89th Div	pneumonia	BH No. 116	87	
9/14/18	Charles E. Rice	Kendallville, IN	Cook	Co E, 22nd Engineers	pneumonia	BH No. 116		Plot E, Row 25, Grave 14
9/17/18	Norene M. Royer	Winchester, ID	Nurse	BH No. 46, Army Nurse Corps	influenza and pneumonia			
9/17/18	Nicholas L. Tilney	Orange, NJ	CPT(civ)	American Red Cross	pneumonia			Plot F, Row 1, Grave 18
9/20/18	Walter R. McCarty	Rochester, NY	2LT	24th Aero Squadron	pneumonia	BH No. 18		
9/22/18	Ernest D. Stout	Portland, OR	CPL	BH No. 46, Medical Dept	disease			
9/23/18	Charles B. Morgan	Springfield, IL	Wagoner	Supply Co, 123rd Field Artillery, 33rd Div	influenza and pneumonia	BH No. 42		
9/28/18	Charlotte A. Cox	Baltimore, MD	Nurse	BH No. 42, Army Nurse Corps	dysentery			Plot F, Row 1, Grave 25
9/29/18	John A. Andrews	Bridgewater, MA	PVT	Co H, 306th Inf, 77th Div	gassed	BH No. 18		
9/30/18	Cornelius W. Gist	Eureka, CA	PVT	637th Aero Supply Squadron	pneumonia	BH No. 116		

Appendix: Servicemen and Women Who Died

Date of Death	Name	Residence	Rank	Unit	Cause of Death	Hospital Unit	Grave Number at U.S. Military Cemetery No. 6	Grave Location at Meuse-Argonne American Cemetery
10/4/18	Marion M. Green	Palmerton, PA	Wagoner	6th Engineer Train, 3rd Div	pneumonia		118	
10/4/18	Charles B. Johnson Jr.	Corsicana, TX	PFC	Co H, 59th Inf, 4th Div	gassed	BH No. 46		
10/4/18	Charles M. Smith	Hartford, CT	PVT	Co G, 308th Inf, 77th Div	wounds (gsw)	BH No. 116	124	
10/5/18	Isadore Harris	Baltimore, MD	PVT	BH No. 42, Medical Dept	accidental explosion			
10/6/18	Emanuel Hodel	Odessa, ND	PVT	Co F, 307th Inf, 77th Div	pneumonia			Plot D, Row 37, Grave 9
10/7/18	Walter E. Caven	Cuchara, CO	PVT	Co H, 110th Inf, 28th Div	wounds	BH No. 18		
10/7/18	Charles O. Hanson	Peoria, IL	PVT	Co D, 139th Inf, 35th Div	wounds	BH No. 116		
10/7/18	John L. Keenan	Philadelphia, PA	CPL	Co K, 313th Inf, 79th Div	wounds (shell)	BH No. 42		
10/7/18	Lawrence V. Kobb	Mishawaka, IN	PFC	Co D, 126th Inf, 32nd Div	wounds		152	Plot C, Row 34, Grave 29
10/7/18	Ima I. Ledford	Hillsboro, OR	Nurse	BH No. 116, Army Nurse Corps	pneumonia			
10/8/18	George C. Wilkinson	Petersburg, VA	CPL	Co H, 22nd Engineers	influenza and pneumonia	BH No. 116		
10/9/18	John J. Curtin	Minneapolis, MN	Private	Co H, 3rd Pioneer Inf	pneumonia	BH No. 46		Plot C, Row 40, Grave 19
10/9/18	Carl F. Lasswell	Rossville, KS	CPL	465th Mtr Truck Co, 417th Mtr Supply Train	disease	BH No. 66		
10/10/18	Isadore Drucker	Evansville, IN	SGT	Co F, 28th Inf, 1st Div	wounds	BH No. 18		
10/10/18	Joseph A. McGrath	Philadelphia, PA	CPL	Co D, 304th, Engineers 79th Div	wounds (gsw)			
10/11/18	John V. Vanaerschot	Farrell, PA	SGT	Co E, 111th Inf, 28th Div	wounds (gsw)		176	
10/13/18	William E. Hamilton	Signal Mountain, TN	PVT	Co C, 117th Engineers, 42nd Div	pneumonia	BH No. 18	197	
10/14/18	Francis M. Ferguson	Rochester, NY	PVT	Co B, 344th Tank Battalion, Tank Corps	pneumonia			Plot A, Row 31, Grave 39

Appendix: Servicemen and Women Who Died

Date of Death	Name	Residence	Rank	Unit	Cause of Death	Hospital Unit	Grave Number at U.S. Military Cemetery No. 6	Grave Location at Meuse-Argonne American Cemetery
10/16/18	David R. James	Hammond, IN	SGT	Co E, 59th Inf, 4th Div	wounds	BH No. 46		
10/17/18	Guy H. Criss	Little Birch, WV	PFC	BH No. 60, Medical Dept	disease			Plot C, Row 39, Grave 21
10/17/18	Terrence P. McGowan	Redstone, MT	PVT	Co B, 308th Inf, 77th Div	pneumonia			Plot C, Row 40, Grave 37
10/18/18	Fred J. Duncan	Centerville, UT	PVT	Batt B, 16th Field Artillery, 4th Div	measles and pneumonia	BH No. 46		Plot B, Row 40, Grave 10
10/18/18	Luther C. Shanks	Paris, KY	PVT	Co K, 16th Inf, 1st Div	wounds	BH No. 42		
10/20/18	Ray Scovel	Libertyville, IA	PVT	Co H, 358th Inf, 90th Div	pneumonia	BH No. 116		
10/21/18	Earl McKenzie	Three Rivers, MI	PFC	Batt C, 60th Artillery, Coast Artillery Corps	pneumonia			Plot E, Row 24, Grave 22
10/22/18	Eric I. Johnson	Escanaba, MI	PVT	Co I, 7th Inf, 3rd Div	dysentery			Plot D, Row 41, Grave 8
10/22/18	Charles I. Morton	Oakfield, ME	PVT	Co A, 26th Inf, 1st Div	pneumonia			
10/24/18	Elwood D. Colton	Evansville, IN	PVT	7th Anti-Aircraft Batt, Coast Artillery Corps	influenza and pneumonia	BH No. 18	312	
10/24/18	George W. Kulp	Cogan House Township, PA	PVT	Co E, 56th Pioneer Inf	meningitis			
10/24/18	Samuel J. Lewis	Raleigh, NC	PVT	7th Anti-Aircraft Batt, Coast Artillery Corps	influenza and pneumonia	BH No. 18		
10/24/18	Harry T. Little	Manchester, OH	PVT	Co B, 16th Inf, 1st Div	pneumonia			Plot A, Row 38, Grave 30
10/24/18	Frank C. Richter	Philadelphia, PA	PVT	Co A, 315th Inf, 79th Div	wounds (gsw)			
10/24/18	Joseph J. Stan	Meadville, PA	SGT	Co E, 15th Machine Gun Batt, 5th Div	wounds (gsw)			
10/25/18	William I. Deardorff	Occoquan, VA	PFC	Batt A, 315th Field Artillery, 80th Div	wounds	BH No. 116		
10/25/18	John R. Higgins	Flemington, NJ	PVT	Co M, 312th Inf, 78th Div	typhoid fever	BH No. 18		
10/26/18	Irvin H. Brown	Lewisburg, PA	PVT	103rd Trench Mortar Batt, 28th Div	pneumonia	BH No. 46		
10/26/18	Robert L. Mawyer	Lynchburg, VA	PVT	Co G, 11th Inf, 5th Div	wounds (gsw)			
10/26/18	Roger M. O'Donnell	Danville, IN	PFC	Co B, 307th Field Signal Batt, 82nd Div	disease			
10/26/18	Joseph Steinberg	New York, NY	PVT	Co B, 114th Inf, 29th Div	wounds (gsw)			
10/27/18	Allsey O. Browne Jr.	New Orleans, LA	PVT	Batt F, 150th Field	disease	BH No. 116		

Appendix: Servicemen and Women Who Died 159

Date of Death	Name	Residence	Rank	Unit	Cause of Death	Hospital Unit	Grave Number at U.S. Military Cemetery No. 6	Grave Location at Meuse-Argonne American Cemetery
10/27/18	Dole M. Smith	Baltimore, MD	PFC	BH No. 42, Medical Dept	influenza and pneumonia		292	
10/27/18	Reuben T. Strom	Chicago, IL	PVT	Co A, 108th Field Signal Batt, 33rd Div	wounds (gsw)			
10/28/18	Chauncey L. Brier	Columbus, MT	PVT	Co B, 362nd Inf, 91st Div	pneumonia	BH No. 42	360	Plot B, Row 38, Grave 39
10/28/18	Harry E. Glass	Prophetstown, IL	CPL	Co G, 47th Inf, 4th Div	gassed			
10/28/18	William Kelley	Baltimore, MD	Wagoner	Supply Co, 313th Inf, 79th Div	gassed			
10/28/18	Anshelm S. Norman	Norway, MI	PVT	Co H, 104th Inf, 26th Div	pneumonia			Plot D, Row 46, Grave 5
10/29/18	Henry J. Regallo	Dos Palos, CA	PFC	Co D, 363rd Inf, 91st Div	wounds			
10/29/18	Harry J. Vandenburg	Grand Rapids, MI	CPL	536th Mtr Truck Co, 426th Mtr Supply Train	pneumonia			
10/30/18	William T. Connor	Indiana	CPL	Hdqrs Co, 364th Inf, 91st Div	pneumonia		284	
10/30/18	Walter W. Kirby	Denver, CO	CPL	Co B, 7th Engineers, 5th Div	wounds (gsw)			
10/30/18	Lucien R. Lovewell	South Lyon, MI	PVT	Co E, 308th Mtr Transport Corps	myocarditis			
10/31/18	Eddie Anderson	Oakland, NE	Wagoner	Supply Co, 4th Inf, 3th Div	pneumonia			Plot D, Row 37, Grave 6
10/31/18	Robert B. Wilcox	Youngsville, PA	PVT	Co B, 313th Machine Gun Batt, 80th Div	wounds (shell)	BH No. 42		
11/1/18	John O. Steffen	Saint Cloud, MN	PVT	Co G, 354th Inf, 89th Div	gassed	BH No. 116		
11/2/18	George B. Ouren	New Rockford, ND	PVT	Supply Co, 39th Inf, 4th Div	pneumonia	BH No. 46		
11/4/18	Cleveland Hicks	Evansville, IN	PVT	Co B, 333rd Inf, 84th Div	influenza and pneumonia	BH No. 42		Plot C, Row 38, Grave 34
11/12/18	Jeannette Bellman	Dayton, OH	Nurse	BH No. 18, Army Nurse Corps	pneumonia typhoid fever			

Appendix: Servicemen and Women Who Died

Date of Death	Name	Residence	Rank	Unit	Cause of Death	Hospital Unit	Grave Number at U.S. Military Cemetery No. 6	Grave Location at Meuse-Argonne American Cemetery
12/8/18	Malcolm P. Law	Kingston, PA	SGT	462nd Aero Squadron	influenza and pneumonia	BH No. 18		Plot H, Row 35, Grave 2
12/12/18	Delbert D. Graves	Carthage, SD	PVT	Co H, 351st Inf, 88th Div	scarlet fever	BH No. 18	422	
1/12/19	David K. O'Brien	Wilton, ND	PFC	Co L, 18th Inf, 1st Div	pneumonia			
1/21/19	Chester W. Brown	Portland, OR	SGT	Batt B, 147th Field Artillery, 41st Div	disease		933	Plot B, Row 40, Grave 21
1/24/19	John W. Jones	Plumerville, AR	PVT	Co D, 508th Engineers	execution		957	
1/26/19	George W. Stocking	St. Paul, MN	PVT	Co C, 60th Engineers	typhoid fever			
1/29/19	Octaviano Lucero	Taos, NM	PFC	Co A, 351st Inf, 88th Div	disease		931	Plot G, Row 29, Grave 19
2/1/19	Andrew Malm	McPherson, KS	PVT	Supply Co, 137th Inf, 35th Div	pulmonary tuberculosis	BH No. 79		Plot A, Row 45, Grave 39
2/5/19	Le Roy J. Burks	Monon, IN	Wagoner	Supply Co, 147th Field Artillery, 41st Div	influenza	BH No. 116		
2/5/19	Frank Fabrycki	Oshkosh, WI	PVT	Co F, 128th Inf, 32nd Div	accident		914	
2/5/19	Claude V. Kime	Ridgway, PA	Secretary	YMCA	pneumonia	BH No. 21	490	
2/7/19	Thomas B. Shaughnessy	Duluth, MN	PVT	Co B, 128th Machine Gun Batt, 35th Div	pneumonia	BH No. 79		
2/10/19	David B. Burris	New York, NY	SGT	Remount Depot, Quarter Master Corps	pneumonia		903	Plot E, Row 26, Grave 8
2/11/19	Earnest F. Bourk	Okoboji, SD	PFC	Co D, 352th Inf, 88th Div	disease	BH No. 60		Plot A, Row 44, Grave 28
2/12/19	Carmelo Chillemi	Albany, NY	PVT	Co M, 21st Engineers (Light Railway)	accidental burns		897	
2/13/19	Frank H. Suit	Indiana	PFC	69th Transportation Corps Co	meningitis	BH No. 81		Plot C, Row 37, Grave 35
2/15/19	Basil L. Kiste	Noblesville, IN	SGT	Unit No. 308, Mtr Repair Department	drowning	BH No. 79	856	
2/20/19	Warren F. Fisherdick	Amherst, MA	SGT	Co E, 16th Engineers	disease	BH No. 79		
3/25/19	Andrew W. Johnson	New York, NY	PFC	Co D, 55th Tel Batt, Signal Corps	septicemia		833	Plot D, Row 41, Grave 13
3/25/19	Herman H. Steinrueck	Chicago, IL	Wagoner	Hdqrs Co, 13th Engineers	disease			
3/28/19	William McKnight	Louisville, KY	CPL	536th Repair Unit	disease			
4/6/19	Donald J. Conover	Asbury Park, NJ	PVT	Co D, 104th Ammunition Train, 29th Div	automobile accident			

Chapter Notes

Chapter One

1. *The National WWI Museum and Memorial: Kansas City, Missouri* 2016, 7–10, 30.
2. Jaffin 1991, 23–24.
3. Hansen 1996, 39–55; American Hospital of Paris. Brave Volunteers & Heroes of the Resistance. https://www.american-hospital.org/the-world-wars/AHP_Brave_Volunteers_and_Heroes_of_the_Resistance.pdf; and American Hospital of Paris. Bearing the Torch. https://www.american-hospital.org/en/american-hospital-of-paris/bearing-the-torch/bearing-the-torch.html; both accessed April 12, 2018.
4. Jaffin 1991, 24–26.
5. *Ibid.*, 26–28; and Carey 2014, 319–327.
6. Carey 2014, 319–327.
7. Nieves 2015, 94.
8. Jaffin 1991, 1, 26–28; and Ford 1927, 19–20.
9. Ford 1927, 127.
10. Jaffin 1991, 70.
11. *On Active Service with Base Hospital 46 U.S.A.* n.d., 99–111.
12. Lynch 1925, 261; and Ford 1927, 318.
13. American Battle Monuments Commission 1938, 437–439.
14. Lynch 1925, 132.
15. Marble 2013, 1.
16. Wever 2016, 1187–1194.
17. Lynch 1925, 105–106, 114, 132.
18. *Ibid.*, 106, 136–141.
19. Ford 1927, 284.
20. Lynch 1925, 126, 142.
21. Marble 2013, 1.
22. *Ibid.*
23. Lynch 1925, 165–166.
24. Marble 2013, 1.
25. Ford 1927, 92.
26. *Ibid.*, 235.
27. *Ibid.*, 257, 474.
28. *Ibid.*, 473–477.
29. *Ibid.*, 473–476.
30. *Ibid.*, 592–596.
31. *Ibid.*, 473–475.
32. *Ibid.*, 5.
33. *Ibid.*, 547.

Chapter Two

1. Mason 2005, 27.
2. *On Active Service with Base Hospital 46 U.S.A.* n.d., 66; Ford 1927, 537; and Sand Stevenson 1976, 54–55.
3. *On Active Service with Base Hospital 46 U.S.A.* n.d., 66.
4. *Ibid.*, 68; and Gavin 1997, 56.
5. *On Active Service with Base Hospital 46 U.S.A.* n.d., 78.
6. Ford 1927, 540, 644–645.
7. *History of Base Hospital No. 18: American Expeditionary Forces (Johns Hopkins Unit)* 1919, 46.
8. *Ibid.*, 14–18, 52.
9. *Ibid.*, 34, 119–120; and Ancestry. Pennsylvania, WWI Veterans Service and Compensation Files, 1917–1919, 1934–1948 for Edwin S Linton. https://www.ancestry.com; accessed December 24, 2017.
10. Former W. & J. Man Honored in Death 1918.
11. Hull 1928, 48.
12. *History of Base Hospital No. 18: American Expeditionary Forces (Johns Hopkins Unit)* 1919, 120; and Ancestry. Lyle Barnes Rich in the Directory of Deceased American Physicians, 1804–1929. https://www.ancestry.com; accessed December 24, 2017.
13. North Dakota Newspaper Association. Willow City American Legion Post 112 Has Honorable History. https://www.ndna.com/ndna-sponsored-web-site/stories/7478/; accessed December 24, 2017.
14. *On Active Service with Base Hospital 46 U.S.A.* n.d., 66–67; and Pottle 1929, 93.
15. American Battle Monuments Commission. Edwin S. Linton. https://www.abmc.gov/node/329534#.WgMADGjWzIU; and American Battle Monuments Commission. Lyle B. Rich. https://www.abmc.gov/node/331054#.WgMB5GjWzIU; both accessed December 24, 2017.
16. *Report of the Surgeon General U.S. Army to the Secretary of War 1919 in Two Volumes: Vol. II* 1919, 1802.
17. Ford 1927, 537–547, 668, 672.
18. *Ibid.*, 241–261, 475, 537.
19. *Ibid.*, 545.
20. Bonk 2011, 8; and Ferrell 2007, 33.
21. *Report of the Surgeon General U.S. Army to the Secretary of War 1919 in Two Volumes: Vol. II* 1919, 1803.
22. Ball 1922, 254–256.
23. Gavin 1997, 107.
24. *Report of the Surgeon General U.S. Army to the Secretary of War 1919 in Two Volumes: Vol. II* 1919, 1950.
25. Ford 1927, 547.
26. *Ibid.*, 645, 668, 672, 734.
27. Ferrell 2007, xi.
28. Wever 2014, 538–546.
29. *Report of the Surgeon General U.S. Army to the Secretary of War 1919 in Two Volumes: Vol. II* 1919, 1803–1804.

30. *Ibid.*, 1804.
31. Ford 1927, 645, 668.
32. *Report of the Surgeon General U.S. Army to the Secretary of War 1919 in Two Volumes: Vol. II* 1919, 1876.
33. *On Active Service with Base Hospital 46 U.S.A.* n.d., 61.
34. Ford 1927, 537–547, 698, 734.
35. *Ibid.*, 545. Notably, Ford also mentions a number of 66,284 patients passing through Bazoilles Hospital Center up to March 31, 1919. See: Ford 1927, 476–477.
36. *The National WWI Museum and Memorial: Kansas City, Missouri* 2016, 4.
37. Ford 1927, 476–477, 544.

The Sound of the Siren

1. *On Active Service with Base Hospital 46 U.S.A.* n.d., 59.
2. *Ibid.*, 155.
3. Sand Stevenson 1976, 48.
4. Ford 1927, 540; and Ancestry. U.S., Army Transport Service, Passenger Lists, 1910–1939 for Alice G. Carr (Incoming). https://www.ancestry.com; accessed January 6, 2018.
5. Out of the Box: Materials and News from Wright State University Libraries' Special Collections & Archives. Alice Carr, WWI Red Cross Nurse. https://www.libraries.wright.edu/community/outofthebox/2015/03/27/alice-carr-wwi-red-cross-nurse/; accessed January 6, 2018.
6. *On Active Service with Base Hospital 46 U.S.A.* n.d., 59, 155; and Ford 1927, 540.
7. Letter from France 1919; and Ancestry. Pennsylvania, WWI Veterans Service and Compensation Files, 1917–1919, 1934–1948 for Searle F Grove. https://www.ancestry.com; accessed January 6, 2018.
8. Nurses Come Unheralded 1919.
9. Ancestry. Pennsylvania, WWI Veterans Service and Compensation Files, 1917–1919, 1934–1948 for Edward Harry Schell. https://www.ancestry.com; accessed January 6, 2018.
10. Lt. Col. Schell Back; Praises 28th's Pluck 1919.

Chapter Three

1. Ford 1927, 545.
2. *On Active Service with Base Hospital 46 U.S.A.* n.d., 95.
3. *History of Base Hospital No. 18: American Expeditionary Forces (Johns Hopkins Unit)* 1919, 116.
4. Ball 1922, 255.
5. Ford 1927, 545.
6. *Ibid.*, 544.
7. Honor Roll of the Reading 1919.
8. American Casualties in Fighting on the French Front 1918.
9. Ball 1922, 292.
10. *Ibid.*, 68, 105.
11. *Ibid.*, 69.
12. *Ibid.*, 105. Captain Ball never mentions specifically that he was assigned to Base Hospital No. 60. He mentions, however, that he went overseas on the troopship *Dante Alighieri* and arrived at Bazoilles-sur-Meuse "about the middle of September." See: Ball 1922, 143, 254. The only hospital at Bazoilles Hospital Center which matches this description is Base Hospital No. 60. See: Ford 1927, 684.
13. Ball 1922, 254; and Ford 1927, 540.
14. Ball 1922, 254–257.
15. Bonk 2011, 8; and Ferrell 2007, 33.
16. Ball 1922, 254.
17. *History of Base Hospital No. 18: American Expeditionary Forces (Johns Hopkins Unit)* 1919, 90–92.
18. Ball 1922, 254–255.
19. Wever 2012, 78–82.
20. Vedder 1917, iii.
21. *Ibid.*, 181.
22. Ball 1922, 257.
23. National Archives at Kansas City, Kansas City, MO. Record Group 120: Records of the American Expeditionary Forces (World War I), 1848–1942, Correspondence of the Hospital Center at Bazoilles, 1918–1919, National Archives Identifier 6636481 (NA KC 6636481), box 2 folder 705 Patients. Adm. of: Failure to record administration of ATS, dated September 23, 1918.
24. *On Active Service with Base Hospital 46 U.S.A.* n.d., 114.
25. Wikipedia. Fluoroscopy. https://en.wikipedia.org/wiki/Fluoroscopy; and Wikipedia. WWI Fluoroscope Operation. https://en.wikipedia.org/wiki/File:WW1_fluoroscope_operation.jpg; both accessed February 28, 2017.
26. Ball 1922, 256.
27. Pottle 1929, 144–145; Walker 2002, 870–876; and Dutkowski 2008, 1998–2003.
28. Whitfield 2015, 421–442.
29. *Ibid.*; and Collections. Rockefeller University Records, Special Events and Activities, War Demonstration Hospital. http://hillelarnold.com/staticAid/collections/100/; accessed February 16, 2017.
30. Wolfe 1928, 498.
31. *Ibid.*, 516.
32. Ball 1922, 256–257.
33. Kalkman n.d.
34. Osgood 2016.
35. Ford 1927, 261.
36. *Ibid.*, 543.
37. *Harvard College Class of 1911: Decennial Report* 1921, 315; and Osgood 2016.
38. Osgood 2016.
39. Sand Stevenson 1976, 45–46.
40. Ball 1922, 257.

Gas! Gas!
Treatment of Gas Cases

1. Osgood 2016.
2. Thompson 2004, 109.
3. *History of Base Hospital No. 18: American Expeditionary Forces (Johns Hopkins Unit)* 1919, 115.
4. *Ibid.*, 50.
5. *On Active Service with Base Hospital 46 U.S.A.* n.d., 61.
6. *Ibid.*, 109–110.
7. Thompson 2004, 109–110.

Chapter Four

1. Ancestry. U.S., World War I Draft Registration Cards, 1917–1918 for James Lawrence Comfort. https://www.ancestry.com; accessed October 11, 2016.
2. BillionGraves. Grave Information for Gertrude Sharp Comfort. https://billiongraves.com/grave/Gertrude-Sharp-Comfort/3846380#/; and BillionGraves. Grave Information for James W. Comfort. https://billiongraves.com/grave/James-W-Comfort/3923041#/; both accessed October 11, 2016.

3. Ancestry. 1910 United States Federal Census for James L Comfort. https://www.ancestry.com; accessed October 11, 2016; and Reported as Missing, Georgian Is Gassed 1918.

4. Ancestry. U.S., World War I Draft Registration Cards, 1917–1918 for James Lawrence Comfort. https://www.ancestry.com; accessed October 11, 2016.

5. Action of District Board No. 2 on Exemption Claims Is Officially Announced 1917.

6. Reported as Missing, Georgian Is Gassed 1918; and email message from Bernadine Lennon to author, dated January 7, 2017, with the honorable discharge record for James L. Comfort # 2284154 Pvt provided by the Clerk of Court's Office, Gwinnet County Courthouse, Lawrenceville, GA.

7. *The Forty-Seventh Infantry: A History, 1917–1918 1919* 1919, 26–28.

8. America's Roll of Honor 1918.

9. Reported as Missing, Georgian Is Gassed 1918.

10. *The Forty-Seventh Infantry: A History, 1917–1918 1919* 1919, 47–52.

11. *Ibid.*, 136.

12. Casualties Reported by Gen. Pershing 1918.

13. *37th Division: Summary of Operations in the World War* 1944, 20.

14. Casualties Reported by Gen. Pershing 1919.

15. Email message from Bernadine Lennon to author, dated January 7, 2017, with the honorable discharge record for James L. Comfort # 2284154 Pvt provided by the Clerk of Court's Office, Gwinnet County Courthouse, Lawrenceville, GA.

16. Find A Grave. James L Comfort. https://www.findagrave.com/memorial/134824494; accessed November 8, 2017.

17. BillionGraves. Grave Information for Pvt Quinlan B Comfort. https://billiongraves.com/grave/Quinlan-B-Comfort/3829618#/; accessed October 12, 2016.

18. BillionGraves. Grave Information for James Lawrence Comfort. https://billiongraves.com/grave/James-Lawrence-Comfort/3846525#/; accessed October 12, 2016.

19. Georgia Death Certificates. Comfort, James L. http://vault.georgiaarchives.org/cdm/ref/collection/gadeaths/id/321741; accessed October 12, 2016. Notably, compared to the dates on his headstone, the certificate of death of James L. Comfort lists slightly discrepant dates of birth and death: February 16, 1892, and August 9, 1927, respectively. Yet, all other information on James L. Comfort on this document is consistent with the other sources.

20. Fred Smith, Much Decorated War Veteran, Dies 1969.

21. *The Official Roster of Ohio Soldiers, Sailors and Marines in the World War 1917–18: Volume XVI* 1928, 16085.

22. *American Decorations: A List of Awards of the Congressional Medal of Honor, the Distinguished-Service Cross and the Distinguished-Service Medal Awarded Under Authority of the Congress of the United States, 1862–1926* 1927, 567.

23. *The Fifth U.S. Division in the World War 1917–1919* 1919, 105.

24. American Casualties in Fighting on the French Front 1918; and Fred Smith, Much Decorated War Veteran, Dies 1969.

25. *American Decorations: A List of Awards of the Congressional Medal of Honor, the Distinguished-Service Cross and the Distinguished-Service Medal Awarded Under Authority of the Congress of the United States, 1862–1926* 1927, 567.

26. Fred Smith, Much Decorated War Veteran, Dies 1969.

27. Ancestry. U.S., World War I Draft Registration Cards, 1917–1918 for Michael Joseph Oconnor. https://www.ancestry.com; and Ancestry. 1930 United States Federal Census for Michal J O Connor. https://www.ancestry.com; both accessed December 12, 2016.

28. The Archives-Museum Branch, the Adjutant General's Office of Massachusetts, Concord, MA. Service card of Michael J. O'Connor; and 327th Infantry Veterans. The 327th Under Fire. History of the 327th Infantry, 82nd Division in the Great World War. http://327infantry.org/files/File/Bastogne/82_in327_hist11.pdf; accessed December 13, 2016. The service card of Michael J. O'Connor lists his age at induction in the U.S. Army on September 20, 1917, as 22 10/12 years. This indicates that his date of birth was around November 1894 which is consistent with the date of birth of November 1, 1894, listed on Michael Joseph O'Connor's draft registration card.

29. 327th Infantry Veterans. The 327th Under Fire. History of the 327th Infantry, 82nd Division in the Great World War. http://327infantry.org/files/File/Bastogne/82_in327_hist11.pdf; accessed December 13, 2016.

30. 327th Infantry Veterans. Roster. 327th Infantry Regiment, 1917–1919. http://327infantry.org/files/regiment_history/327th_Roster.pdf; accessed December 13, 2016.

31. Ancestry. U.S., World War II Draft Registration Cards, 1942 for Michael Joseph O'Connor. https://www.ancestry.com; accessed December 13, 2016.

32. The Archives-Museum Branch, the Adjutant General's Office of Massachusetts, Concord, MA. Service card of Michael J. O'Connor.

33. Ancestry. U.S., World War II Draft Registration Cards, 1942 for Michael Joseph O'Connor. https://www.ancestry.com; accessed December 13, 2016.

34. Ancestry. 1930 United States Federal Census for Michal J O Connor. https://www.ancestry.com; accessed December 12, 2016.

35. BillionGraves. Grave Information for Michael J O'Connor. https://billiongraves.com/grave/Michael-J-OConnor/7479731#/; accessed December 14, 1916; and email message from Michele McCarthy to author, dated December 14, 2016, with funeral details for Michael J. O'Connor from Athy Memorial Home, Worcester, MA.

Treatment of Wounded German Prisoners of War

1. Osgood 2016.
2. *On Active Service with Base Hospital 46 U.S.A.* n.d., 62.
3. Osgood 2016.
4. Sand Stevenson 1976, 46–47.

Chapter Five

1. Ford 1927, 545.
2. Sand Stevenson 1976, 48.
3. van Bergen 2009, 140.
4. Ford 1927, 545.
5. Warren's Home Page. Grandpa's World War I Diary. http://e.wa.home.mindspring.com/wwidiary/; accessed April 27, 2017.
6. *On Active Service with Base Hospital 46 U.S.A.* n.d., 66.
7. Ford 1927, 545.
8. *Ibid.*
9. Wever 2014, 538–546.

10. *Sons of Men: Evansville's War Record 1920*, 45–47, 85–86.
11. *Ibid.*, 45–47; *Gold Star Honor Roll* 1921, 634; and Find A Grave. Elwood Digby Colton. https://www.findagrave.com/memorial/20558664; accessed December 17, 2017.
12. *Gold Star Honor Roll* 1921, 639; and American Battle Monuments Commission. Cleveland Hicks. https://www.abmc.gov/node/331014#.WlsFsqjibIU; accessed January 14, 2018.
13. *Sons of Men: Evansville's War Record 1920*, 85–86.
14. Ford 1927, 645.
15. American Battle Monuments Commission. Search ABMC Burials and Memorials. https://www.abmc.gov/database-search; accessed May 15, 2017.
16. NA KC 6636481, box 2 folder 383.6 Enemy Prisoners of War: The Report of Death. Enemy Prisoner of War, dated November 7, 1918.
17. Ford 1927, 545.
18. Wever 2014, 538–546.
19. *On Active Service with Base Hospital 46 U.S.A.* n.d., 61.
20. *Ibid.*, 111.
21. Wever 2014, 538–546.
22. *On Active Service with Base Hospital 46 U.S.A.* n.d., 111.
23. *Ibid.*, 61.
24. *Ibid.*, 111.
25. Grist 1979, 1632–1633.
26. *History of Base Hospital No. 18: American Expeditionary Forces (Johns Hopkins Unit)* 1919, 111–117 and Ford 1927, 537–540.
27. *History of Base Hospital No. 18: American Expeditionary Forces (Johns Hopkins Unit)* 1919, 116.
28. Guy Zimmerman's Web Page. Charles Landry Wells WWI Diary. http://guyzimmerman.com/CWells.pdf; accessed May 17, 2017.
29. Sand Stevenson 1976, 48–49.
30. Byerly 2005, 114–116.
31. Lengel 2008, 193.
32. NA KC 6636481, box 1 folder 211 Nurses. 1918 – 2\10\19: Request Return of Nurses, dated September 23, 1918.
33. Osgood 2016.
34. Dock 1922, 1482; and Kalkman n.d.
35. Dock 1922, 1479; and Mason 2005, 69.
36. Strausstown Roots. Jeanette Belleman. http://www.bergergirls.com/getperson.php?personID=I250264&tree=Strausstown; accessed May 19, 2017.
37. Sand Stevenson 1976, 48.
38. *On Active Service with Base Hospital 46 U.S.A.* n.d., 61; and *History of Base Hospital No. 18: American Expeditionary Forces (Johns Hopkins Unit)* 1919, 111.
39. Sand Stevenson 1976, 48.
40. *History of Base Hospital No. 18: American Expeditionary Forces (Johns Hopkins Unit)* 1919, 116–117.

Convalescent Camp No. 2

1. Ford 1927, 127.
2. *Ibid.*, 259–287.
3. *Ibid.*, 540–546.

Chapter Six

1. Oregon Health & Science University, Portland, OR. Historical Collections & Archives, Grace Phelps Papers, Coll. No. 2010–005 (OHSU GPP), box 2 folder 3: caption to undated photo showing the Meuse valley and Bazoilles Hospital Center.
2. Ford 1927, 540.
3. *On Active Service with Base Hospital 46 U.S.A.* n.d., 109.
4. *Oregon Boys in the War* 1918, 70–73.
5. Ancestry. Oregon, Biographical and Other Index Card File, 1700s-1900s for Henry Andrews Ladd. https://www.ancestry.com; accessed November 13, 2016.
6. Deaths 1941.
7. OHSU GPP, box 1 folder 7: letter from Phelps to Royer, dated September 18, 1918; and Love Tragedy of World War Related by Veteran 1927.
8. 5,212 War Dead Brought Home on Transport 1921.
9. 11 Coming Back in Caskets for Burial in Old Home Town 1921.
10. Burial of Nurse 1921.
11. Private collection author.
12. Ancestry. U.S., Army Transport Service, Passenger Lists, 1910–1939 for James V Lewis (Outgoing). https://www.ancestry.com; accessed April 26, 2017.
13. Rinaldi 2004, 177.
14. Ancestry. U.S., Army Transport Service, Passenger Lists, 1910–1939 for James V Lewis (Incoming). https://www.ancestry.com; accessed April 26, 2017.
15. Ancestry. James Lewis in the U.S., Department of Veterans Affairs BIRLS Death File, 1850–2010. https://www.ancestry.com; accessed April 26, 2017.
16. Ancestry. U.S., World War II Draft Registration Cards, 1942 for James Varus Lewis. https://www.ancestry.com; accessed April 26, 2017.
17. Ancestry. California, San Joaquin, County Public Library Obituary Index, 1850–1991 for James Varus Lewis. https://www.ancestry.com; accessed April 26, 2017.
18. Find A Grave. James Varus Lewis. https://www.findagrave.com/memorial/54809418; accessed November 8, 2017.

Chapter Seven

1. *History of the U.S.S. Leviathan* n.d., 11, 32, 218.
2. *Ibid.*, 31–36; and Crosby 2003, 126.
3. *Ibid.*, 39–49.
4. *Ibid.*, 56, 219.
5. *Ibid.*, 91, n.p. (*U. S. S. Leviathan* Statistics of Numbers Carried).
6. Ford 1927, 540.
7. *History of the U.S.S. Leviathan* n.d., 92.
8. *Ibid.*, 159.
9. Crosby 2003, 126–127.
10. *History of the U.S.S. Leviathan* n.d., 92.
11. *Ibid.*, 157.
12. *Ibid.*, 92.
13. *Ibid.*, 158–159.
14. *Ibid.*, 92.
15. *Ibid.*, 163.
16. *Ibid.*, 153–156.
17. Crosby 2003, 127.
18. *Ibid.*, 158, 161.
19. *Ibid.*, 160–161; and Crosby 2003, 132.
20. *History of the U.S.S. Leviathan* n.d., 162.
21. *Ibid.*, 93.
22. Sand Stevenson 1976, 17–21, 29, 33; and Shiller 2014, 11–15.
23. Sand Stevenson 1976, 33–34, 40.
24. *Ibid.*, 51.
25. *Ibid.*, 36–37.
26. *History of the U.S.S. Leviathan* n.d., 91–93, n.p.

(*U. S. S. Leviathan* Statistics of Numbers Carried); and Crosby 2003, 134–135.
  27. Ford 1927, 688; and *Buffalo County Biographical History* 2002, 68–70.
  28. Nellie G. Galliher from San Francisco, California, served with Base Hospital No. 62 and, like Eileen L. Forrest, travelled to France on board the *U.S.S. Leviathan* on its ninth overseas trip. She died of pleural pneumonia "on the day she reached France" at the age of 33. See: Ancestry. U.S., Army Transport Service, Passenger Lists, 1910–1939 for Nellie G Galliher (Outgoing). https://www.ancestry.com; and Ancestry. California, World War I Death Announcements, 1918–1921 for Nellie G Galliher. https://www.ancestry.com; both accessed May 6, 2017.
  29. Sand Stevenson 1976, 37–38, 40.
  30. Eileen Forrest 1920; *Buffalo County Biographical History* 2002, 68–70; and email message from Le Anne Loesel to author, dated May 15, 2017.
  31. Overseas League to Erect Memorial for Woman War Victims 1922.
  32. *Buffalo County Biographical History* 2002, 68–70.
  33. Sand Stevenson 1976, 38–46.
  34. *History of the U.S.S. Leviathan* n.d., 93–94, n.p. (*U. S. S. Leviathan* Statistics of Numbers Carried).
  35. Chamberlain 1926, 350.
  36. Barry 2008, 1427–1434.
  37. Crosby 2003, 139–140.

War Is Over

1. Sand Stevenson 1976, 51.
2. Osgood 2016.

Chapter Eight

  1. *Names and Addresses : Officers, Nurses and Enlisted Personnel Base Hospital 116 A.E.F.* n.d., n.p.; and Ford 1927, 734.
  2. The photo album does not specifically mention its original compiler. The author presumes that the album belonged to Major Theodore J. Abbott because the first endpaper of the book holds a single photo depicting Major Abbott. Furthermore, the album holds a postcard addressed to Major Abbott as well as a picture portraying four officers of which all but Major Abbott are named in pencil on the photo.
  3. Email message from David Lilburne to author, dated April 3, 2016.

Christmas Overseas

1. Sand Stevenson 1976, 52–54.
2. Osgood 2016.

Chapter Nine

  1. Ancestry. U.S., World War I Draft Registration Cards, 1917–1918 for Frederick Loeffel. https://www.ancestry.com; Find A Grave. Alexander John Loeffel. https://www.findagrave.com/memorial/44539243; and Find A Grave. Rosina Bini Loeffel. https://www.findagrave.com/memorial/44539290; all accessed November 8, 2017.
  2. Ancestry. U.S., World War I Draft Registration Cards, 1917–1918 for Frederick Loeffel. https://www.ancestry.com; accessed October 16, 2016.
  3. Ancestry. Pennsylvania, WWI Veterans Service and Compensation Files, 1917–1919, 1934–1948 for Frederick Loeffel. https://www.ancestry.com; accessed October 16, 2016.
  4. First Detail in New Quota of Selectives Leaves City to Train at Fort Thomas 1918.
  5. Ancestry. Pennsylvania, WWI Veterans Service and Compensation Files, 1917–1919, 1934–1948 for Frederick Loeffel. https://www.ancestry.com; accessed October 16, 2016.
  6. Ibid.
  7. Lengel 2008, 92–95.
  8. Ancestry. U.S., Army Transport Service, Passenger Lists, 1910–1939 for Fredk. Loeffle (Incoming); and Ancestry. Pennsylvania, WWI Veterans Service and Compensation Files, 1917–1919, 1934–1948 for Frederick Loeffel; both accessed February 20, 2018.
  9. Ancestry. Pennsylvania, WWI Veterans Service and Compensation Files, 1917–1919, 1934–1948 for Frederick Loeffel. https://www.ancestry.com; accessed February 20, 2018.
  10. Bailey 1929, 167.
  11. Email message from Jim Shetler to author, dated February 17, 2018, with Dixmont admission and discharge records of Frederick Loeffel provided by the Pennsylvania State Archives, Harrisburg, PA.
  12. Rhein 1919, 71.
  13. Bailey 1929, 52.
  14. Weed 1923, 575.
  15. Email message from Jim Shetler to author, dated February 17, 2018, with Dixmont admission and discharge records of Frederick Loeffel provided by the Pennsylvania State Archives, Harrisburg, PA; and Dixmonthospital.com. History. http://www.dixmonthospital.com/History.html; accessed February 21, 2018.
  16. Ancestry. 1930 United States Federal Census for Fred Loeffel; Ancestry. 1940 United States Federal Census for Fred Loeffel.. https://www.ancestry.com; and VA Maryland Health Care System. History of the Perry Point VA Medical Center. https://www.maryland.va.gov/about/History_of_the_Perry_Point_VA_Medical_Center.asp; all accessed February 21, 2018.
  17. Loeffel 1961; and email message from Jim Shetler to author, dated December 27, 2017, with the Maryland State Department of Health Certificate of Death for Frederick Loeffel provided by the Maryland State Archives, Annapolis, MD.
  18. Ancestry. Pennsylvania, Veterans Burial Cards, 1777–2012 for Frederick Loeffel. https://www.ancestry.com; and Find A Grave. Frederick Loeffel. https://www.findagrave.com/memorial/44539274; both accessed November 8, 2017. Notably, his veterans burial card, certificate of death and the headstone of his grave mention a date of birth of November 6, 1891, which is inconsistent with the date of November 9, 1892, mentioned on his draft registration card and his veterans service and compensation file. However, as both the veterans service and compensation file and the veterans burial card list Army Service Number 2705744, there is no doubt that it concerns the same person.
  19. Bailey 1929, 405.
  20. Ibid., 276.
  21. Ibid., 51, 405–408.
  22. Ford 1927, 734.
  23. Ancestry. U.S., World War II Draft Registration Cards, 1942 for Harry H McQuigg. https://www.ancestry.com; accessed April 18, 2017. Notably, his World War I draft registration card lists his date of birth as March 17, 1891. Ancestry. U.S., World War I Draft Registration Cards, 1917–1918 for Harry McQuigg. https://www.ancestry.com; accessed April 18, 2017.

24. Ancestry. U.S., World War I Draft Registration Cards, 1917–1918 for Harry McQuigg. https://www.ancestry.com; accessed April 18, 2017.
25. Email message from Bernadine Lennon to author, dated March 26, 2017, with the honorable discharge record for Harry H. McQuigg # 1967589 Pvt provided by the Wayne County Recorder, County Administration Building, Wooster, OH.
26. Email message from Dave McQuigg to author, dated March 14, 2017.
27. Email message from Bernadine Lennon to author, dated March 26, 2017, with the honorable discharge record for Harry H. McQuigg # 1967589 Pvt provided by the Wayne County Recorder, County Administration Building, Wooster, OH.
28. Ancestry. U.S., Army Transport Service, Passenger Lists, 1910–1939 for Harry McQuigg (Outgoing). https://www.ancestry.com; accessed April 19, 2017.
29. Wikipedia. 83rd Infantry Division (United States). https://en.wikipedia.org/wiki/83rd_Infantry_Division_(United_States); accessed April 19, 2017.
30. Email message from Bernadine Lennon to author, dated March 26, 2017, with the honorable discharge record for Harry H. McQuigg # 1967589 Pvt provided by the Wayne County Recorder, County Administration Building, Wooster, OH.
31. Wikipedia. Runner (Soldier). https://en.wikipedia.org/wiki/Runner_(soldier); accessed April 19, 2017.
32. National Personnel Records Center (Military), National Archives at St. Louis, St. Louis, MO. Records on Harry H. McQuigg provided by Golden Arrow Military Research, St. Louis, MO, on April 5, 2017.
33. *United States Army in the World War, 1917–1919: General Orders, GHQ, AEF, Volume 16* 1992, 378.
34. Email message from Dave McQuigg to author, dated March 14, 2017.
35. Email message from Bernadine Lennon to author, dated March 26, 2017, with the honorable discharge record for Harry H. McQuigg # 1967589 Pvt provided by the Wayne County Recorder, County Administration Building, Wooster, OH.
36. Email message from Dave McQuigg to author, dated March 10, 2017.
37. Crosby 2003, 160.
38. National Personnel Records Center (Military), National Archives at St. Louis, St. Louis, MO. Records on Harry H. McQuigg provided by Golden Arrow Military Research, St. Louis, MO, on April 5, 2017.
39. Ancestry. U.S., Army Transport Service, Passenger Lists, 1910–1939 for Harry McQuigg (Incoming). https://www.ancestry.com; accessed April 19, 2017.
40. Email message from Bernadine Lennon to author, dated March 26, 2017, with the honorable discharge record for Harry H. McQuigg # 1967589 Pvt provided by the Wayne County Recorder, County Administration Building, Wooster, OH.
41. Email message from Dave McQuigg to author, dated March 13, 2017.
42. Harry McQuigg, Mail Carrier 1966.
43. Email messages from Dave McQuigg to author, dated 10, 13 and March 14, 2017.
44. Ancestry. Harry H McQuigg in the Ohio, Deaths, 1908–1932, 1938–2007. https://www.ancestry.com; accessed April 19, 2017.
45. Find A Grave. Harry Horace McQuigg. https://www.findagrave.com/memorial/124655928; accessed November 8, 2017.
46. Email messages from Dave McQuigg to author, dated July 24 and August 28, 2017.
47. Ancestry. U.S., World War I Draft Registration Cards, 1917–1918 for Morgan J Magnews. https://www.ancestry.com; accessed March 18, 2017.
48. National Personnel Records Center (Military), National Archives at St. Louis, St. Louis, MO. Records on Morgan J. Magness provided by Golden Arrow Military Research, St. Louis, MO, on 2 and March 11, 2017.
49. Judson n.d., 2.
50. *Roster of 62nd Engineers, 4th Ry. Div. 13th G. D. Z. of A., American Ex. Forces, France: 1918–1919* 1919, 1–2.
51. *Ibid.*; and National Personnel Records Center (Military), National Archives at St. Louis, St. Louis, MO. Records on Morgan J. Magness provided by Golden Arrow Military Research, St. Louis, MO, on 2 and March 11, 2017.
52. Wever 2014, 538–546.
53. National Personnel Records Center (Military), National Archives at St. Louis, St. Louis, MO. Records on Morgan J. Magness provided by Golden Arrow Military Research, St. Louis, MO, on 2 and March 11, 2017.
54. Ford 1927, 547, 698.
55. National Personnel Records Center (Military), National Archives at St. Louis, St. Louis, MO. Records on Morgan J. Magness provided by Golden Arrow Military Research, St. Louis, MO, on 2 and March 11, 2017.
56. *Ibid.*
57. Intermountain Obituaries 1971. This obituary of Morgan J. Magness in *The Salt Lake Tribune* lists an erroneous age of death at 81.

Review of the Personnel by General Pershing

1. Sand Stevenson 1976, 93–97.
2. Osgood 2016.

Chapter Ten

1. Captain at Dallas Tells of Hanging Soldier in France 1921; Graves Service Official Denies Hubbard Story 1922; and Williams 2010, 172.
2. West 1919, 100–102.
3. Osgood 2016.
4. *Ibid.*
5. Ford 1927, 540.
6. West 1919, 100–102.
7. Major Opie Weeps on Witness Stand 1922.
8. *On Active Service with Base Hospital 46 U.S.A.* n.d., 66–67; and Pottle 1929, 93.
9. Army Rumors 1922; and Williams 2010, 172.
10. Williams 2010, 172.
11. Watson Says Soldiers Were Hanged in France without Court-martial 1921; and Senate Orders Inquiry into Army Hangings 1921.
12. Ford 1927, 540.
13. Conwell Describes Hanging 1921.
14. *Ibid.*
15. Says Bodies of Three Men Hung Were Found in Cemetery in France 1922.
16. D.C. Men in N.Y. Hospitals 1919.
17. Captain at Dallas Tells of Hanging Soldier in France 1921.
18. Blacks Hanged after Trials, Captain Avers 1921.
19. Secretary of War Hits at U.S. Senator 1921.
20. Coughlin 1939, n.p.
21. The Watson Charges Probe 1922.
22. 3 Soldiers Had Ropes around Neck 1922.

23. The Watson Charges Probe 1922; Saw Bodies with Rope about Necks 1922; and Tells of Hangings in France 1922.
24. The Watson Charges Probe 1922.
25. More Officers Deny Watson's Charges 1922; and Bryant and Peck 2009, 735.
26. Soldiers Buried Noose on Neck, Records Disclose 1922; and West Point Association of Graduates. Samuel J. Heidner 1913. http://apps.westpointaog.org/Memorials/Article/5141/; accessed April 17, 2017.
27. Wrong Bodies Not Sent Say 3 Witnesses 1922; and Soldier Bodies Buried Without a Rope and Cap 1922.
28. Graves Service Official Denies Hubbard Story 1922.
29. Burial Methods Investigated by Senate Committee 1922.
30. Army Rumors 1922.
31. Hickory Hill. Statesman. http://www.hickory-hill.org/statesman; and New Georgia Encyclopedia. Thomas E. Watson (1856–1922). http://www.georgiaencyclopedia.org/articles/history-archaeology/thomas-e-watson-1856-1922; both accessed April 17, 2017.
32. Finds Soldier Hanging Allegations Baseless 1923.
33. Army Rumors 1922.
34. Hangings Cheered by French 1922.
35. Bryant and Peck 2009, 735.
36. Ancestry. Pennsylvania, WWI Veterans Service and Compensation Files, 1917–1919, 1934–1948 for Charles E Chambers. https://www.ancestry.com; accessed September 28, 2016.
37. American Battle Monuments Commission. Charles E. Chambers. https://www.abmc.gov/node/334431#.WPPsg4iLTIW; accessed April 17, 2017.
38. National Archives at College Park, College Park, MD. Record Group 92: Records of the Office of the Quartermaster General, 1774–1985, Card Register of Burials of Deceased American Soldiers, 1917–1922, National Archives Identifier 6943087, box 48 G.R.S. Form 13 for Jones John Wesley.

Chapter Eleven

1. JHU Collections. Explore WWI Flag. http://course-exhibits.library.jhu.edu/2015/Spring/jgree115/AS14010601/exhibits/show/690/explore#; and JHU Collections. Metadata WWI Flag. http://course-exhibits.library.jhu.edu/2015/Spring/jgree115/AS14010601/items/show/690; both accessed December 4, 2015.
2. *History of Base Hospital No. 18: American Expeditionary Forces (Johns Hopkins Unit)* 1919, 10–12; and Ford 1927, 540, 644–645.
3. Johns Hopkins Nursing. Letters from the Front. http://magazine.nursing.jhu.edu/2005/04/letters-from-the-front/; accessed December 4, 2015.
4. JHU Collections. Explore WWI Flag. http://course-exhibits.library.jhu.edu/2015/Spring/jgree115/AS14010601/exhibits/show/690/explore#; accessed December 4, 2015.
5. *Illustrated Catalogue of Standard Surgical Instruments and Allied Lines* n.d., 17.
6. Wolfe 1928, 493–524.
7. *Ibid.*
8. Wikipedia. Motor Transport Corps. https://en.wikipedia.org/wiki/Motor_Transport_Corps; accessed December 2, 2015.
9. Ford 1927, 540.
10. *On Active Service with Base Hospital 46 U.S.A.* n.d., 27, 37, 38, 87, 159–160.
11. *Ibid.*, 16–17, 37, 41, 90–94, 96.
12. Wikipedia. Fluid Ounce. https://en.wikipedia.org/wiki/Fluid_ounce; accessed May 2, 2016.
13. *Illinois Glass Co. Bottles of Every Description: Diamond Products, General Catalogue "A."* n.d., 12–17; Lockhart 2005, 54–60; Glass Bottle Marks. "Diamond I" or "I Inside a Diamond" Mark Seen on Antique Bottles. http://www.glassbottlemarks.com/diamond-i-or-i-inside-a-diamond-mark-seen-on-antique-bottles/; and Society for Historical Archaeology. Bottle Typing/Diagnostic Shapes: Medicinal/Chemical/Druggist Bottles. http://www.sha.org/bottle/medicinal.htm#Oval Druggists; both accessed November 27, 2015.
14. NA KC 6636481, box 2 folder 383.6 Enemy Prisoners of War (November 10, 2016; personal observation by author).
15. *On Active Service with Base Hospital 46 U.S.A.* n.d., 67.
16. NA KC 6636481, box 2 folder 383.6 Enemy Prisoners of War: Report of Death, dated October 14, 1918; Landesarchiv Baden-Württemberg, Abt. Hauptstaatsarchiv Stuttgart, M 430/3 Personalakten III; and Der I. Weltkrieg 1914–1918: Teil 33, 2015.
17. OHSU GPP, box 3: notebook of Chief Nurse Grace Phelps with details on the service of the nurses of Base Hospitals Nos. 46 and 81.
18. The National WWI Museum and Memorial: display of personal items of Nurse Ruth Regina Shields in Memory Hall (November 11, 2016; personal observation by author).
19. American Battle Monuments Commission. Meuse-Argonne American Cemetery. https://abmc.gov/cemeteries-memorials/europe/meuse-argonne-american-cemetery#.WVwRGIjyi00; accessed July 5, 2017.
20. Ancestry. Charlotte A Cox in the Maryland Military Men, 1917–1918. https://www.ancestry.com; Arlington National Cemetery Website. Mary Gavin, Lieutenant Colonel, United States Army. http://www.arlingtoncemetery.net/mgavin.htm; and West Virginia Division of Culture and History. West Virginia Veterans Database Record Detail. http://www.wvculture.org/history/wvmemory/vetdetail.aspx?Id=12155; all accessed July 5, 2017.
21. American Battle Monuments Commission. Charlotte A. Cox. https://www.abmc.gov/node/335320#.WViUFIjyjIU; accessed July 5, 2017.
22. American Casualties 1918; Ancestry. U.S., World War I Draft Registration Cards, 1917–1918 for Guy Harley Criss. https://www.ancestry.com; and American Battle Monuments Commission. Guy H. Criss. https://www.abmc.gov/node/331042#.WVyAdIjyjIU; both accessed July 5, 2017.
23. American Battle Monuments Commission. Meuse-Argonne American Cemetery Visitor Brochure. https://abmc.gov/sites/default/files/publications/Meuse-Argonne%20508_R3-26-2015.pdf; accessed July 5, 2017.
24. Ancestry. Connecticut, Military Questionnaires, 1919–1920 for Lawrence Thomas Hager. https://www.ancestry.com; and Hoover Institution Library & Archives. Digital Collections. The Convalescent Entertainers. http://digitalcollections.hoover.org/objects/12790/the-convalescent-entertainers-10-whiz-bangs-back-from-the; both accessed June 26, 2017.
25. Evans 1921, 176.
26. *History of Base Hospital No. 18: American Expeditionary Forces (Johns Hopkins Unit)* 1919, 27–30, 132–134; *On Active Service with Base Hospital 46 U.S.A.* n.d., 162–163; and The "Whiz Bangs" Are Home Again 1919.
27. *On Active Service with Base Hospital 46 U.S.A.* n.d., 162–163; and Ancestry. Pennsylvania, WWI Veter-

ans Service and Compensation Files, 1917–1919, 1934–1948 for John J Belco. https://www.ancestry.com; accessed June 29, 2017.

28. The "Whiz Bangs" Are Home Again 1919; Ancestry. U.S., World War I Draft Registration Cards, 1917–1918 for Lawrence Thomas Hager; and Ancestry. Connecticut, Military Questionnaires, 1919–1920 for Lawrence Thomas Hager. https://www.ancestry.com; both accessed June 26, 2017.

29. Wears Dead Man's Eyebrow n.d.

30. The "Whiz Bangs" Are Home Again 1919.

31. *On Active Service with Base Hospital 46 U.S.A.* n.d., 157–163.

32. The "Whiz Bangs" Are Home Again 1919.

33. *On Active Service with Base Hospital 46 U.S.A.* n.d., 162–163.

34. Liveliest Group of Invalids in Europe Make Wounded Forget Their Troubles 1919; and The "Whiz Bangs" Are Home Again 1919.

35. Kendrew 1919, 20; The "Whiz Bangs" Are Home Again 1919; and Evans 1921, 176.

36. Liveliest Group of Invalids in Europe Make Wounded Forget Their Troubles 1919.

37. Ancestry. U.S., Army Transport Service, Passenger Lists, 1910–1939 for Charles A Speidel (Incoming). https://www.ancestry.com; accessed June 28, 2017.

38. Ancestry. U.S., American Red Cross Nurse Files, 1916–1959 for Gertrude Hayden Bowling. https://www.ancestry.com; accessed March 15, 2018.

39. *History of Base Hospital No. 18: American Expeditionary Forces (Johns Hopkins Unit)* 1919, 21.

40. *Ibid.*, 87.

41. Nurses Were "Shock Team" 1919.

42. Hopkins Nurses Land 1919.

43. *On Active Service with Base Hospital 46 U.S.A.* n.d., 123.

44. News, announcements, and insights from OHSU Historical Collections & Archives. Thanksgiving at Base Hospital 46, 1918. http://ohsu-hca.blogspot.nl/2015/11/thanksgiving-at-base-hospital-46-1918.html; accessed April 19, 2018.

45. *Songs of the Soldiers and Sailors U.S.* 1917.

46. Email message from Greg Donaldson to author, dated December 2, 2015.

47. Kimberly Jensen's Blog. Eleanor Donaldson, R.N.: The Base Hospital Nurses Club Part I. http://kimberlyjensenblog.blogspot.nl/2015/03/eleanor-donaldson-rn-base-hospital.html; accessed December 30, 2015.

48. Ford 1927, 672, 700.

49. Ford 1927, 672.

50. *On Active Service with Base Hospital 46 U.S.A.* n.d., 38, 180.

51. Email message from Dustin Farris to author, dated January 12, 2016.

52. U.S. Militaria Forum. WW1 Advanced Service Supply Patch. http://www.usmilitariaforum.com/forums/index.php?/topic/198001-ww1-advanced-service-supply-patch/; accessed January 12, 2016.

53. Wikipedia. RMS Empress of Scotland (1906). https://en.wikipedia.org/wiki/RMS_Empress_of_Scotland_(1906); accessed December 30, 2015.

54. Kimberly Jensen's Blog. Eleanor Donaldson and "Our Trip Home" Part I. http://kimberlyjensenblog.blogspot.nl/2015/06/eleanor-donaldson-and-our-trip-home.html; accessed December 30, 2015.

55. Degrees Given To-Day 1898; and U.S. Militaria Forum. WW1 Army Medical Corps Col. Elmer Dean Distinguished Service Medal. http://www.usmilitariaforum.com/forums/index.php?/topic/168238-ww1-army-medical-corps-col-elmer-dean-distuished-service-medal/; accessed January 1, 2016.

56. Recruits Back Out 1898.

57. Of Interest to the Pacific Coast 1900.

58. Floyd Medals. Army Distinguished Service Medal, numbered "1767." http://www.floydmedals.com/order/exec/frmProductDetails.aspx?abs=1&productid=NDQ5MQ==&CatID=MQ==&1=1; accessed January 1, 2016.

59. Wikipedia. Mexican Border Service Medal. https://en.wikipedia.org/wiki/Mexican_Border_Service_Medal; accessed January 1, 2016.

60. U.S. Militaria Forum. WW1 Army Medical Corps Col. Elmer Dean Distinguished Service Medal. http://www.usmilitariaforum.com/forums/index.php?/topic/168238-ww1-army-medical-corps-col-elmer-dean-distuished-service-medal/; accessed January 1, 2016.

61. Ford 1927, 656–658.

62. *Ibid.*, 537–547.

63. U.S. Militaria Forum. WW1 Army Medical Corps Col. Elmer Dean Distinguished Service Medal. http://www.usmilitariaforum.com/forums/index.php?/topic/168238-ww1-army-medical-corps-col-elmer-dean-distuished-service-medal/; accessed January 1, 2016.

64. *American Decorations: A List of Awards of the Congressional Medal of Honor, the Distinguished-Service Cross and the Distinguished-Service Medal Awarded Under Authority of the Congress of the United States, 1862–1926* 1927, 695.

65. U.S. Militaria Forum. WW1 Army Medical Corps Col. Elmer Dean Distinguished Service Medal. http://www.usmilitariaforum.com/forums/index.php?/topic/168238-ww1-army-medical-corps-col-elmer-dean-distuished-service-medal/; accessed January 1, 2016.

66. *On Active Service with Base Hospital 46 U.S.A.* n.d., 66–67.

67. *On Active Service with Base Hospital 46 U.S.A.* n.d., 152.

68. *On Active Service with Base Hospital 46 U.S.A.* n.d., 66–67.

69. *Gold Star Honor Roll* 1921, 227.

70. NA KC 6636481, box 2 folder 687 Cemeteries: letter from Dinan to Commanding Officer, dated January 1, 1919; and *Ibid.*: memorandum No. 2 from Hdqrs. Hospital Center, APO. #731, dated January 2, 1919.

71. 3 Soldiers Had Ropes around Neck 1922.

72. Wikipedia. 88th Infantry Division (United States). https://en.wikipedia.org/wiki/88th_Infantry_Division_(United_States); accessed February 12, 2018.

73. Find A Grave. Delbert Dee Graves. https://www.findagrave.com/memorial/118195565; accessed February 12, 2018.

74. Ancestor Soup. Delbert Dee Graves, World War I. http://ancestorsoup.blogspot.co.at/2009/11/delbert-dee-graves-world-war-i.html; accessed February 12, 2018; and email messages from Karen Seeman to author, dated 11 and February 13, 2018.

Bibliography

Primary Sources

Books

American Battle Monuments Commission. *American Armies and Battlefields in Europe: A History, Guide and Reference Book*. Washington, D.C.: Government Printing Office, 1938.

American Decorations: A List of Awards of the Congressional Medal of Honor, the Distinguished-Service Cross and the Distinguished-Service Medal Awarded Under Authority of the Congress of the United States, 1862–1926. Washington, D.C.: Government Printing Office, 1927.

Bailey, P., Williams, F.E., Komora, P.O., Salmon, T.W., and Fenton, N. *The Medical Department of the United States Army in the World War, Volume X: Neuropsychiatry*. Washington, D.C.: Government Printing Office, 1929.

Blatt, H. *Sons of Men: Evansville's War Record*. Evansville, IN: Abe P. Madison, 1920.

Chamberlain, W.P., and Weed, F.W. *The Medical Department of the United States Army in the World War, Volume VI: Sanitation*. Washington, D.C.: Government Printing Office, 1926.

Coughlin, C.E. *Senator William E. Borah—No Blood Profits*. Royal Oak, MI: n.p., 1939.

Dock, L.L., Pickett, S.E., Noyes, C.D., Clement, F.F., Fox, E.G., and van Meter, A.R. *History of American Red Cross Nursing*. New York: The Macmillan Company, 1922.

Evans, J.W., and Harding, G.L. *Entertaining the American Army: The American Stage and Lyceum in the World War*. New York: Association Press, 1921.

Ford, J.H. *The Medical Department of the United States Army in the World War, Volume II: Administration American Expeditionary Forces*. Washington, D.C.: Government Printing Office, 1927.

The Fifth U.S. Division in the World War 1917–1919. Washington, D.C.: The Society of the Fifth Division, 1919.

The Forty-Seventh Infantry: A History, 1917–1918 1919. Saginaw, MI: Press of Seemann & Peters, 1919.

Gold Star Honor Roll: A Record of Indiana Men and Women Who Died in the Service of the United States and the Allied Nations in the World War, 1914–1918. Indianapolis: The Indiana Historical Commission, 1921.

Harvard College Class of 1911: Decennial Report. Boston: The Four Seas Company, 1921.

History of Base Hospital No. 18: American Expeditionary Forces (Johns Hopkins Unit). Baltimore, MD: Base Hospital 18 Association, 1919.

History of the U.S.S. Leviathan: Cruiser and Transport Forces, United States Atlantic Fleet. New York: The Brooklyn Eagle Job Department, n.d.

Illinois Glass Co. Bottles of Every Description: Diamond Products, General Cataloque "A." n.p., n.d.

Illustrated Catalogue of Standard Surgical Instruments and Allied Lines. Union Hill, NJ: Hudson Surgical Co., n.d.

Judson, W.W., Emmerich, J.L., and Remy, H. *History of Camp De Grasse, Saint-Pierre-Des-Corps, France: 1918–1919*. Tours, France: Deslis Frères et Cie, n.d.

Lynch, C., Ford, J.H., and Weed, F.W. *The Medical Department of the United States Army in the World War, Volume VIII: Field Operations*. Washington, D.C.: Government Printing Office, 1925.

Mason, V.R. *Dear Ginny: Letters to My Wife*. Bloomington, IN: Xlibris Corporation, 2005.

Names and Addresses: Officers, Nurses and Enlisted Personnel Base Hospital 116 A.E.F. N.p., n.d.

The Official Roster of Ohio Soldiers, Sailors and Marines in the World War 1917–18: Volume XVI. Columbus, OH: The F.J. Heer Printing Co., 1928.

On Active Service with Base Hospital 46 U.S.A. Portland, OR: Arcady Press, n.d.

Oregon Boys in the War. Portland, OR: Glass & Prudhomme Co., 1918.

Pottle, F.A. *Stretchers: The Story of a Hospital Unit on the Western Front*. New Haven, CT: Yale University Press, 1929.

Report of the Surgeon General U.S. Army to the Secretary of War 1919 in Two Volumes: Vol. II.

Washington, D.C.: Government Printing Office, 1919.

Roster of 62nd Engineers, 4th Ry. Div. 13th G. D. Z. of A., American Ex. Forces, France: 1918–1919. Auxerre, France: Bourguignon, 1919.

Sand, Stevenson S. *Lamp for a Soldier: The Caring Story of a Nurse in World War I.* Bismarck: North Dakota State Nurses' Association, 1976.

Songs of the Soldiers and Sailors U.S. Washington, D.C.: Government Printing Office, 1917.

37th Division: Summary of Operations in the World War. Washington, D.C.: Government Printing Office, 1944.

Thompson, H.S. *Trench Knives and Mustard Gas: With the 42nd Rainbow Division in France.* College Station: Texas A&M University Press, 2004.

United States Army in the World War, 1917–1919: General Orders, GHQ, AEF, Volume 16. Washington, D.C.: Center of Military History United States Army, 1992.

Vedder, E.B. *Medical War Manual No. 1: Sanitation for Medical Officers.* Philadelphia, PA: Lea & Febiger, 1917.

Weed, F.W. *The Medical Department of the United States Army in the World War, Volume V: Military Hospitals in the United States.* Washington, D.C.: Government Printing Office, 1923.

West, W.B., *The Fight for the Argonne: Personal Experiences of a "Y" Man.* New York: Abingdon Press, 1919.

Wolfe, E.P. *The Medical Department of the United States Army in the World War, Volume III: Finance and Supply.* Washington, D.C.: Government Printing Office, 1928.

Magazines

Ball, C.R. The Experiences of a Civilian Doctor in the Army, at Home and Abroad. *The Medical Pickwick*, 1922: 8: 68–72, 105–110, 140–148, 179–184, 216–220, 254–257, 292–295, 330–335, 353–360.

Hull C., and West, C.J. Funds Available in the United States for the Support and Encouragement of Research in Science and its Technologies. *Bulletin of the National Research Council* No. 66 (November 1928): 48.

Kendrew, E.G. In Paris. *Variety* 54, No. 10 (1919): 20.

Rhein, J.H.W. Psychopathic Reactions to Combat Experiences in the American Army. *American Journal of Insanity* 76, No. 1 (1919): 71–78.

Newspapers

3 Soldiers Had Ropes Around Neck. *Independence Daily Reporter.* January 4, 1922: 1.

11 Coming Back in Caskets for Burial in Old Home Town. *The Oregon Daily Journal.* June 1, 1921: 4.

5,212 War Dead Brought Home on Transport. *New York Tribune.* May 19, 1921: 6.

Action of District Board No. 2 on Exemption Claims Is Officially Announced. *The San Bernardino Daily Sun.* August 31, 1917: 2.

American Casualties. *The Pittsburgh Post.* November 27, 1918: 8.

American Casualties in Fighting on the French Front. *The Washington Post.* October 16, 1918: 4.

American Casualties in Fighting on the French Front. *The Washington Post.* November 17, 1918: 8.

America's Roll of Honor. *The Atlanta Constitution.* September 18, 1918: 6.

Army Rumors. *The Indianapolis News.* January 7, 1922: 6.

Blacks Hanged After Trials, Captain Avers. *Oklahoma Leader.* November 5, 1921: 1.

Burial Methods Investigated by Senate Committee. *The Houston Post.* January 18, 1922: 2.

Burial of Nurse. *Shawano County Journal.* June 16, 1921.

Captain at Dallas Tells of Hanging Soldier in France. *The Galveston Daily News.* November 5, 1921: 1.

Casualties Reported by Gen. Pershing. *Official U.S. Bulletin.* November 21, 1918: 21.

Casualties Reported by Gen. Pershing. *Official U.S. Bulletin.* February 26, 1919: 38.

Conwell Describes Hanging. *New York Times.* November 4, 1921: 12.

D.C. Men in N.Y. Hospitals. *The Washington Post.* March 31, 1919: 3.

Deaths. *New York Times.* June 28, 1941.

Degrees Given To-Day. *The Philadelphia Times.* June 8, 1898: 8.

Eileen Forrest. *The Mondovi Herald.* August 6, 1920: n.p.

Finds Soldier Hanging Allegations Baseless. *The Indianapolis News.* March 2, 1923: 30.

First Detail in New Quota of Selectives Leaves City to Train at Fort Thomas. *The Pittsburgh Post.* May 3, 1918: 2.

Former W. & J. Man Honored in Death. *The Pittsburgh Gazette Times.* June 4, 1918: 7.

Fred Smith, Much Decorated War Veteran, Dies. *Springfield Daily News.* December 13, 1969: 8.

Graves Service Official Denies Hubbard Story. *The Washington Times.* January 17, 1922: 2.

Hangings Cheered by French. *The Washington Times.* January 5, 1922: 1.

Harry McQuigg, Mail Carrier. *Wooster Daily Record.* July 12, 1966: 2.

Honor Roll of the Reading. *The Reading Eagle.* October 5, 1919: 17.

Hopkins Nurses Land. *The Baltimore Sun.* February 26, 1919: 7.

Intermountain Obituaries. *The Salt Lake Tribune.* October 25, 1971: 31.

Letter from France. *The Fulton Democrat.* February 6, 1919: 1.

Lt. Col. Schell Back; Praises 28th's Pluck. *The Evening News*. April 28, 1919: 7.
Liveliest Group of Invalids in Europe Make Wounded Forget Their Troubles. *The Sandusky Register*. March 23, 1919: 19.
Loeffel. *Pittsburgh Post-Gazette*. August 20, 1961: 40.
Love Tragedy of World War Related by Veteran. 1927-dated, unpaginated newspaper cutting (Oregon Health & Science University, Portland, OR. Historical Collections & Archives, Grace Phelps Papers, Coll. No. 2010–005, box 2 folder 4).
Major Opie Weeps on Witness Stand. *The Oregon Daily Journal*. January 5, 1922: 19.
More Officers Deny Watson's Charges. *New York Times*. January 12, 1922: 9.
Nurses Come Unheralded. *The Oregonian*. April 28, 1919: 7.
Nurses Were "Shock Team." *The Baltimore Sun*. March 7, 1919: 8.
Of Interest to the Pacific Coast. *The San Francisco Call*. February 22, 1900: 2.
Overseas League to Erect Memorial for Woman War Victims. *The Springfield Daily Leader*. November 10, 1922: 10.
Recruits Back Out. *The St. Paul Globe*. December 21, 1898: 3.
Reported as Missing, Georgian Is Gassed. *The Atlanta Constitution*. September 19, 1918: 7.
Saw Bodies with Rope About Necks. *The Abilene Daily Reporter*. January 4, 1922: 1.
Says Bodies of Three Men Hung Were Found in Cemetery in France. *The Olean Evening Times*. January 4, 1922: 3.
Secretary of War Hits at U.S. Senator. *Logansport Pharos-Tribune*. November 5, 1921: 1.
Senate Orders Inquiry into Army Hangings. *New York Tribune*. November 2, 1921: 11.
Soldier Bodies Buried Without a Rope and Cap. *The Charlotte News*. January 17, 1922: 1.
Soldiers Buried Noose on Neck, Records Disclose. *The Atlanta Constitution*. January 18, 1922: 14.
Tells of Hangings in France. *Coshocton Tribune*. January 4, 1922: 8.
The Watson Charges Probe. *Arkansas City Daily Traveler*. January 4, 1922: 1.
The "Whiz Bangs" Are Home Again. *Bridgeport Herald*. June 15, 1919: n.p.
Watson Says Soldiers Were Hanged in France Without Court-martial. *Gastonia Daily Gazette*. November 1, 1921: 1.
Wears Dead Man's Eyebrow. Undated, unpaginated newspaper cutting (Ancestry. Connecticut, Military Questionnaires, 1919–1920 for Lawrence Thomas Hager. https://www.ancestry.com).
Wrong Bodies Not Sent Say 3 Witnesses. *The Anniston Star*. January 17, 1922: 1.

Unpublished

Kalkman, L.M., U.S. Army Nurse. *Personal Account of Louise Kalkman's Experiences as an Army Nurse During World War I*. Collection U.S. Army Medical Department Museum, San Antonio, TX.
Osgood, H., M.D., First Lieut., Reserve Medical Corps. *World War I Letters and Diaries*. Edited by Lawrence Osgood, 2016.

Secondary Sources

Books

Bonk, D. *St Mihiel 1918: The American Expeditionary Forces' Trial by Fire*. Oxford: Osprey Publishing, 2011.
Bryant, C.D., and Peck, D.L. *Encyclopedia of Death and the Human Experience*. Thousand Oaks, CA: SAGE Publications, 2009.
Buffalo County Biographical History: Celebrating 150 Years, 1853–2003. Paducah, KY: Turner Publishing Company, 2002.
Byerly, C.R. *Fever of War: The Influenza Epidemic in the U.S. Army During World War I*. New York: New York University Press, 2005.
Crosby, A.W. *America's Forgotten Pandemic: The Influenza of 1918*. New York: Cambridge University Press, 2003.
Ferrell, R.H. *America's Deadliest Battle: Meuse-Argonne, 1918*. Lawrence: University Press of Kansas, 2007.
Gavin, L. *American Women in World War I: They Also Served*. Niwot: University Press of Colorado, 1997.
Hansen, A.J. *Gentlemen Volunteers: The Story of the American Ambulance Drivers in the First World War*. New York: Arcade Publishing, 1996.
Jaffin, J.H. *Medical Support for the American Expeditionary Forces in France During the First World War*. Fort Leavenworth, KS: U.S. Army Command and General Staff College; 1991 (master's thesis).
Lengel, E.G. *To Conquer Hell: The Meuse-Argonne, 1918*. New York: Henry Holt and Company, 2008.
Marble, S. *Skilled and Resolute: A History of the 12th Evacuation Hospital and the 212th MASH, 1917–2006*. Fort Sam Houston, TX: Borden Institute U.S. Army Medical Department Center & School, 2013.
The National WWI Museum and Memorial: Kansas City, Missouri. Marceline, MO: Donning Company Publishers, 2016.
Nieves, J., and O'Malia, D. "Organization, Cohesion and Well-Trained Men: George W. Crile, Harvey W. Cushing and U.S. Base Hospitals in Europe During WWI." In: *Glimpsing Modernity: Military Medicine in World War I*, edited by S.C.

Craig and D.C. Smith. Newcastle upon Tyne: Cambridge Scholars Publishing, 2015.

Rinaldi, R.A. *The U.S. Army in World War I Orders of Battle: Ground Units, 1917–1919*. United States: Tiger Lily Publications, 2004.

van Bergen, L. *Before My Helpless Sight: Suffering, Dying and Military Medicine on the Western Front, 1914–1918*. Farnham, England: Ashgate, 2009.

Williams, C.L. *Torchbearers of Democracy: African American Soldiers in the World War I Era*. Chapel Hill: University of North Carolina Press, 2010.

Magazines

Barry, J.M., Viboud C., and Simonsen, L. Cross-Protection Between Successive Waves of the 1918–1919 Influenza Pandemic: Epidemiological Evidence from U.S. Army Camps and from Britain. *Journal of Infectious Diseases* 198 (2008): 1427–1434.

Carey, M.E. Major Harvey Cushing's Difficulties with the British and American Armies during World War I. *Journal of Neurosurgery* 121 (2014): 319–327.

Dutkowski, P., de Rougemont O., and Clavien, P-A. Alexis Carrel: Genius, Innovator and Ideologist. *American Journal of Transplantation* 8 (2008): 1998–2003.

Grist, N.R. Pandemic Influenza 1918. *British Medical Journal* 6205 (1979): 1632–1633.

Der I. Weltkrieg 1914–1918: Teil 33. *Mitteilungsblatt Oedheim*. March 4, 2015: 4–5.

Lockhart, B., Lindsey B., Whitten D., and Serr, C. The Dating Game: The Illinois Glass Company. *Bottles and Extras* 16 (2005): 54–60.

Shiller, J. Lamp for a Soldier—The Story of a WWI Nurse. *American Association for the History of Nursing Bulletin* No. 109 (Spring 2014): 11–15.

Walker, L.G., Jr. Carrel's War Research Hospital at Compiegne: Prototype of a Research Facility at the Front. *Journal of the American College of Surgeons* 195 (2002): 870–876.

Wever, P.C. The U.S. Army Medical Belt for Front Line First Aid: A Well-Considered Design That Failed the Medical Department During the First World War. *Military Medicine* 181 (2016): 1187–1194.

Wever, P.C., and van Bergen L. Death from 1918 Pandemic Influenza During the First World War: A Perspective from Personal and Anecdotal Evidence. *Influenza and Other Respiratory Viruses* 8 (2014): 538–546.

Wever, P.C., and van Bergen L. Prevention of Tetanus During the First World War. *Medical Humanities* 38 (2012): 78–82.

Whitfield, N. Surgical Skills Beyond Scientific Management. *Medical History* 59 (2015): 421–442.

Internet

American Battle Monuments Commission. Charles E. Chambers. https://www.abmc.gov/node/334431#.WPPsg4iLTIW

American Battle Monuments Commission. Charlotte A. Cox. https://www.abmc.gov/node/335320#.WViUFIjyjIU

American Battle Monuments Commission. Cleveland Hicks. https://www.abmc.gov/node/331014#.WlsFsqjibIU

American Battle Monuments Commission. Edwin S. Linton. https://www.abmc.gov/node/329534#.WgMADGjWzIU

American Battle Monuments Commission. Guy H. Criss. https://www.abmc.gov/node/331042#.WVyAdIjyjIU

American Battle Monuments Commission. Lyle B. Rich. https://www.abmc.gov/node/331054#.WgMB5GjWzIU

American Battle Monuments Commission. Meuse-Argonne American Cemetery. https://abmc.gov/cemeteries-memorials/europe/meuse-argonne-american-cemetery#.WVwRGIjyi00

American Battle Monuments Commission. Meuse-Argonne American Cemetery Visitor Brochure. https://abmc.gov/sites/default/files/publications/MeuseArgonne%20508_R3-26-2015.pdf

American Battle Monuments Commission. Search ABMC Burials and Memorials. https://www.abmc.gov/database-search

American Hospital of Paris. Bearing the Torch. https://www.american-hospital.org/en/american-hospital-of-paris/bearing-the-torch/bearing-the-torch.html

American Hospital of Paris. Brave Volunteers & Heroes of the Resistance. https://www.american-hospital.org/the-world-wars/AHP_Brave_Volunteers_and_Heroes_of_the_Resistance.pdf

Ancestor Soup. Delbert Dee Graves, World War I. http://ancestorsoup.blogspot.co.at/2009/11/delbert-dee-graves-world-war-i.html

Ancestry. https://www.ancestry.com

Arlington National Cemetery Website. Mary Gavin, Lieutenant Colonel, United States Army. http://www.arlingtoncemetery.net/mgavin.htm

BillionGraves. Grave Information for Gertrude Sharp Comfort. https://billiongraves.com/grave/Gertrude-Sharp-Comfort/3846380#/

BillionGraves. Grave Information for James Lawrence Comfort. https://billiongraves.com/grave/James-Lawrence-Comfort/3846525#/

BillionGraves. Grave Information for James W. Comfort. https://billiongraves.com/grave/James-W-Comfort/3923041#/

BillionGraves. Grave Information for Michael J. O'Connor. https://billiongraves.com/grave/Michael-J-OConnor/7479731#/

BillionGraves. Grave Information for Pvt. Quinlan

Bibliography

B. Comfort. https://billiongraves.com/grave/Quinlan-B-Comfort/3829618#/

Collections. Rockefeller University Records, Special Events and Activities, War Demonstration Hospital. http://hillelarnold.com/staticAid/collections/100/

Dixmonthospital.com. History. http://www.dixmonthospital.com/History.html

Find a Grave. Alexander John Loeffel. https://www.findagrave.com/memorial/44539243

Find a Grave. Delbert Dee Graves. https://www.findagrave.com/memorial/118195565

Find a Grave. Elwood Digby Colton. https://www.findagrave.com/memorial/20558664

Find a Grave. Frederick Loeffel. https://www.findagrave.com/memorial/44539274

Find a Grave. Harry Horace McQuigg. https://www.findagrave.com/memorial/124655928

Find a Grave. James L. Comfort. https://www.findagrave.com/memorial/134824494

Find a Grave. James Varus Lewis. https://www.findagrave.com/memorial/54809418

Find a Grave. Rosina Bini Loeffel. https://www.findagrave.com/memorial/44539290

Floyd Medals. Army Distinguished Service Medal, numbered "1767." http://www.floydmedals.com/order/exec/frmProductDetails.aspx?abs=1&productid=NDQ5MQ==&CatID=MQ==&1=1

Georgia Death Certificates. Comfort, James L. http://vault.georgiaarchives.org/cdm/ref/collection/gadeaths/id/321741

Glass Bottle Marks. "Diamond I" or "I Inside a Diamond" Mark Seen on Antique Bottles. http://www.glassbottlemarks.com/diamond-i-or-i-inside-a-diamond-mark-seen-on-antique-bottles/

Guy Zimmerman's Web Page. Charles Landry Wells WWI Diary. http://guyzimmerman.com/CWells.pdf

Hickory Hill. Statesman. http://www.hickory-hill.org/statesman

Hoover Institution Library & Archives. Digital Collections. The Convalescent Entertainers. http://digitalcollections.hoover.org/objects/12790/the-convalescent-entertainers-10-whiz-bangs-back-from-the

JHU Collections. Explore WWI Flag. http://course-exhibits.library.jhu.edu/2015/Spring/jgree115/AS14010601/exhibits/show/690/explore#

JHU Collections. Metadata WWI Flag. http://course-exhibits.library.jhu.edu/2015/Spring/jgree115/AS14010601/items/show/690

Johns Hopkins Nursing. Letters from the Front. http://magazine.nursing.jhu.edu/2005/04/letters-from-the-front/

Kimberly Jensen's Blog. Eleanor Donaldson and "Our Trip Home" Part I. http://kimberlyjensenblog.blogspot.nl/2015/06/eleanor-donaldson-and-our-trip-home.html

Kimberly Jensen's Blog. Eleanor Donaldson, R.N.: The Base Hospital Nurses Club Part I. http://kimberlyjensenblog.blogspot.nl/2015/03/eleanor-donaldson-rn-base-hospital.html

New Georgia Encyclopedia. Thomas E. Watson (1856–1922). http://www.georgiaencyclopedia.org/articles/history-archaeology/thomas-e-watson-1856–1922

News, Announcements, and Insights from OHSU Historical Collections & Archives. Thanksgiving at Base Hospital 46, 1918. http://ohsu-hca.blogspot.nl/2015/11/thanksgiving-at-base-hospital-46-1918.html

North Dakota Newspaper Association. Willow City American Legion Post 112 Has Honorable History. https://www.ndna.com/ndna-sponsored-web-site/stories/7478/

Out of the Box: Materials and News from Wright State University Libraries' Special Collections & Archives. Alice Carr, WWI Red Cross Nurse. https://www.libraries.wright.edu/community/outofthebox/2015/03/27/alice-carr-wwi-red-cross-nurse/

Society for Historical Archaeology. Bottle Typing/Diagnostic Shapes: Medicinal/Chemical/Druggist Bottles. http://www.sha.org/bottle/medicinal.htm#Oval Druggists

Strausstown Roots. Jeanette Belleman. http://www.bergergirls.com/getperson.php?personID=I250264&tree=Strausstown

327th Infantry Veterans. Roster. 327th Infantry Regiment, 1917–1919. http://327infantry.org/files/regiment_history/327th_Roster.pdf

327th Infantry Veterans. The 327th Under Fire. History of the 327th Infantry, 82nd Division in the Great World War. http://327infantry.org/files/File/Bastogne/82_in327_hist11.pdf

U.S. Militaria Forum. WW1 Advanced Service Supply Patch. http://www.usmilitariaforum.com/forums/index.php?/topic/198001-ww1-advanced-service-supply-patch/

U.S. Militaria Forum. WW1 Army Medical Corps Col. Elmer Dean Distinguished Service Medal. http://www.usmilitariaforum.com/forums/index.php?/topic/168238-ww1-army-medical-corps-col-elmer-dean-distuished-service-medal/

VA Maryland Health Care System. History of the Perry Point VA Medical Center. https://www.maryland.va.gov/about/History_of_the_Perry_Point_VA_Medical_Center.asp

Warren's Home Page. Grandpa's World War I Diary. http://e.wa.home.mindspring.com/wwidiary/

West Point Association of Graduates. Samuel J. Heidner 1913. http://apps.westpointaog.org/Memorials/Article/5141/

West Virginia Division of Culture and History. West Virginia Veterans Database Record Detail. http://www.wvculture.org/history/wvmemory/vetdetail.aspx?Id=12155

Wikipedia. 83rd Infantry Division (United States). https://en.wikipedia.org/wiki/83rd_Infantry_Division_(United_States)

Wikipedia. 88th Infantry Division (United States). https://en.wikipedia.org/wiki/88th_Infantry_Division_(United_States)

Wikipedia. Fluid Ounce. https://en.wikipedia.org/wiki/Fluid_ounce

Wikipedia. Fluoroscopy. https://en.wikipedia.org/wiki/Fluoroscopy

Wikipedia. Mexican Border Service Medal. https://en.wikipedia.org/wiki/Mexican_Border_Service_Medal

Wikipedia. Motor Transport Corps. https://en.wikipedia.org/wiki/Motor_Transport_Corps

Wikipedia. RMS Empress of Scotland (1906). https://en.wikipedia.org/wiki/RMS_Empress_of_Scotland_(1906)

Wikipedia. Runner (Soldier). https://en.wikipedia.org/wiki/Runner_(soldier)

Wikipedia. WWI Fluoroscope Operation. https://en.wikipedia.org/wiki/File:WW1_fluoroscope_operation.jpg

Index

Numbers in *bold italics* indicate pages with illustrations

Abbott, MAJ Theodore J. 1, **96–103**
Advance Section **12**, 13, 17, 39, 47, **61**, **147**, 148
AEF University 114
Aix-les-Bains 145
Albert I, Prince of Monaco 145
Allan, Chief Nurse Jessie P. 93
Allentown State Hospital 109
Allerey-sur-Saône 17
American Ambulance Field Service 9
American Ambulance Hospital 7, **8**, 9, **46**
American Graves Registration Service 127–128
American Hospital of Paris 7, 9
American National Red Cross 7, 9, 71, 78, 81, **106**, 141
Angers 17, 34, 117
anti-tetanus serum 13, 38, 42, **44–45**, 46
Antwerp 13
Argonne Forest **19**
Armistice Day 10, 17, 33, 68, 76, 93–94, **95**, 108
Army Ambulance Service Jazz Band 145
Army Nurse Corps 35, 65, 90, 141

Baccarat 54, **55**, 56
Ball, CPT Charles R. 30, 38, 40, **41**, 44, 46, 48, 52
Base Sections **12**, 13, 17
Base Hospital No. 2 10
Base Hospital No. 4 7,9, **10–11**
Base Hospital No. 5 10
Base Hospital No. 10 10
Base Hospital No. 12 10
Base Hospital No. 18 18, 21, **22–24**, 25, 28, **29**, 31, **32**, 33, 37–39, **49**, **53**, 54, **70**, 72–73, **75**, 76, 124, 132, **133**, 144, **146–147**, 152
Base Hospital No. 21 10
Base Hospital No. 23 91
Base Hospital No. 30 149
Base Hospital No. 42 25, 28, **29**, 31, 33, **35**, **71**, 76, 123, **140**, 141, **142**, 143
Base Hospital No. 46 **21–22**, 25, 28, **29–30**, 31, 33, 37, **39**, **50**, 54–55, 65, **72**, 73–75, 79–80, **81–83**, 124, **135–137**, **141**, 144, **145**, 146, **147–148**, **150**, 151
Base Hospital No. 53 107
Base Hospital No. 59 **117**
Base Hospital No. 60 25, **29**, 30–31, 33, 35, 37, 40, **41**, 49, 51, 65, 68, 74, 75–76, 86–88, **90**, **92**, 93–94, **104**, 105, 118–119, 123, 143
Base Hospital No. 62 86–87, 89, 92
Base Hospital No. 65 91
Base Hospital No. 66 25, 74, **138**
Base Hospital No. 79 25, **29**, 33, **34–36**, 49, 51, 76, **116**, 117, 123
Base Hospital No. 81 **4**, 25, **29**, 31, 33, 48, **84**, **111**, 123, 147
Base Hospital No. 116 **4**, 25, **27**, 28, **29**, 30, **31**, **33**, 34, **45**, 50, **51**, 54, **55**, 67, **69**, 74–76, 94–95, **96–97**, **105**, 106, 108, **111**, 118, 120, **121**, 123, 135
Base Hospital No. 117 111
battalion aid station 13
Battle of St. Mihiel **19**, 30, 38, **39**, 41, 60, 63, **83**, 112
Battle of the Marne 28, 38, **39**
Bauer, PFC Charles W. 145, **146**
Bazoches-sur-Vesles 57
Beau Désert 17
Beaune 17, 114
Belco, CPL John J. **146**
Bellman, Nurse Jeannette **75**
Benson, MAJ Robert L. 124
Berg, Nurse Anna C. 81

Berlin University 67
Bernécourt 16
Bertrichamps 15
Bézu-le-Guéry 54
Binnig, *Leutnant* Sebastian **140–141**
Bordeaux 17
Bowling, Nurse Gertrude H. **146–147**
Bowman, Bert **146**
Brandegee, Sen. Frank B. 128
Brest 13, 17, 57, 85, **87**, 89–90, **91–92**, 94, 114, 147, **148**
bronchitis **116**, 117
Brown, Nurse Margaret L. 90
Byam, PFC John W. **146**

camp hospital 15, 76–78
Cannes 17
Carlisle, 2LT Cecil A. 20
Carrel, Dr. Alexis 47
Carrel-Dakin treatment 38, 47, **48–49**
center laboratory 1, 49–50, **51–52**, 74, 95
Chambers, PVT Charles E. 124, 128, **130–131**
Chamonix 145
Château de Bazoilles-sur-Meuse 21, **22**, 24, **32**, 49, 124
Château-Thierry **39**, 55, 79, **101**
Cherbourg 116
Christmas 74, **104–106**
Clermont-Ferrand 17
Clostridium perfringens 39
Clostridium tetani 42
Cohn, PFC Asger G. 126
Colton, PVT Elwood D. **70**
Comfort, PVT James L. 57, **58–60**
Commercy 74
Committee on Medical Preparedness 9
Compiègne 47

175

Index

Connantre 116
Convalescent Camp No. 2 18, 25, 26, 33, *76-77*
The Convalescent Entertainers *144-146*
Conwell, PFC J. Danby 125-126
cooties *see* lice
Corgas, Surgeon General William C. 9
Cornay *63*
Coupal, Chaplain Frederick P 106
Cox, Nurse Charlotte A. *142*, 143
Crile, COL George W. 9-10, *11*
Criss, PFC Guy H. *143*
Crohn's disease 114
Cushing, COL Harvey 9
Cuxhaven 86

Dakin, Dr. Henry 47
Dakin's solution 38, 47, *48-49*
Dale, LTC H.L. 119
Davis, LTC W.R. 56
Dean, COL Elmer A. 31, *149*, 150
DeBaun, 1LT Albert T. 93
Dehelly, Georges 47
dementia praecox 108-109, 112
Dijon 50
Dinan, Chaplain Thomas A. 81, 151
Dixmont Hospital for the Insane 109
Domrémy-la-Pucelle 18, 74
Donaldson, Chief Nurse Eleanor 2, *147-148*, *150*
Donner Jameson, Mia 30
dressing station 13, *15*, 30, 42, 44, 144
dysentery 50, 68, *142*, 143

Ellwangen an der Jagst 140
epilepsy 112
evacuation chain 7, 13, *14*, 38, 44, 51
evacuation hospital 13, 15, 23, 30, 44, 50, 56, 143; No. 2 54, *55*; No. 6 125-126; No 21 33, 76

Fatland, Vida L. *50*
field hospital 13, 42, 44; No. 1 54; No. 353 *16*
field medical card 42, *43*, 46
fluoroscopy *46*, 47
Forrest, Nurse Eileen L. 2, 86, 92-93
Franz Ferdinand, Archduke of Austria 7

Galliher, Nurse Nellie G. 92
gas gangrene 39, *40*, *140*, 141
Gazzola, PVT Valentino 145, *146*
General Hospital No. 9 10
George V, King of the United Kingdom 10
Getz, PFC Lawrence 24
Ghormley, PFC Ralph K. *24*
Grandpré 144
Graves, PVT Delbert D. 2, *152*, 153
Grenoble 145
Grove, PFC Searle Fairfax 37

Hager, PVT Lawrence T. 144-145, *146*
Haig, MAJ 90
Hall, PFC George H. *146*
Harley, CPT 51
Harvard University 9-10, 50
Heidner, MAJ Samuel J. 128
Hicks, PVT Cleveland 70, *71*
Holloway, Agatha *50*
Hoskinson, 1LT Carl M. 126
hospital train 12, 15, 38, 40, *41*, 52-53, 56, 65, *66*, 67, 75, 136, 144; No. 61 *98*
Hubbard, Rufus P. *127*, 128
Hyères 17

Illinois Glass Company 137, *138-139*
influenza *see* Spanish flu
influenza A subtype H1N1 virus 70
Intermediate Section *12*, 13,17, 33

Jacobson, CPL Donald. L. 128
Joan of Arc 18, 74
Johns Hopkins Unit 21, *22*, 24, 132, *133*
Johns Hopkins University 21, 23, *24*, 132, *133*, 136
Johnson, SGT Adolph C. *36*
Jones, PVT John W. 128, 130-131
Juilly 9

Kackley, PVT Harry K. 135
Kalkman, Nurse Louise 2, 48, 75
Kerhuon 17
Kerhuon Hospital Center 86, *92-93*
Kiste, SGT Basil L. 151

Ladd, PVT Henry A. 79, *80*
Lakeside Hospital 7, 9
Lamb, COL Edwin E. 128
Lambézellec 91-92
Landernau 91
Langres 17
Lavelle, 1LT Thomas E. 101
Ledford, Nurse Ima 75
Le Havre 63
Le Mans 84
leukemia 59
USS *Leviathan* 86, *87-92*, 94
Lewis, PVT James V. *84-85*
Leyendecker, J.C. *88*
lice 23, 41, 137
Liffol-le-Grand 18, 26, *76-77*, 117
Limoges 17
Linton, PFC Edwin S. 24, *25*
Liverpool 62, 116
Loeffel, PVT Frederick 108, *109-111*, 112

Magness, PVT Morgan J. 115, *116-118*
Mangan, LT Louis 56
Mars Hospital Center *16*, 34
Mars-sur-Allier *16*, 17, 34
Martindale, PFC Joseph W. *24*
Mayer, PFC William F. *24*

McCown, 1LT Arthur C. 79-80
McCrae, LTC John 81
McFee, PFC William F. *24*
McGrath, CPL Joseph A. 39, *40*
McKee, PVT Mayne W. *146*
McQuigg, PVT Harry H. 2, *112-115*
measles 31, 68
Medical Reserve Corps 23
Meekins, PFC Gilbert E. *24*
meningitis 68, 138
Menton 17
Mesves Hospital Center 17
Mesves-sur-Loire 17
Meuse-Argonne American Cemetery 24, *25*, *71*, 72, 127, 130, *131*, *142-143*, 144, 151
Meuse-Argonne Offensive 18, *19*, 31, 38, *39*, 51, 60, *63*, 73-74, 108, 140, 142, 144
Meuse River 18, *19*, 29, 71, 79, *123*, 124, *150*, 151
Monte Carlo 145
Morgan, PFC Hugh J. *24*
mortality rate 68-70, 73, 91
mumps 31, 78
mustard gas 52, *55*, 56-57, *58*, 59, 112

Nantes 17, 34, 117-118, 120, *121*
Nantillois 39, *40*
Naval Hospital No. 5 91
Neufchâteau 18, *19*, 25, 74, 94, 95, 111, 118, *120*, 122, 124, *138*; Military Cemetery of Neufchâteau *141*
Neuilly *46*
neuropsychiatric department 17, *29*, 31, 33, 108-109, *111*, 112
neurosis 111-112
Newhall, CPT (civ) 106
Nice 17
Nimes *146*
Noble, PFC William D. *24*
Northwestern University 10

O'Connor PVT Michael J. 2, 62, *63-65*
Orléans 17
Orr, PFC Victor M.W. 145, *146*
Osgood, 1LT Howard 1, 50, *51*, 54, 67, 74, 94-95, *101*, 104, 106, 118, 120, 123

Palmer, 1LT Dorwin L. *135*
Paris *8*, 13, 80, 106, *144*, 145
Pasteur Lyceum 7
Pennsylvania Hospital 10
Périgueux 17
Pershing, CINC John J. 10, *25*, 75, 107, 118, *119-121*, 126
Phelps, Chief Nurse Grace 80, *81-82*, 147
phosgene gas 54-55
Pierce, PVT 54
Pinkney, Reverend 93
pleurisy 59
pneumococcus 50
pneumonia 50, 56, 68, *69-72*, 73-

Index

76, 78, 80, *82–83*, 89, 91, 93, 105, 114
Porter, CPT Irving D. 126, 128
Presbyterian Hospital 10
prisoners of war *45*, 46, 65, *66*, 67, *72*, *140*, 151
Provisional Base Hospital No. 1 *32*, 33
psychopathic state 112
psychosis 108–110, 112

Quain, LTC Eric P. 104
Quain, Miss Eric P. 104

Rimaucourt 17, 117
Rimaucourt Hospital Center *117*
Riviera Hospital Center 17
Rockefeller Institute for Medical Research 47
Romagne-sous-Montfaucon 24, *25*, *71*, 72, 127, 130, *131*, *142–143*, 151
Rosenfeld, 1LT Arthur S. *136–137*
Rotterdam 13
Rouen 10
Royat 149
Royer, Master Engineer Ed. 81
Royer, Nurse Norene M. 80–81, *82–83*

St. Nazaire 17, 112, 120, 132, 147
Saint-Pierre-des-Corps 116
Saint-Raphaël 17
Saint-Sébastien-sur-Loire 121
St. Vincent's Hospital 141
Sand, Nurse Sarah 35, 51–52, 65, 74–75, *90*, 92–94, *104*, 105, 118
Sanitary Train 13, *16*, 83
Sarajevo 7
Savenay 17
scarlet fever 24, 68, *152*
Schell, LTC Edward H. 37
schizophrenia *see* dementia praecox
Seidler, 1LT Victor B. 120

Services of Supply *12*, 13, 17, 47, *147*, 148
shell shock *see* neurosis
Shields, Nurse Ruth R. *141*, 142
Skene, MAJ William H. 147–148
Smith, SGT Fred 60, *61–62*
Southampton 63
Spanish flu 18, 31, 68, *69–72*, 73–76, 78, 86, 88–89, *90*, 91, *92*, 94, 114, 117
Speidel, SGT Charles A. *146*
Stanford University 136
Steglich, *Soldat* Emil *72*
Stelsel, PVT Garret *135*
Stout, CPL Ernest D. 124
Swan, Dr. J.M. 9

tetanus 39, 42, 44
Thanksgiving Day 74, *146*
Thompson, 2LT Hugh S. 54, 56
tonsillitis 78
Toul 17, 74
Toul Hospital Center 34
Tours *12*, 17
tuberculosis 78
type A hospital *26*, 28
typhoid fever 24, 50, 68

ulcerative colitis 114
U.S. Army General Hospital No. 28 109
U.S. Army Medical Corps 23, 40, *41*, 136
U.S. Military Cemetery No. 6 39, *70*, 71–72, 82, *83*, *103*, 124, 140, 143, *150–152*, 156–160
U.S. Veterans' Hospital No. 42 109, *110*
U.S. Veterans' Hospital No. 62 59
University of Maryland 25
University of Oregon 25, 136
University of Pennsylvania 9, 149

Val Marconi *see* Gazzola, PVT Valentino

Vaterland see USS *Leviathan*
venereal diseases 68, 148
Verdun 18, 70
Vesle River 57
Veterans Administration Hospital 62
Vichy 17
Viéville 60, *61*
Vittel-Contrexéville 17
Vittel-Contrexéville Hospital Center 56
Vosges mountains 18, 126

Walker, COL John B. 95
Walton, Nurse Julia A. 52, 94
War Demonstration Hospital 47
War Department 42, 47, 57, *61*, *81*, 106, 129
Washington University 10
Watson, Sen. Thomas E. 122, *125*, 126–128, *129*
Watson inquiry 128, *129*, 130; Senatorial committee 122, 126–128, *129*
Wayman, PVT Conrad L. 145, *146*
Wells, PVT Charles L. 74
West, U.S. Army chauffeur William B. 122
Western Reserve University 9
Wilhelm, Crown Prince of Germany 65, 95
Wilhelm II, Kaiser of Germany 95
Wilson, President Woodrow 7, 9–10
wound bacteriology division 1, 50, *51*

X-rays 23, 28, *46*, 47, 135

Y.M.C.A. *see* Young Men's Christian Association
Youland, 1LT William E. 95, 101
Young Men's Christian Association *144*, 145–146